Student Handbook and Solutions Manual

Harry Nickla

Concepts *of* Genetics

NINTH EDITION

William S. Klug
The College of New Jersey

Michael R. Cummings
Illinois Institute of Technology

Charlotte A. Spencer
University of Alberta

Michael A. Palladino
Monmouth University

With contributions by

Sarah M. Ward,
Colorado State University

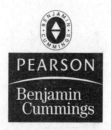

PEARSON

Benjamin
Cummings

San Francisco Boston New York
Cape Town Hong Kong London Madrid Mexico City
Montreal Munich Paris Singapore Sydney Tokyo Toronto

Executive Editor: Gary Carlson
Project Editor: Leata Holloway
Managing Editor: Michael Early
Production Supervisor: Camille Herrera
Production Management and Composition: Prepare Inc.
Cover Production: Richard Whitaker
Illustrators: Prepare Inc.
Manufacturing Buyer: Michael Penne
Text and Cover Printer: Bradford & Bigelow

Cover Photo Credit: Cottonwoods (Populus deltoids) in snowstorm, Heber City, Utah, USA. Cottonwoods are also
known as necklace poplars. RGK Photography/Stone Collection.

ISBN 10-digit: 0-321-54460-9
       13-digit: 978-0-321-54460-5

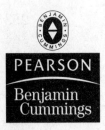

PEARSON
Benjamin
Cummings

3 4 5 6 7 8 9 10—**B&B**—12 11 10 09
www.pearsonhighered.com

Contents

How to Increase Your Chances of Success in Genetics:

1. Attend Class.
2. Read the Book.
3. Do the Assigned Problems.
4. Don't Cram.
5. Study When There Are No Tests.
6. Develop Confidence from Effort.
7. Set Disciplined Study Goals.
8. Learn Concepts.
9. Be Careful with Old Exams.
10. Don't "Second Guess" the Teacher.

A first course in genetics can be a humbling experience for many students. The intent of this book is to help you understand introductory genetics as presented in the text *Concepts of Genetics* (9th edition). It is possible that the lowest grades received in one's major, or even in one's undergraduate career, may be in genetics. It is not unusual for some students to become frustrated with their own inability to succeed in genetics. Teachers recognize this frustration as they field the following types of student comments.

"I studied all the material but failed your test."

"I must have a mental block to it. I just don't get it. I just don't understand what you are asking."

"Where did you get that question? I didn't see anything like that in the book or in my notes."

"This is the first test I have *ever* failed."

"I helped three of my friends last night and I got the lowest grade."

"I am getting a 'D' in your course and I have never received less than a 'B' in my whole life."

"I stayed up all night studying for your exam and I still failed."

Similar to Algebra

Think back to the first time you encountered "word problems" in your first algebra class. How many times did you ask yourself, your parents, or your teacher the following classic question?

> "I hate word problems. I just can't understand them, and why do I need to learn this anyway? I'll never use it."

At that time you had two choices: drop out and be afraid of problem solving for the rest of your life (which unfortunately happens too often); or regroup, seek help, strip away distractions, and focus on learning something new and powerful. Because you are taking genetics, you probably succeeded in algebra, perhaps with difficulty at first, and you will probably succeed in genetics.

In algebra you were forced to convert something real and dynamic (two trains leaving at different times from different stations at different speeds—when do they meet?) to a somewhat abstract formula that can be applied to an infinite number of similar problems. In genetics you will again learn something new. It will involve the conversion of something real and dynamic (genes, chromosomes, hereditary elements, gamete formation, gene splicing, and evolution) to an array of general concepts (similar to mathematical formulas), which will allow you to predict the outcome of an infinite number of presently known and yet to be discovered phenomena relating to the origin and maintenance of life.

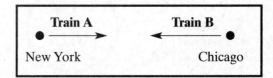

Mental Pictures and Symbols

When working almost any "word" problem it is often helpful to make a simple drawing, which relates, in space, the primary participants. From that drawing one can often predict or estimate a likely outcome. A mathematical formula and its solution provide the precise outcome. To understand genetics, it is often helpful to make drawings of the participants whether they be crosses ($Aa \times Aa$), gametes (A or a), or the interactions of molecules (anticodon with codon).

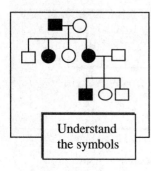

Understand the symbols

As with algebra, symbols used to represent a multitude of structures, movements, and interactions are abstract, informative, and fundamental to understanding the discipline. It is the set of symbols and their interrelationships that comprise the concepts that make up the framework of genetics. Test questions and problems exemplify the concepts and may be completely unfamiliar to the student. Nevertheless, they refer directly to the basic concepts of genetics.

Attendance and Attention Are Mandatory

Because many professors do not take attendance in lectures, some students will likely opt to take a day off now and then. Unless those students are excellent readers and excellent students in general, continual absences will usually result in failure.

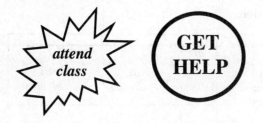

attend class GET HELP

Remember how difficult it was to set up and understand the first algebra word problem on your own? It is likely that your ultimate source of understanding came from the course instructor. While using the text is important in your understanding of genetics, the teacher can walk you through the concepts and strategies much more efficiently than a text because a text is organized in a sequential manner. A good teacher can "cut and paste" an idea from here and there as needed.

To benefit from the wisdom of the instructor, the student must concentrate during the lecture session rather than sit passively taking notes, assuming that he or she can figure out the ideas at a later date. Too often the student is unable to relate to notes passively taken weeks before. In addition, the instructor will not be able to cover all the material in the text. Some parts will be emphasized and others may be omitted entirely.

There is no magic formula for understanding genetics or any other discipline of significance. Learning anything, especially at the college level, requires time, patience, and confidence. First, a student must be willing to focus on the subject matter for an hour or so each day over the entire semester (quarter, trimester, etc.). Study time must be free of distractions and framed by realistic goals.

The student must be patient and disciplined, studying even when no assignments are due and no tests are looming.

> *Since it is the instructor who writes and grades the tests, who is in a better position to prepare the students for those tests?*

The majority of successful students are willing to read the text ahead of the lecture material, spend time thinking about the concepts and examples, and work as many sample problems as possible. They study for a period of time, stop, and then return to review the most difficult areas. They do not try to cram information into marathon study sessions a few nights before the examinations. Although they may get away with that practice on occasion, more often than not, understanding the concepts in genetics requires more mature study habits and preparation.

Perhaps a Different Way of Thinking

Because the acquisition of problem-solving abilities requires that students rely on new and important ways of seeing things rather than memorizing the book and notes, some students find the transition more difficult than others. Some students are more able to deal in the abstract, concept-oriented framework than others. Students who have 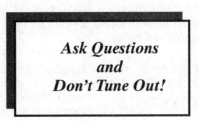 typically relied on "pure memory" for their success will find a need to focus on concepts and problem solving. They may struggle at first, just as they may have struggled with the first word problem in algebra. But the reward for their struggle is intellectual growth. That is what college is supposed to stimulate. With such growth will come an increased ability to solve a variety of problems beyond genetics. Problem solving is a process, a style, that can be applied to many disciplines. Few people are actually born with the touch of synthetic brilliance. Success comes from probing deeply into a few areas to see how problems are approached in a given discipline. Then, because problems are usually approached in a fairly consistent manner, a given problem-solving approach can often be applied to a variety of activities.

Read ahead. You have been told that it is important to read the assigned material before attending lectures. This allows you to make full use of the information provided in the lecture and to concentrate on those areas that are unclear in the readings. You are often given an opportunity to ask questions. Your questions will be received much more favorably if you can state that after reading the book and listening to

the lecture a particular point is still unclear. It is very likely that your question will be quickly dealt with to your benefit and the benefit of others in the class.

Ask Questions and Don't Tune Out!

How to Study

Genetics is a science that involves symbols (A, b, p), structures (chromosomes, ribosomes, plasmids), and processes (meiosis, replication, translation) that interact in a variety of ways. Models describe the manner in which hereditary units are made, how they function, and how they are transmitted from parent to offspring. Because many parts of the models interact in both time and space, genetics cannot be viewed as a discipline filled with facts that should be memorized. Rather, one must be, or become, comfortable with seeking to understand not only the components of the models but also the way the models work.

Time, Work, Patience

One can memorize the names and shapes of all the parts of an automobile engine, but without studying the interrelationships among the parts in time and space, one will have little understanding of the real nature of the engine. It takes time, work, and patience to see how an engine works, and it will take time, work, and patience to understand genetics.

Don't cram. A successful tennis player does not learn to play tennis overnight; similarly, you cannot expect to learn genetics under the pressure of night-long cramming. It will be necessary for you to develop and follow a realistic study schedule for genetics as well as the other courses you are taking. It is important that you organize your study periods into intensive, but short, sessions each day throughout the entire semester (or quarter or trimester). Because genetics tests often require you to think "on the spot," it is very important that you get a good night's sleep before each test. Avoid caffeine on the evening before the test because a clear, rested, well-prepared mind will be required.

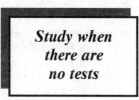

Study when there are no tests

Study goals. The instruction of genetics is often divided into large conceptual units. A test usually follows each unit. It will be necessary for you to study genetics on a routine basis long before each test. To do so, set specific study goals. Adhere to these goals and do not let examinations in one course interfere with the study goals of another course. Notice that each course being taken is handled in the same way—study ahead of time and don't cram.

Study each subject at least every other day—especially when there are no tests!

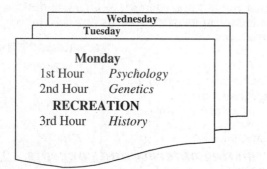

Wednesday			
Tuesday			
Monday			
1st Hour	*Psychology*		
2nd Hour	*Genetics*		
RECREATION			
3rd Hour	*History*		

Develop a Realistic Monthly Schedule

M	T	W	T	F	S	S
			Ch1	Ch2	Ch3	
		Ch4	Ch5			
				Exam #1		
	Ch6					
		Ch7			Ch8	

Develop a Plan for the Semester or Quarter

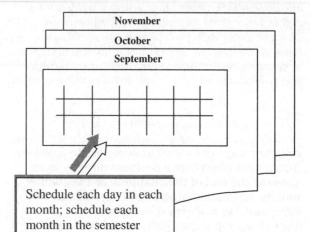

November

October

September

Schedule each day in each month; schedule each month in the semester

Work the assigned problems. The basic concepts of genetics are quite straightforward, but there are many examples that apply to these concepts. To help students adjust to the variety of examples and approaches to concepts, instructors often assign practice problems from the back of each chapter. If your instructor has assigned certain problems, finish working them *at least* one week before each examination. Before starting a set of problems, read the chapter carefully and consider the information presented in class.

Suggestions for working problems:

(1) Work the problem without looking at the answer. Commit each answer to paper!

(2) Check your answer in this book.

(3) If incorrect, work the problem again.

(4) If still incorrect, you don't understand the concept.

(5) Re-read your lecture notes and the text.

(6) Work the problem again.

(7) If you still don't understand the solution, mark it, and go to the next problem.

In your next study session, return to those problems that you have marked. Expect to make mistakes and learn from those mistakes. Sometimes what is difficult to see one day may be obvious the next. If you are still having problems with a concept, schedule a meeting with your instructor. The problem can usually be cleared up in a few minutes.

You will notice that in this book, I have presented the solution to each problem. I provide different ways of looking at some of the problems. Instructors often take a problem directly from those at the end of the chapters, or they will modify an existing problem. Reversing the "direction" of a question is a common approach. Instead of giving characteristics of the parents and asking for characteristics of the offspring, the question may provide characteristics of the offspring and ask for particulars on the parents. Think as you work the problems.

Separate examples from concepts. As mentioned earlier, genetics boils down to a few (perhaps 15 to 20) basic concepts. However, many examples apply to those concepts. Too often students have trouble separating examples from the concepts. Notice that in the "Sample Test" section in this book, I have made such separations clear. Examples allow you to picture, in concrete terms, various phenomena but they do not exemplify each phenomenon or concept in its entirety.

Be careful when using old examinations. Often it is customary for students to request or otherwise obtain old examinations from previous students. Such a practice is loaded with pitfalls. First, students often, albeit unconsciously, find themselves "second guessing" about

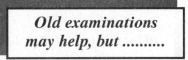

Old examinations may help, but ....

questions on an upcoming examination. They forget that usually an examination only tests you on a subset of the available information in a section. Therefore, entire "conceptual areas" may be available that have not appeared on recent exams.

Often the reproductions of old examinations are of poor quality (having been copied and passed around repeatedly), and it is difficult to determine whether the answer provided is correct. In addition, if a question has the same general structure as one on a previous examination, but is modified, students often provide an answer for the "old" question rather than the one being asked. Granted, it is of value to see the format of each question and the general emphasis of previous examinations, but remember that each examination is potentially a new production capable of covering areas that have not been tested before. This is especially likely in a course such as genetics where the material changes very rapidly.

> *Don't try to figure out what will be asked. Study all the material as well as possible.*

Structure of This Book

The intent of this book is to help you understand the concepts of genetics as given in the text, and most likely in the lectures, and then to apply these concepts to the solution of all problems and questions at the ends of each chapter. Rather than merely provide you with the solutions to the problems, I have tried to walk you through each component of each question so that you can see where information is obtained and how it can be applied in the solution. At the beginning of each chapter is a section that relates general concept areas to particular problems. This should help you practice certain conceptual areas as needed.

Vocabulary: Organization and listing of terms and concepts.

Understanding the vocabulary of a discipline is essential to understanding the discipline. Throughout the text you will find terms in bold print. Such terms generally refer to structures or substances, processes/methods, and concepts. I have separated these terms and *other important terms* into these categories.

> ***Structures and Substances***
> ***Processes/Methods***
> ***Concepts***

Those terms or concepts that require special explanation or are more complex or intimately related to other terms are denoted with a code (**F2.1**, **F23.2**, etc.) that refers you to the figures immediately following each *Concepts* section of this book.

Use the listings as checklists to make certain that you understand the meaning of each term in each chapter. Also, a given term's category will help you begin to understand whether it refers to a structure or substance, a process or method, or a more general concept. Notice that the various terms are not redefined. It is important that you use the text for the original definitions.

> *Understand the words and phrases of the discipline.*

Concepts. In the section *Vocabulary: Organization and Listing of Terms and Concepts,* you will find a section called *Concepts* , which may be followed by a simple sketch or two to help you focus on a particular concept. Such sketches are oversimplifications, and you should fill in the details by examining the textbook and the lecture notes.

Solved problems. Each problem at the end of each chapter is solved from a beginner's point of view. Many of the answers to the questions and problems will refer you to the text. Be certain that you fully understand the solution to each of the questions suggested or assigned by your instructor.

Supplemental questions. A series of solved sample test questions supplements the questions provided in the text and helps you determine your level of preparation. These sample test questions are located at the end of this book. Concepts relating to each question as well as common errors are presented in boxes before and after each answer.

> *Supplemental Questions*
> *Concepts*
> *Comprehensive Solution*
> *Common Errors*

Chapter 1: Introduction to Genetics

Concept Areas	Corresponding Problems
Mendelism	1, 3, 4
Homologous Chromosomes	6
Chromosome Theory of Inheritance	1, 2, 6
Central Dogma of Genetics	5, 7, 8, 9
Model Organisms and Methods	10, 14
Genetics and Social Issues	11, 12, 13, 15, 16, 17

Vocabulary: Organization and Listing of Terms and Concepts

Historical

Genetics

  Mendel (1866)

  Rediscovery (1900)

    Correns

  Avery, MacLeod, McCarty (1944)

  Watson and Crick (1953)

Structures and Substances

Model Organisms

  Escherichia coli

  Saccharomyces cerevisiae

  Neurospora crassa

  Caenorhabditis elegans

  Arabidopsis thaliana

  Danio rerio

Gene

  allele

  phenotype

  genotype

  protein

Bacteriophage (phage)

Genetic material

  DNA (deoxyribonucleic acid)

RNA (ribonucleic acid)

nucleotide

  A, T, G, C

amino acids (20)

messenger RNA

ribosome

transfer RNA

enzymes

  restriction enzymes

energy of activation

Sickle cell anemia

  α, β

Dolly

Transgenic organism

DNA (chip) microarray

Processes/Methods

deCode

Mitosis, Meiosis

Transcription

Translation

  ribosome, tRNA

Coding

  complementarity, hydrogen bonds

1

Chapter 1 Introduction to Genetics

Transmission genetics

Molecular genetic analysis

   sequencing

   genomics

   recombinant DNA technology

   gene therapy

Genetics and Society

Human Genome Project

   human genetic engineering

   cloning

Concepts

Genealogy in Iceland

Genetics

   variation, alleles

   genotype, phenotype

Chromosome

   diploid number (2n)

   haploid number

   homologous chromosomes

Chromosome theory of inheritance

Genetic variation

   gene mutations

Genetic information

   genetic code

   protein synthesis

Central dogma of genetics

Human Genome Project

Model organisms

Genetics and social issues

F1.1 Simple diagram of the relationships among major components of the *Trinity of Molecular Genetics*.

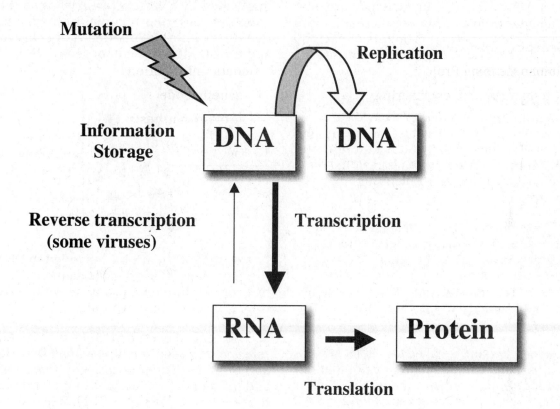

Solutions to Problems and Discussion Questions

1. Mendel proposed that traits are passed from one generation to the next by following certain predictable patterns. He hypothesized that traits in peas are controlled by discrete units, which are now called genes. He also suggested that factors occur in pairs and that members of each gene pair separate from each other during gamete formation.

2. Based on the parallels between Mendel's model of heredity and the behavior of chromosomes, the chromosome theory of inheritance emerged. It states that inherited traits are controlled by genes residing on chromosomes that are transmitted by gametes.

3. The genotype of an organism is defined as the specific allelic or genetic constitution of an organism, often the allelic composition of one or a limited number of genes under investigation. The observable feature of those genes is called the phenotype.

4. A gene variant is called an allele. Many such variants can be found in a population, but for a diploid organism, only two such alleles can exist in any given individual.

5. Genes possess a variety of functions. Since proteins can contain up to 20 different amino acids, each being structurally unique, a vast amount of functional variation is possible. In addition, proteins can engage in a variety of enzymatic activities. DNA is made up of only six different components (sugar, phosphate, and four bases) arranged in a rather monotonous, linear fashion. It seems likely that proteins, given their cellular abundance and versatility, should be the genetic material.

6. *Genes*, linear sequences of nucleotides, usually exert their influence by producing proteins through the processes of transcription and translation. Genes are the functional units of heredity. They sometimes associate with proteins to form *chromosomes*. During the cell cycle, chromosomes (and therefore genes) are duplicated by a variety of enzymes so that daughter cells inherit copies of the parental hereditary information. Genes of eukaryotes and prokaryotes are composed of DNA.

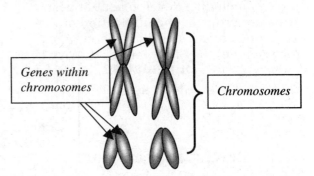

7. Genetic information is encoded in DNA by the sequence of bases. This sequence is transcribed into RNA products, which are then translated into proteins.

8. The central dogma of molecular genetics refers to the relationships among DNA, RNA, and proteins. The processes of *transcription* and *translation* are integral to understanding these relationships (see F1.1). Because DNA and RNA are discrete chemical entities, they can be isolated, studied, and manipulated in a variety of experiments that define modern genetics.

9. If a protein chain is 5 amino acids long, at each position there can be 20 amino acids; therefore, there would be 20^5 different possible combinations.

10. Restriction enzymes (endonucleases) cut double-stranded DNA at particular base sequences. Often, short single-stranded overhangs are generated so that ends from one fragment can anneal with ends from another (assuming the same enzyme is used). When a vector is cleaved with the same enzyme, complementary ends are created so that ends, regardless of their origin, can be combined and ligated to form intact double-stranded structures. Such recombinant forms are often useful for industrial, research, and/or pharmaceutical efforts.

11. In the last 40 years, human traditional transmission, cytological, and molecular genetics have provided an understanding of many aspects of both plant and animal biology including development of pest-resistant crops and identification of hazardous organisms in our food (*E. coli*, for example). Recently, biotechnology has allowed genes to be moved in a variety of ways to generate transgenic plants. Such plants can be engineered to increase their ecological breadth, disease resistance, and/or nutrient value. Wheat, rice, corn, beans, and cassava are being modified to enhance nutritional value by increasing vitamin and mineral content.

12. The United States Supreme Court ruled in 1980 that unique transgenic plants and animals can be patented. Supporters of organismic patenting argue that it is needed to encourage innovation and to help recoup the costs of discovery. Capital investors assume that there is a likely chance that their investments will yield positive returns. Others argue that natural substances should not be privately owned and that once owned by a small number of companies, free enterprise will be stifled.

Individuals and companies needing vital, but patented, products may have limited access. Such, concentration of products may reduce genetic variation as farmers are forced to grow limited varieties of crops.

13. Some mechanism should be in place to protect the investments of individuals and institutions that develop needed and useful products. However, both ethical and economic safeguards need to be developed to ensure that relatively free and fair access exists when vital issues are in question. Any mechanism needs to protect investors as well as consumers.

14. Model organisms are not only useful but necessary for understanding genes that influence human diseases. Given that genetic/molecular systems are highly conserved across broad phylogenetic lines, what is learned in one organism is usually applied to all organisms. In addition, most model organisms have peculiarities, such as ease of growth, genetic understanding, or abundant offspring, that make them straightforward and especially informative in genetic studies.

15. This question is open to many "answers" depending on the individual. Although it may be difficult to put yourself in this position, consider not only what your decision would be but also why you would make such a decision. Often, as a person ages, his or her perspective changes; for instance, how would the possibility of children influence their decision?

16. Safeguards should probably include tests for allergenicity, environmental impact, and likelihood of cross-pollination. In addition, concern would increase if such a crop contained antibiotic-resistant genetic markers and genes conferring toxicity to pests. While genetic labeling is not required in the United States, in the interest of the consumer, one might consider labeling such products as genetically modified. On a broader scale, one might reduce vulnerability by using multiple suppliers (if available) and help minimize the domination of the world food supply by a few companies.

17. Such groups seek to reclaim community involvement and decision making in governmental and industrial applications of biotechnology. They consider that profit-driven motives may compromise benefits that such technology may provide. They question the safety of genetically modified organisms to human health and ecological harmony, not to mention biotechnical applications to weapons development.

Chapter 2: Mitosis and Meiosis

Vocabulary: Organization and Listing of Terms and Concepts

Structures and Substances

Cells

  plasma membrane

  cell wall

    cellulose, peptidoglycan

  capsule

  Diplococcus pneumoniae

    cell coat

    AB, MN antigens

  histocompatibility antigens

  receptor molecules

  nucleus, nucleoid

  genetic material (DNA)

  genes

  chromatin

  histones

  chromosomes

    nucleolus

    nucleolar organizer (NOR)

  cytoplasm

    organelles

    cytosol

    endoplasmic reticulum (ER)

ribosomes

cytoskeleton

mitochondria

chloroplasts

centrosome

basal body

centrioles, spindle fibers

microtubules

microfilaments

  tubulin-derived

  actin-derived

tubulin

kinetochore

Chromosomes

  chromatin

  chromomere

  centromere

  metacentric

  submetacentric

  acrocentric

  telocentric

  p arm, *q* arm

  karyotype

locus (loci)

sex-determining chromosomes

X, Y

Mitosis

zygotes

centrosome

kinetochore

spindle fibers

chromatid

sister chromatid

metaphase plate

daughter chromosome

molecular motors

cell plate

middle lamella

cell furrow

checkpoints

G1/S

G2/M

M

kinase

cyclin

cdc mutations

Meiosis

synapse

bivalent

synaptonemal complex

Saccharomyces cerevisiae

ZP1

central elements

lateral elements

tetrad

dyad

monad

sister chromatids

nonsister chromatids

chiasma (chiasmata)

spermatogonium

primary spermatocyte

secondary spermatocyte

spermatid

spermatozoa (sperm)

oogonium

primary oocyte

secondary oocyte

first polar body

ootid

second polar body

ova (ovum)

Microspore

male gametophyte

Megaspore

female gametophyte

Processes/Methods

Oxidative phases of cell respiration

Photosynthesis

Karyokinesis

Cytokinesis

Mitosis

Cell cycle

cytokinesis

interphase

S phase (replication)

G1, G2, G0, M

checkpoints

prophase

prometaphase

metaphase

anaphase

telophase

Meiosis

  reductional

  equational

  prophase I

    leptonema

      homology search

      rough pairing

    zygonema

    pachynema

      synapsis

    diplonema

    diakinesis (terminalization)

  metaphase I

  anaphase I

    disjunction, nondisjunction

  telophase I

    random segregation

    independent assortment

Meiosis II

  prophase II

  metaphase II

  anaphase II

  telophase II

Spermatogenesis

Spermiogenesis

Oogenesis

First meiotic division

Second meiotic division

Nondisjunction

Sexual reproduction

  reshuffle chromosomes

  provides for crossing over and variation

Alternation of generations

  sporophyte

  gametophyte

Folded-fiber model

Concepts

Prokaryotic

Eukaryotic

Endosymbiont hypothesis

Homologous chromosomes (F2.2)

  diploid number ($2n$) (F2.1)

  loci, locus (F2.2)

  haploid genome (haploid number, n)

    biparental inheritance

    alleles (F2.2)

Crossing over

Mitosis (F2.3)

  identical daughters

  equivalent genetic information

Meiosis (F2.4)

  produces haploid gametes or spores

  reshuffles genetic combinations (chromosomes)

  genetic recombination (crossing over)

  constant amount of genetic material

  production of variation

Alternation of generations

Nondisjunction

Fertilization

  reconstitution of genetic material

Segregation

Independent assortment

Primary nondisjunction (meiosis I)

Secondary nondisjunction (meiosis II)

Alternation of generations

Sexual reproduction

F2.1 Diagram illustrating relationships among stages of interphase. Also illustrated are chromosomes, chromosome number, and structure in an organism with a diploid chromosome number of 4 ($2n = 4$). Individual chromosomes cannot be seen at interphase; therefore the chromosomes pictured here are hypothetical. In mitosis there is no change in chromosome number, even though the DNA content doubles during the S phase. The chromosomes become doubled structures as a result of S phase.

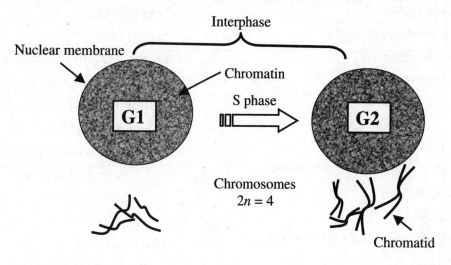

F2.2 Important nomenclature referring to chromosomes and genes in an organism where the diploid chromosome number is 4 ($2n = 4$). There are two pairs of chromosomes: one large metacentric and one small telocentric. Sister chromatids are identical to each other, whereas homologous chromosomes are similar to each other in terms of overall size, centromere location, function, and other factors described in the text.

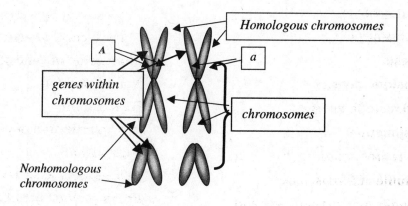

F2.3 Illustration of chromosomes of mitotic cells in an organism with a chromosome number of 4 ($2n = 4$).

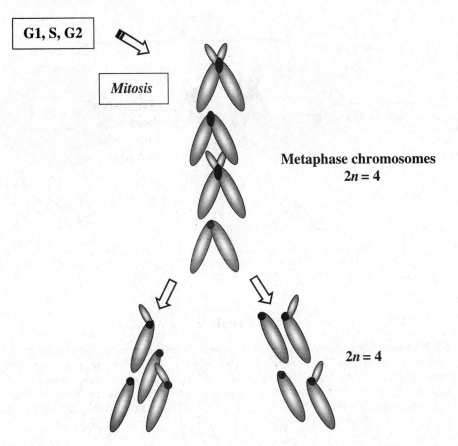

G1, S, G2

Mitosis

Metaphase chromosomes
$2n = 4$

$2n = 4$

F2.4 Illustration of chromosomes of meiotic cells in an organism with a chromosome number of 4 ($2n = 4$).

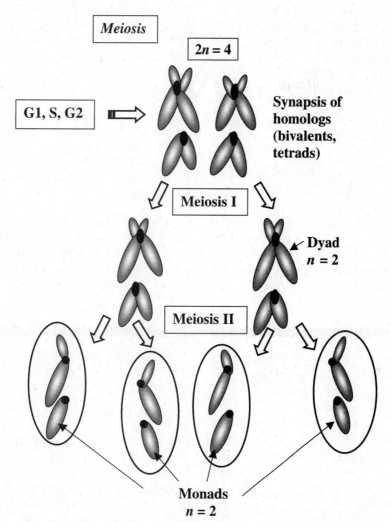

Solutions to Problems and Discussion Questions

1. (a) During interphase of the cell cycle (mitotic and meiotic), chromosomes are not condensed and are in a genetically active, spread out form. In this condition, chromosomes are not visible as individual structures under the microscope (light or electron). See F2.1 for a sketch of what *chromatin* might look like. Chromatin contains the genetic material that is responsible for maintaining hereditary information (from one cell to daughter cells and from one generation to the next) and production of the phenotype.

(b) The *nucleolus (pl. nucleoli)* is a structure that is produced by activity of the nucleolar organizer region in eukaryotes. Composed of ribosomal DNA and protein, it is the structure for the production of ribosomes. Some nuclei have more than one *nucleolus*. Nucleoli are not present during mitosis or meiosis because in the condensed state of chromosomes, there is little or no RNA synthesis.

(c) The *ribosome* is the structure where various RNAs, enzymes, and other molecular species assemble the primary sequence of a protein. That is, amino acids are placed in order as specified by messenger RNA. Ribosomes are relatively nonspecific in that virtually any ribosome can be used in the translation of any mRNA. The structure and function of the ribosome will be described in greater detail in later chapters of the text.

(d) The *mitochondrion (pl. mitochondria)* is a membrane-bound structure located in the cytoplasm of eukaryotic cells. It is the site of oxidative phosphorylation and production of relatively large amounts of ATP. It is the trapping of energy in ATP that drives many important metabolic processes in living systems.

(e) The *centriole* is a cytoplasmic structure involved (through the formation of spindle fibers) in the migration of chromosomes during mitosis and meiosis—primarily in animal cells.

(f) The *centromere* serves as an attachment point for sister chromatids (see F2.3, F2.4) and a region where spindle fibers attach to chromosomes (kinetochore). The centromere divides during mitosis and meiosis II, thus aiding in the partitioning of chromosomal material to daughter cells. Failure of centromeres or spindle fibers to function properly may result in nondisjunction.

2. One of the most important concepts to be learned from this chapter is the relationship that exists among chromosomes in a single cell. Chromosomes that are homologous share many properties including:

Overall length: Look carefully at the figures on the preceding page to see that each cell, prior to anaphase I, contains two chromosomes in which a homolog is of approximately the same overall length.

Position of the centromere (metacentric, submetacentric, acrocentric, telocentric): Again, look carefully at F2.2 and F2.3. Notice in each that if there is one metacentric chromosome, there will be another metacentric chromosome.

Banding patterns: Using various cytological techniques, we can induce bands in chromosomes. Homologous chromosomes of pair #1, for example, will have the same banding pattern. Although the overall length of chromosome pairs #16 and #17 appears to be the same, the banding patterns of these nonhomologous chromosomes will be different.

Sister chromatids have identical banding patterns, as would be expected since sister chromatids are, with the exception of mutation, identical copies of each other. We would expect that homologous chromosomes would have banding patterns that are very similar (but not identical) because homologous chromosomes are genetically similar but not genetically identical.

Type and location of genes: Notice in F2.2 that a locus signifies the location of a gene along a chromosome. What that really means is that for each characteristic specified by a gene, like blood type, eye color, and skin pigmentation, there are genes located along chromosomes. The *order* of such loci is identical in homologous chromosomes, but the genes themselves, while being in the same order, may not be identical. Look carefully at the inset (box) in the upper portion of F2.2 and note the alternative forms of genes, *A* and *a*, at the same location along the chromosome. *A* and *a* are located at the same place and specify the same *characteristic* (eye color, for example), but they are slightly different manifestations of eye color (*brown* vs. *blue*, for example). Just as an individual may inherit gene *A* from the father and gene *a* from the mother, each zygote inherits one homolog of each pair from the father and one homolog of each pair from the mother.

Autoradiographic pattern: Homologous chromosomes tend to replicate during the same time of S phase.

Diploidy is a term often used in conjunction with the symbol $2n$. It means that both members of a homologous pair of chromosomes are present. Refer to F2.1 in this book. Notice that during mitosis, the normal chromosome complement is $2n$, or diploid. In humans, the diploid chromosome number is 46, while in *Drosophila melanogaster* it is 8. The text lists the *haploid* chromosome number for a variety of species.

Notice that in humans and flies, the haploid chromosome number is one-half the diploid number. This applies to other organisms as well. However, it is very important to realize that *haploidy* specifically refers to the fact that each haploid cell contains *one chromosome of each homologous pair of chromosomes.*

Compare the nuclear contents of a spermatid and a cell at zygonema in the text. Note that each spermatid contains one member of each of the original chromosome pairs (seen at zygonema). Haploidy is usually symbolized as *n*.

The change from a diploid ($2n$) to haploid (n) occurs during *reduction division* when tetrads become dyads during meiosis I. Referring to the number of human chromosomes, the primary spermatocyte ($2n = 46$) becomes two secondary spermatocytes, each with $n = 23$.

3. As you examine the criteria for *homology* in question 2, you can see that overall length and centromere position are but two factors required for homology. Most importantly, genetic content in nonhomologous chromosomes is expected to be quite different. Other factors including banding pattern and time of replication during S phase would also be expected to vary among nonhomologous chromosomes.

4. Because a major section of Chapter 2 deals with mitosis, it would be best to deal with this question by reading the appropriate section in the text and examining corresponding figures. Understanding mitosis and all the related terms is essential for an understanding of genetics. Several sample test questions at the end of this book will help you determine your understanding of mitosis.

5. The first sentence tells you that $2n = 16$ and it is a question about mitosis. Since each chromosome in prophase is doubled (having gone through an S phase) and is visible at the end of prophase, there should be 32 chromatids. Because the centromeres divide and what were previously sister chromatids migrate to opposite poles during anaphase, 16 chromosomes should be moving to each pole. If you refer to F2.2, you will see an example with $2n = 4$, and you will observe that there are four doubled chromosomes in prophase. Notice that eight chromatids are visible at late prophase.

6. Refer to the text figures for an explanation. Notice the different anaphase shapes of chromosomes as they move to the poles: (a) metacentric, (b) submetacentric, (c) acrocentric, and (d) telocentric. Your understanding of these structures will be determined by several of the sample test questions at the end of this book. Notice that the centromere is placed in the middle for a metacentric chromosome and at one end for a telocentric chromosome.

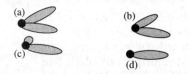

7. Because of a cell wall around the plasma membrane in plants, a cell plate, which was laid down during anaphase, becomes the middle lamella where primary and secondary layers of the cell wall are deposited.

8. Carefully read the section on mitosis and cell division in the text. Major divisions of the cell cycle include interphase and mitosis. Interphase is composed of four phases: G1, G0, S, and G2. During the S phase, chromosomal DNA doubles. Karyokinesis involves nuclear division, whereas cytokinesis involves division of the cytoplasm. Refer to F2.1 for information pertaining to the interphase, and see the text figures for a diagram of mitosis. Notice that, in contrast to meiosis, there is no pairing of homologous chromosomes in mitosis and that the chromosome number does not change.

9. Not necessarily, if crossing over occurs in meiosis I, then the chromatids in the secondary oocyte are not identical. Once they separate during meiosis II, unlike chromatids they reside in the ootid and the second polar body.

10. Compared with mitosis, which maintains a chromosomal constancy, meiosis provides for a reduction in chromosome number and an opportunity for exchange of genetic material between homologous chromosomes. In mitosis no change takes place in chromosome number or kind in the two daughter cells, whereas in meiosis numerous potentially different haploid (*n*) cells are produced. During oogenesis, only one of the four meiotic products is functional; however, all four of the meiotic products of spermatogenesis are potentially functional.

11. (a) *Synapsis* is the point-by-point pairing of homologous chromosomes during prophase of meiosis I.

(b) *Bivalents* are those structures formed by the synapsis of homologous chromosomes. In other words, two chromosomes (and four chromatids) make up a bivalent. If an organism has a diploid chromosome number of 46, then there will be 23 bivalents in meiosis I.

(c) *Chiasmata* is the plural form of chiasma and refers to the structure, when viewed microscopically, of crossed chromatids. Notice how the figures in the text show the exchange of chromatid pieces in diplonema and diakinesis.

(d) *Crossing over* is the exchange of genetic material between chromatids. Also called recombination, it is a method of providing genetic variation through the breaking and rejoining of chromatids.

(e) *Chromomeres* are bands of chromatin that look different from neighboring patches along the length of a chromosome.

(f) Examine F2.1 in this book. Notice that *sister chromatids* are "post-S phase" structures of replicated chromosomes. Sister chromatids are genetically identical (except where mutations have occurred) and are originally attached to the same centromere. Identify sister chromatids in the figures in the text. Note that sister chromatids separate from each other during anaphase of mitosis and anaphase II of meiosis.

(g) *Tetrads* are synapsed homologous chromosomes thereby composed of four chromatids. There are as many tetrads as the haploid chromosome number.

(h) Actually, each tetrad is made of two dyads that separate from each other during anaphase I of meiosis. Note that *dyads* are composed of two chromatids joined by a centromere.

(i) At anaphase II of meiosis, the centromeres divide and the sister chromatids (*monads*) go to opposite poles.

12. Sister chromatids are genetically identical, except where mutations may have occurred during DNA replication. Nonsister chromatids are genetically similar if they are on homologous chromosomes or genetically dissimilar if on nonhomologous chromosomes. If crossing over occurs, then chromatids attached to the same centromere will no longer be identical.

13. During meiosis I, the chromosome number is reduced to haploid complements. This is achieved by synapsis of homologous chromosomes and their subsequent separation. It would seem that it is more mechanically difficult for genetically identical daughters to form from mitosis if homologous chromosomes are paired. By having chromosomes unpaired at metaphase of mitosis, only centromere division is required for daughter cells to eventually receive identical chromosomal complements.

14. Look carefully at F2.4 in this book and notice that for a cell with 4 chromosomes, there are two tetrads, each comprised of a homologous pair of chromosomes.

(a) If there are 16 chromosomes, there should be 8 tetrads.

(b) Also note that, after meiosis I and in the second meiotic prophase, there are as many dyads as there are pairs of chromosomes. There will be 8 dyads.

(c) Because the monads migrate to opposite poles during meiosis II (from the separation of dyads), there should be 8 monads migrating to *each* pole.

15. Examine appropriate figures in the text. Notice that major differences include the sex in which each occurs and that the distribution of cytoplasm is unequal in oogenesis, but considered to be equal in the products of spermatogenesis. Chromosomal behavior is the same in spermatogenesis and oogenesis except that the nuclear activity in oogenesis is "off-center," thereby

producing first and second polar bodies by unequal cytoplasmic division. Each spermatogonium and primary spermatocyte produces four spermatids, whereas each oogonium and primary oocyte produces one ootid. Because early development occurs in the absence of outside nutrients, the unequal distribution of cytoplasm in oogenesis likely evolved to provide sufficient information and nutrients to support development until the transcriptional activities of the zygotic nucleus begin to provide products. Polar bodies probably represent nonfunctional by-products of such evolution.

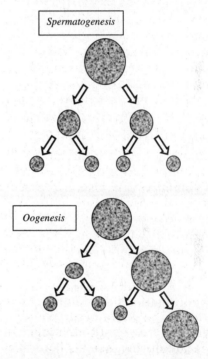

16. This answer contains several parts. First, through independent assortment of chromosomes at anaphase I of meiosis, daughter cells (secondary spermatocytes and secondary oocytes) may contain different sets of maternally and paternally derived chromosomes. Examine the accompanying diagram. Notice that the maternally and paternally derived chromosomes may align in several ways. Can you calculate the probability of all the maternally derived chromosomes going to the "right-hand" pole? Second, crossing over, which happens at a much higher frequency in meiotic cells as compared with mitotic cells, allows maternally and paternally derived chromosomes to exchange segments, thereby increasing the likelihood that daughter cells (that is, secondary spermatocytes and secondary oocytes) are genetically unique.

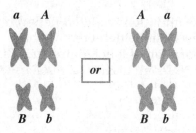

Notice that there are two different orientations of tetrads in meiosis. Independent assortment of nonhomologous chromosomes adds to genetic variability. Daughter cells resulting from the process of mitosis are usually genetically identical.

17. This question specifically tests your understanding of meiosis and the behavior of chromosomes during anaphase. In this question you must first visualize the alignment of the three homologous chromosome pairs—C1/C2, M1/M2, and S1/S2—in mitosis where there is no synapsis of homologous chromosomes.

C1
M1
C2
M2
S1
S2

(a) After mitosis, when sister chromatids have migrated to opposite poles, each daughter cell will be genetically identical and have the same chromosomal content as the parent cell: C1/C2, M1/M2, and S1/S2.

(b) The first meiotic metaphase will have the following configuration:

XX
XX
X X

Label each chromosome according to the symbols in part **(a)** above

(c) For the haploid products of the cell in part (b), there are eight possibilities, depending on the alignment of the homologous chromosomes:

X C1 or C2

X M1 or M2

X S1 or S2

During Meiosis II, the centromeres divide and send a chromatid from each chromosome to the resulting gametes.

18. If there are 8 combinations possible for part (c) in the previous problem, there will be 16 combinations with the addition of another chromosome pair.

19. As you first read this question, think about an animal with $n = 6$; therefore, there will be six tetrads. The question concerns one of these tetrads as it passes normally through meiosis I, but one dyad undergoes secondary nondisjunction. Secondary nondisjunction occurs during the second meiotic division.

(a) The mature ovum should contain $n + 1$ chromosomes: the five chromosomes from normal disjunction and two (from one dyad) from the nondisjunctional chromosome.

(b) The second polar body did not receive one of the six monads it would normally receive, so it should have five monads (which are chromosomes).

(c) When the normal sperm with its n chromosome number combines with an $n + 1$ ovum, it will produce a zygote with $2n + 1$, or 13 chromosomes. This condition is termed *trisomy*.

20. One-half of each tetrad will have a maternal homolog: $(1/2)^{10}$.

21. (a) Although the molecular processes involved in crossing over likely occur earlier, crossing over is known to have occurred by pachynema.

(b) *Synapsis* begins at zygonema with continuation of the homology search and when homologous chromosomes align in a

16

point-by-point fashion to form bivalents or tetrads. More intimate pairing (synapsis) is completed during pachynema.

(c) Chromosomes begin to condense at the earliest stage of prophase I, leptonema.

(d) *Chiasmata* are clearly visible at diplonema.

22. In angiosperms, meiosis results in the formation of microspores (male) and megaspores (female), which give rise to the haploid male and female gametophyte stage. Micro- and megagametophytes produce the pollen and the ovules, respectively. Following fertilization, the sporophyte is formed.

23. The transition from chromatin to individual chromosomes occurs at the beginning of mitosis (or meiosis). During this time, chromatin fibers fold up and condense into the typical mitotic chromosome. The *folded-fiber model* depicts this transition.

24. The folded-fiber model is based on each chromatid consisting of a single fiber wound like a skein of yarn. Each fiber consists of DNA and protein. A coiling process occurs during the transition of interphase chromatin into more condensed chromosomes during prophase of mitosis or meiosis. Such condensation leads to a 5000-fold contraction in the length of the DNA within each chromatid. The transition is at the end of interphase and the beginning of prophase when the chromosomes are in the condensation process. This eventually leads to the typically shortened and "fattened" metaphase chromosome.

25. They would probably be homologous chromosomes and contain similar (but not identical) genetic information. Their centromeres would most likely be in the same position relative to chromosome arm lengths and any physical characteristics such as secondary constrictions or bands would be similar. They would have a similar sequence of nitrogenous bases and would

most likely replicate synchronously during the S phase of the cell cycle.

26. (a) When somatic cells from the same species are examined they contain the same number of chromosomes and the lengths, and centromere placements of nearly all such chromosomes can be matched into pairs.

(b) The initiation and completion of DNA synthesis can be detected by the incorporation of labeled precursors into DNA. DNA content in a G2 nucleus is twice that of a G1 nucleus.

(c) If the fibers comprising the mitotic chromosomes are loosened, they reveal fibers like those of interphase chromatin. Electron microscopic observations indicate that mitotic chromosomes are in varying states of extensively folded structures derived from chromatin.

27. Duplicated chromosomes A^m, A^p, B^m, B^p, C^m, and C^p will align at metaphase, with the centromeres dividing and sister chromatids going to opposite poles at anaphase.

28. Side-by-side alignment of A^m, A^p, B^m, B^p, C^m, and C^p will occur in various arrangements at metaphase I. Eight possible combinations of products will occur at the completion of anaphase: A^m, B^p, C^m, for example (each with sister chromatids). In other words, after meiosis I, the two product cells will be as follows: A^m or A^p, B^m or B^p, C^m or C^p.

29. As long as you have accounted for eight possible combinations in the previous problem, no new ones will be added in this problem.

30. Eight ($2 \times 2 \times 2$) combinations are possible.

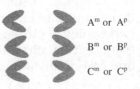

A^m or A^p

B^m or B^p

C^m or C^p

31. See the products of nondisjunction of chromosome *C* at the end of meiosis I, as follows:

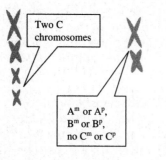

At the end of meiosis II, assuming that, as the problem states, the *C* chromosomes separate as dyads instead of monads during meiosis II, you would have monads for the A and B chromosomes and dyads (from the cell on the left) for both *C* chromosomes as one possibility.

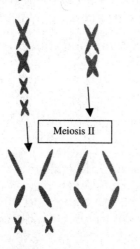

32. Taking this question exactly as it is described—nondisjunction of the *C* chromosome at meiosis I and dyad separation at meiosis II—you will end up, after fertilization, with the following combinations under the conditions described in Problem 31.

zygote 1:   two copies of chromosome *A*
two copies of chromosome *B*
three copies of chromosome *C*

zygote 2:   two copies of chromosome *A*
two copies of chromosome *B*
one copy of chromosome *C*

33. (a) The chromosome number in the somatic tissues of the hybrid would be the summation of the haploid numbers of each parental species: 7 + 14 = 21.

(b) If the G1 DNA content of *Elymus* is 25.5 pg and that of *Secale* is 16.8 pg, the amount of DNA contributing to the somatic cells of the hybrid will be 12.75 pg and 8.4 pg, respectively. Since a metaphase cell has double the amount of DNA as a G1 somatic cell, each metaphase nucleus of the hybrid should have 42.3 pg of DNA.

(c) Given that no homologous chromosome pairing occurs at metaphase I, one would expect 21 univalents and random 1×0 separation of chromosomes at anaphase I. That is, there would be a random separation of univalents to either pole at anaphase I usually leading to inviable haploid cells and thus sterility.

34. The following answers assume a normal chromosomal composition of the mother.

(a) If there were two dyads of chromosome 21 in the first polar body, the secondary oocyte would completely lack chromosome 21. The resulting zygote would have one copy of chromosome 21 (from the father) and two copies of all the other chromosomes.

(b) If the polar body lacked chromosome 21, the secondary oocyte would have two dyads and the resulting zygote would have three number 21 chromosomes (Down syndrome), two coming from the mother and one coming from the father.

(c) The secondary oocyte would have a dyad and a monad from chromosome 21. Depending on how the monad partitioned at meiosis II, you would have either a normal chromosome 21 complement (the zygote that did not receive the monad) or a chromosome 21 trisomy in which the zygote received two number 21 chromosomes from the mother and one from the father.

Chapter 3: Mendelian Genetics

Concept Areas	Corresponding Problems
Mendel's Model	3, 5, 11, 12, 13, 14, 16, 37, 45
Monohybrid Crosses	1, 2, 4, 6, 18, 19, 20, 21, 22, 26, 27, 34, 38
Dihybrid Crosses	7, 8, 9, 10, 15, 23, 32, 40, 41
Trihybrid Crosses	17, 28, 29, 30
Independent Assortment	16, 28
Probability	31, 33, 34, 35, 36, 38, 42, 43, 46
Chi-Square Analysis	24, 25, 37, 44
Pedigree Analysis	26, 27, 33, 37

Vocabulary: Organization and Listing of Terms and Concepts

Historical

Mendelian Genetics (Gregor Mendel)

   Pisum sativum (1865)

   units of heredity (particulate)

Rebirth (1900)

   Hugo DeVries

   Karl Correns

   Erich Tschermak

Punnett squares

Pascal's triangle

Structures and Substances

Unit factors, Genes

Alleles

Processes/Methods

Transmission genetics

   true-breeding, "bred true"

   monohybrid cross

   selfing, self-fertilizing

   reciprocal cross

testcross

parental generation (P_1)

first filial generation (F_1)

second filial generation (F_2)

ratios

   3:1, 1:1

   1:2:1

   9:3:3:1, 1:1:1:1

   27:9:9:9:3:3:3:1

product law

   2^n (n = haploid chromosome number)

sum law

   conditional probability

binomial theorem

   $(a + b)^n$

dihybrid cross (two-factor cross)

trihybrid cross (three-factor cross)

forked-line (branch diagram) method

Statistical testing (analysis)

   predicted occurrences

proportions

sample size

chance deviation

random fluctuations

null hypothesis

measured (observed) values

predicted values

goodness of fit

chi-square analysis (χ^2)

degrees of freedom

probability value (p)

   reject the null hypothesis

   fail to reject the null hypothesis

   0.05 probability value

Pedigree

sibs, sibship line

monozygotic (identical) twins

dizygotic (fraternal) twins

   propositus, propositi

Concepts

Unit factors in pairs (F3.1)

Dominance/recessiveness (F3.1)

Symbolism (F3.2, F3.3)

Segregation

Phenotype

Genotype

Homozygous (homozygote)

Heterozygous (heterozygote)

Independent assortment

Genotypic ratio

Variation of a continuous nature

Variation of a discontinuous nature

Chromosome theory of heredity

Diploid number

Probability

Statistical testing

F3.1 Illustration of the union of maternal and paternal genes (*A* and *a*) to give two genes in the zygote. Mendelian "unit factors" occur in pairs in diploid organisms. Dominant genes are often given the uppercase letter as the symbol, while the lowercase letter is often used to symbolize the recessive gene.

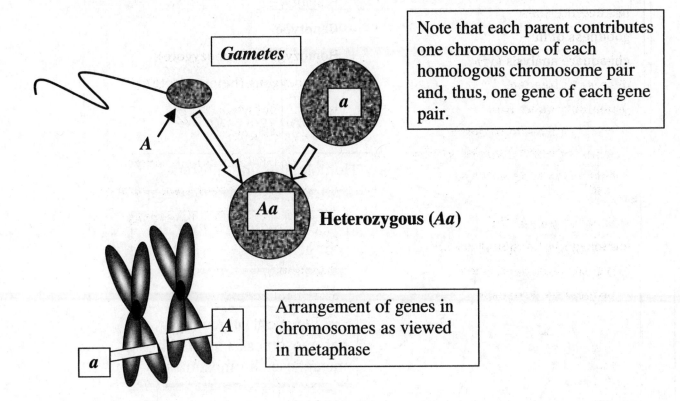

Gametes

a

Note that each parent contributes one chromosome of each homologous chromosome pair and, thus, one gene of each gene pair.

A

Aa   **Heterozygous (*Aa*)**

A

a

Arrangement of genes in chromosomes as viewed in metaphase

F3.2 Critical symbolism associated with genes and chromosomes. Below two different gene pairs (*Aa* and *Bb*) are positioned on nonhomologous chromosomes. Note that with two different gene pairs two different characteristics may be involved, such as seed shape (*A* and *a*) and seed color (*B* and *b*).

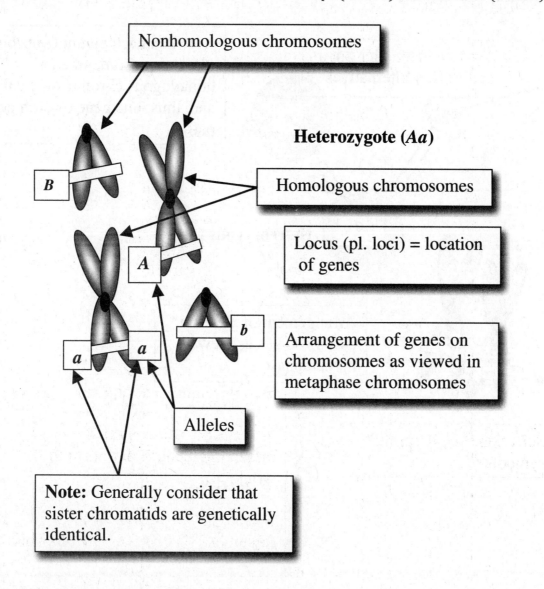

Nonhomologous chromosomes

Heterozygote (*Aa*)

B

Homologous chromosomes

A

Locus (pl. loci) = location of genes

b

a   a

Arrangement of genes on chromosomes as viewed in metaphase chromosomes

Alleles

Note: Generally consider that sister chromatids are genetically identical.

F3.3 One of the most important concepts in this chapter is illustrated in this figure. Two gene pairs (*W* and *B*) are presented, each representing a different characteristic: seed shape (*W* or *w*) and seed color (*B* or *b*). Different gene pairs may influence completely different characteristics (as indicated here) or the same characteristics (described in Chapter 4).

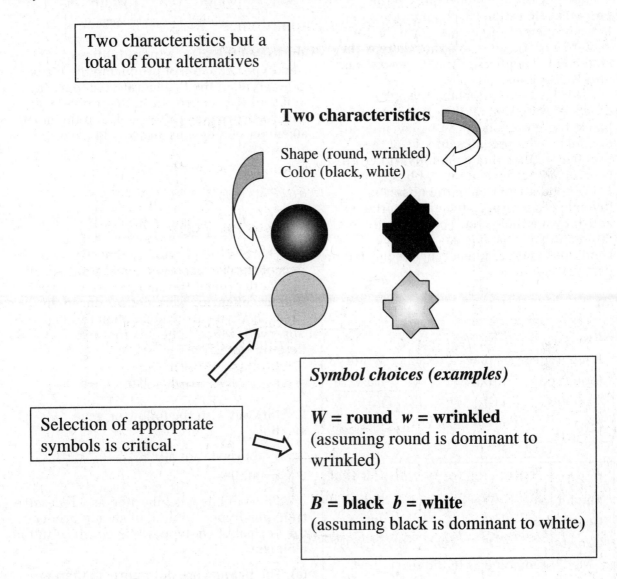

Two characteristics but a total of four alternatives

Two characteristics

Shape (round, wrinkled)
Color (black, white)

Selection of appropriate symbols is critical.

Symbol choices (examples)

W = **round** *w* = **wrinkled**
(assuming round is dominant to wrinkled)

B = **black** *b* = **white**
(assuming black is dominant to white)

Solutions to Problems and Discussion Questions

1. Several points surface in the first sentence of this question. First, two alternatives (black and white) of one characteristic (coat color) are being described; therefore, a monohybrid condition exists.

Second, are the guinea pigs in the parental generation (P_1) homozygous or heterozygous? Notice in the introductory sentence of the question, that there is the statement "members of the P_1 generation are homozygous."

Third, which is dominant, *black* or *white*? Note that all the offspring are black; therefore, black can be considered dominant. The second sentence of the problem verifies that a monohybrid cross is involved because of the 3/4 black and 1/4 white distribution in the offspring. Referring to appropriate figures in the text, and knowing that genes occur in pairs in diploid organisms, one can write the genotypes and the phenotypes requested in part (a) as follows:

(a)

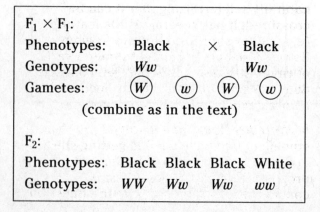

(b) Since *white* is a recessive gene (to *black*), each white guinea pig must be homozygous, and a cross between two white guinea pigs must produce all white offspring.

white	×	white
ww		*ww*

(c) Recall the various possibilities of the genotypes capable of producing the black phenotype in the F_2 generation in part (a): *WW* and *Ww*. In Cross 1 in the problem, all black offspring are observed, and the most likely parental genotypes would be as follows:

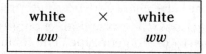

There is the possibility that black guinea pigs of the *Ww* genotype could produce all black offspring if the sample size was such that *ww* offspring were not produced. In Cross 2, a typical 3:1 Mendelian ratio is observed, which indicates that two heterozygotes were crossed:

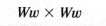

2. Start out with the following gene symbols:

A = normal (not albino)
a = albino

Since albinism is inherited as a recessive trait, genotypes *AA* and *Aa* should produce the normal phenotype, while *aa* will result in albinism.

(a) The parents are both normal; therefore, they could be either *AA* or *Aa*. The fact that they produce an albino child requires that each parent provides an *a* gene to the albino child; thus, the parents must both be heterozygous (*Aa*).

(b) To start out, the normal male could have either the *AA* or *Aa* genotype. The female must be *aa*. Since all the children are normal, one would consider the male to be *AA* instead of *Aa*. However, the male could be *Aa*. Under that circumstance, the likelihood of having six children all normal is 1/64.

(c) To start out, the normal male could have either the *AA* or *Aa* genotype. The female must be *aa*. The fact that half of the children are normal and half are albino indicates a typical "testcross" in which the *Aa* male is mated to the *aa* female.

(d)

The 1:1 ratio of albino to normal in the last generation theoretically results because the mother is *Aa* and the father is *aa*.

3. *Unit Factors in Pairs:* It is important to see that each time a phenotype (normal or abnormal) is being stated, genotypes are symbolized as pairs of genes: *AA*, *Aa*, or *aa*. Review F3.2 to understand the need to assign appropriate symbols to genes.

Dominance and Recessiveness: Because the gene for normal pigmentation is completely dominant over the gene for albinism (*a* is fully recessive), it is necessary first to consider whether normally pigmented individuals in the problem were homozygous normal (*AA*) or heterozygous (*Aa*). By looking at the frequency of expression of the recessive gene in the offspring (in *aa* individuals), one can often determine an *Aa* type from an *AA* type.

Segregation: During gamete formation when homologous chromosomes move to opposite poles, paired elements (genes) separate from each other.

4. While it is very difficult, if not impossible, to know exactly how Mendel made the step from his "monohybrid results" to his postulates, he was able to develop a model with several important components or postulates. First, organisms contained **unit factors** for various traits. Second, if these **factors occurred in pairs**, there existed the possibility that some organisms would "breed true" if homozygous, while others would not (heterozygotes). If one "factor" of a pair had a **dominant influence** over the other, then he could explain how two organisms, looking the same, could be genetically different (homozygous or heterozygous). Third, if the **paired elements separate (segregate)** from each other during gamete formation and if gametes combine at random, he could account for the 3:1 ratios in the monohybrid crosses. The fourth postulate, independent assortment, cannot be demonstrated by a monohybrid cross because two gene pairs must be involved to do so.

Three excellent books provide insight into Mendel's life and the context of his discoveries: Carlson, E. A. 1966. *The Gene: A Critical History.* Philadelphia: W. B. Saunders; Sturtevant, A. H. 1965. *A History of Genetics.* New York: Harper and Row; Voeller, B. R. 1968. *The Chromosome Theory of Inheritance.* New York: Appleton-Century-Crofts.

5. *Pisum sativum* is easy to cultivate. It is naturally self-fertilizing, but it can be crossbred. It has several visible features (e.g., tall or short, red flowers or white flowers) that are consistent under a variety of environmental conditions, yet contrast due to genetic circumstances. Seeds could be obtained from local merchants.

6. With any "long" and involved problem, students often have trouble getting started in the right direction and seeing the problem through to the necessary conclusions. First, read the entire question and see that you are to determine (1) the pattern of inheritance for "checkered and plain," and (2) the gene symbols and genotypes of all the parents and offspring. Notice that reference is made to one characteristic, *pattern*, with two alternatives, checkered vs. plain.

We should consider this to be a monohybrid condition unless complications arise. We are to use the respective offspring from the P_1 cross (F_1 progeny a, b, and c) in a series of F_1 crosses, d through g. Approach the problem by first assigning *probable* genotypes to the P_1 crosses, and then, where there is ambiguity, such as cross (a), use the F_1 crosses for clarification.

Assignment of symbols:

P = checkered; p = plain. Checkered is tentatively assigned the dominant function because in a casual examination of the data, especially cross (b), we see that checkered types are more likely to be produced than plain types.

Cross (a):

$$PP \times PP \quad \text{or} \quad PP \times Pp$$

Notice in cross (d) that the checkered offspring, when crossed to plain, produce only checkered F_2 progeny and in cross (g) when crossed to checkered still produce only checkered progeny. From this additional information, one can conclude that in the progeny of cross (a) there are no heterozygotes and the original cross must have been $PP \times PP$.

Cross (b):

$$PP \times pp$$

This assignment seems reasonable because among 38 offspring, no plain types are produced. In addition, we would expect all the F_1 progeny to be heterozygous and if crossed to plain, as in cross (e), to produce approximately half checkered and half plain offspring. In cross (f) we would expect such heterozygotes to produce a 3:1 ratio, which is observed.

Cross (c): Because all the offspring from this cross are plain, there is no doubt that the genotype of both parents is pp.

Genotypes of all individuals:

		F_1 Progeny	
	P_1 Cross	Checkered	Plain
(a)	$PP \times PP$	PP	
(b)	$PP \times pp$	Pp	
(c)	$pp \times pp$		pp
(d)	$PP \times pp$	Pp	
(e)	$Pp \times pp$	Pp	pp
(f)	$Pp \times Pp$	PP, Pp	pp
(g)	$PP \times Pp$	PP, Pp	

7. In the first sentence you are told that two *characteristics* are being studied: seed shape and cotyledon color. Expect, therefore, this to be a dihybrid situation with *two gene pairs* involved. One also sees the possible alternatives of these two characteristics: *seed shape*—wrinkled vs. round; *cotyledon color*—green vs. yellow. After reading the second sentence, you can predict that the gene for round seeds is dominant to that for wrinkled seeds and that the gene for yellow cotyledons is dominant to the gene for green cotyledons.

Symbolism:

w = wrinkled seeds g = green cotyledons
W = round seeds G = yellow cotyledons

P_1:

$$WWGG \times wwgg$$

Parents are considered to be homozygous for two reasons. First, in the introductory sentence, just after PROBLEMS AND DISCUSSION QUESTIONS, there is the statement "members of the P_1 generation are homozygous." Second, notice that the only offspring are those with round seeds and yellow cotyledons.

Gametes produced: One member of each gene pair is "segregated" to each gamete.

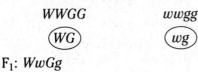

WWGG   wwgg

F$_1$: *WwGg*

F$_1$ × F$_1$:

WwGg × WwGg

Gametes produced: Under conditions of independent assortment, there will be four (2^n, where *n* = number of heterozygous gene pairs) different types of gametes produced by each parent.

Punnett Square:

	WG	Wg	wG	wg
WG	WWGG	WWGg	WwGG	WwGg
Wg	WWGg	WWgg	WwGg	Wwgg
wG	WwGG	WwGg	wwGG	wwGg
wg	WwGg	Wwgg	wwGg	wwgg

Collecting the phenotypes according to the dominance scheme presented above gives the following:

9/16 *W_G_* round seeds, yellow cotyledons
3/16 *W_gg* round seeds, green cotyledons
3/16 *wwG_* wrinkled seeds, yellow cotyledons
1/16 *wwgg* wrinkled seeds, green cotyledons

Notice that a dash (_) is used in instances where, because of dominance, it makes no difference as to the dominant/recessive status of the allele.

Forked, or branch diagram:

Seed shape	Cotyledon color	Phenotypes
3/4 round	3/4 yellow ⟹	9/16 round, yellow
	1/4 green ⟹	3/16 round, green
1/4 wrinkled	3/4 yellow ⟹	3/16 wrinkled, yellow
	1/4 green ⟹	1/16 wrinkled, green

8. *WWgg* = 1/16

9. Symbolism as before:

w = wrinkled seeds	*g* = green cotyledons
W = round seeds	*G* = yellow cotyledons

Examine each characteristic (seed shape vs. cotyledon color) separately.

(a) Notice a 3:1 ratio for seed shape; therefore, *Ww* × *Ww*; and no green cotyledons, therefore, *GG* × *GG* or *GG* × *Gg*. Putting the two characteristics together gives

WwGG × WwGG
or
WwGG × WwGg

(b) Notice a 1:1 ratio for seed shape (8/16 wrinkled and 8/16 round) and a 3:1 ratio for cotyledon color (12/16 yellow and 4/16 green). Therefore, the answer is

wwGg × WwGg

(c) The offspring occur in a typical 9:3:3:1 ratio. Therefore, the F$_2$ plants have the doubly heterozygous genotypes of

WwGg × WwGg

(d) This is a typical 1:1:1:1 testcross (or backcross) ratio and will signify that one parent is doubly heterozygous, while the other is fully homozygous recessive. The answer is

WwGg × wwgg

10. A testcross involves a cross of an organism with an unknown genotype to a fully homozygous recessive organism. In Problem 9, (d) fits this description.

11. Because independent assortment may be defined as one gene pair segregating independently of another gene pair, one would need at least two gene pairs in order to demonstrate independent assortment.

12. Mendel's four postulates are related to the following diagram.

(1) Factors occur in pairs. Notice *A* and *a*.

(2) Some genes have dominant and recessive alleles. Notice *A* and *a*.

(3) Alleles segregate from each other during gamete formation. When homologous chromosomes separate from each other at anaphase I, alleles will go to opposite poles of the meiotic apparatus.

(4) One gene pair separates independently from other gene pairs. Different gene pairs on the same homologous pair of chromosomes (if far apart) or on nonhomologous chromosomes will separate independently from each other during meiosis.

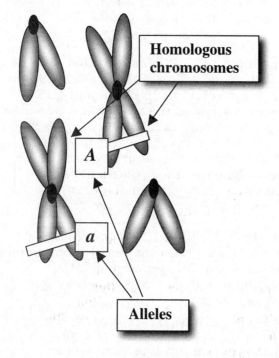

Homologous chromosomes

A

a

Alleles

13. Carefully re-read the answer to Question 2 in Chapter 2. Briefly, the factors that specify chromosomal homology are the following:

overall length
position of the centromere
banding patterns
*type and location of genes** *
autoradiographic pattern

*Functional basis for homologous chromosome designation

14. Homozygosity refers to a condition in which both genes of a pair are the same (i.e., *AA* or *GG* or *hh*), whereas heterozygosity refers to the condition in which members of a gene pair are different (i.e., *Aa* or *Gg* or *Bb*). Homozygotes produce only one type of gamete, whereas heterozygotes will produce 2^n types of gametes where n = number of heterozygous gene pairs (assuming independent assortment).

15. Two characteristics are presented here: body color and wing length. First, assign meaningful gene symbols.

Body color	Wing length
E = gray body color	*V* = long wings
e = ebony body color	*v* = vestigial wings

(a)

P₁:

$$EEVV \times eevv$$

F₁: *EeVv* (gray, long)

F₂: This will be the result of a Punnett square with 16 boxes as in the text.

Phenotypes	Ratio	Genotypes	Ratio
gray, long	9/16	*EEVV*	1/16
		EEVv	2/16
		EeVV	2/16
		EeVv	4/16
gray, vestigial	3/16	*EEvv*	1/16
		Eevv	2/16
ebony, long	3/16	*eeVV*	1/16
		eeVv	2/16
ebony, vestigial	1/16	*eevv*	1/16

(b)

P$_1$:

$$EEvv \times eeVV$$

F$_1$: It is important to see that the results from this cross will be exactly the same as those in part (a) above. The only difference is that the recessive genes are coming from both parents rather than from one parent only as in (a). The F$_2$ ratio will also be the same as (a). When you have genes on the autosomes (not X-linked), independent assortment, complete dominance, and no gene interaction (see later) in a cross involving double heterozygotes, the offspring ratio will be 9:3:3:1.

(c)

P$_1$:

$$EEVV \times EEvv$$

F$_1$: *EEVv* (gray, long)

F$_2$: Notice that all the offspring will have gray bodies and you will get a 3:1 ratio of long to vestigial wings. You should see this before you even begin working through the problem. Even though this cross involves two gene pairs it will give a "monohybrid" type of ratio because one of the gene pairs is homozygous (body color) and one gene pair is heterozygous (wing length).

Phenotypes	Ratio	Genotypes	Ratio
gray, long	3/4	*EEVV*	1/4
		EEVv	2/4
gray, vestigial	1/4	*EEvv*	1/4

NOTE: After working through this problem, it is important that you try to work similar problems without constructing the time-consuming Punnett squares, especially if each problem asks for phenotypic rather than genotypic ratios.

16. The general formula for determining the number of kinds of gametes produced by an organism is 2^n where n = number of *heterozygous* gene pairs.

(a) 4: *AB, Ab, aB, ab*
(b) 2: *AB, aB*
(c) 8: *ABC, ABc, AbC, Abc, aBC, aBc, abC, abc*
(d) 2: *ABc, aBc*
(e) 4: *ABc, Abc, aBc, abc*
(f) $2^5 = 32$

ABCDE	*aBCDE*
ABCDe	*aBCDe*
ABCdE	*aBCdE*
ABCde	*aBCde*
ABcDE	*aBcDE*
ABcDe	*aBcDe*
ABcdE	*aBcdE*
ABcde	*aBcde*
AbCDE	*abCDE*
AbCDe	*abCDe*
AbCdE	*abCdE*
AbCde	*abCde*
AbcDE	*abcDE*
AbcDe	*abcDe*
AbcdE	*abcdE*
Abcde	*abcde*

Notice that there is a pattern that can be used to write these gametes so that fewer errors will occur.

17. (a) When examining this cross

$$AaBbCc \times AaBBCC$$

expect there to be eight different kinds of gametes from one parent (*AaBbCc*), and two different kinds from the other (*AaBBCC*). Therefore, there should be 16 kinds (genotypes) of offspring (8 × 2).

Gametes: Gametes:

ABC
ABc
AbC
Abc
aBC
aBc
abC
abc

ABC
aBC

Offspring:

Genotypes	Ratio	Phenotypes
AABBCC	(1/16)	
AABBCc	(1/16)	
AABbCC	(1/16)	
AABbCc	(1/16)	A_B_C_ = 12/16
AaBBCC	(2/16)	
AaBBCc	(2/16)	
AaBbCC	(2/16)	
AaBbCc	(2/16)	
aaBBCC	(1/16)	
aaBBCc	(1/16)	
aaBbCC	(1/16)	aaB_C_ = 4/16
aaBbCc	(1/16)	

(b) There will be four kinds of gametes for the first parent (*AaBBCc*) and two kinds of gametes for the second parent.

Gametes:

ABC
ABc
aBC
aBc

Gametes:

aBC
aBc

Offspring:

Genotypes	Ratio	Phenotypes
AaBBCC	1/8	A_BBC_ = 3/8
AaBBCc	2/8	
AaBBcc	1/8	A_BBcc = 1/8
aaBBCC	1/8	aaBBC_ = 3/8
aaBBCc	2/8	
aaBBcc	1/8	aaBBcc = 1/8

(c) There will be eight (2^n) different kinds of gametes from each of the parents, and therefore a 64-box Punnett square. Doing this problem by the forked-line method helps considerably.

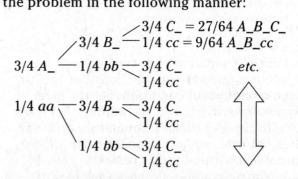

Simply multiply through each component to arrive at the final genotypic frequencies.

For the phenotypic frequencies, set up the problem in the following manner:

3/4 A_ ⟨ 3/4 B_ ⟨ 3/4 C_ = 27/64 A_B_C_
       ⟨   ⟨ 1/4 cc = 9/64 A_B_cc
       ⟨ 1/4 bb ⟨ 3/4 C_   etc.
                 ⟨ 1/4 cc

1/4 aa ⟨ 3/4 B_ ⟨ 3/4 C_
       ⟨   ⟨ 1/4 cc
       ⟨ 1/4 bb ⟨ 3/4 C_
                 ⟨ 1/4 cc

18. In the first reading of this question one should consider that one characteristic is involved: seed color. Given that information and the F_2 progeny of 6022 yellow and 2001 green, a monohybrid condition is suspected. In addition, of the 519 self-fertilized, yellow-seeded plants, 166 bred true while the others produced a 3:1 ratio of yellow to green. This is what would be expected because approximately 1/3 of the yellow F_2 plants should be homozygous, while 2/3 of the yellow F_2 plants should be heterozygous.

Set up the symbols as follows: G = yellow seeds, g = green seeds. We know that the gene for yellow seeds is dominant to that for green seeds because the F_1 is all yellow, not green.

Phenotypes	Genotypes
P_1: Yellow × green	$GG \times gg$
F_1: all yellow	Gg
F_2: 6022 yellow	1/4 GG; 2/4 Gg
2001 green	1/4 gg

Of the yellow F_2 offspring, notice that 1/3 of them are GG and 2/3 are Gg. If you selfed the 1/3 GG types, then all the offspring (the 166) would breed true, whereas the others (353, which are Gg) should produce offspring in a 3:1 ratio when selfed.

$$GG \times GG$$
$$= \text{all } GG$$
$$Gg \times Gg$$
$$= 1/4\ GG;\ 2/4\ Gg;\ 1/4\ gg$$

19. Because only one characteristic is being dealt with in this problem (coat color) and a 3:1 ratio is mentioned in the second sentence, one can initially consider this to be a monohybrid condition. Set the gene symbols as W = black, w = white.

One hundred black animals could be all WW, all Ww, or a mixture (WW, Ww). When the WW individuals are crossed to ww, all the offspring will be black, which is what occurred in 94 of the cases. All these black offspring would be heterozygous and would be expected to produce a 3:1 ratio when intercrossed. In those cases where a 1:1 ratio resulted, the parents must have been Ww. The cross would be as follows:

P_1:

$$Ww \times ww$$

F_1:

$$1/2\ Ww,\ 1/2\ ww$$

If one were to cross the black and white guinea pigs from the above cross, again the offspring would produce 1/2 black and 1/2 white as above.

20. In reading this question, notice that two characteristics are being considered: seed color (yellow, green) and seed shape (round, wrinkled). At this point you should be able to do this problem without writing down each of the steps. The F_1 can be considered to be a double heterozygote (with round and yellow being dominant). See the cross this way:

Symbols:

Seed shape	Seed color
W = round	G = yellow
w = wrinkled	g = green

P_1: $WWgg \times wwGG$

F_1: $WwGg$ cross to $wwgg$
(which is a typical testcross)

The offspring will occur in a typical 1:1:1:1 as

1/4 $WwGg$ (round, yellow)
1/4 $Wwgg$ (round, green)
1/4 $wwGg$ (wrinkled, yellow)
1/4 $wwgg$ (wrinkled, green)

Again, at this point it would be very helpful if you could do such simple problems by inspection.

21. This question deals with the definition of dominance/recessiveness. Notice that there are only two alleles (one gene pair) and three phenotypes associated with the problem: normal, "minor" anemia, and "major" anemia. Under a monohybrid model, the heterozygote is distinguishable from either homozygote that does not fit the definition of dominance. One would conclude that no dominance is involved and incomplete dominance exists (see Chapter 4).

22. Since these are F_2 results from monohybrid crosses, a 3:1 ratio is expected for each. Referring to the text, one can easily set up the analysis.

(a)

Expected ratio	Observed (o)	Expected (e)
3/4	882	885.75
1/4	299	295.25

Expected values are derived by multiplying the expected ratio by the total number of organisms.

$$\chi^2 = \Sigma(o - e)^2/e = .064$$

By looking at the χ^2 table with 1 degree of freedom (because there were two classes—therefore, $n - 1$ or 1 degree of freedom), we find a probability (*p*) value between 0.9 and 0.5.

We would therefore say that there is a "good fit" between the observed and expected values. Notice that as the deviations between the observed and expected values increase, the value of χ^2 increases. So the higher the χ^2 value, the more likely it is that the null hypothesis will be rejected.

(b)

Expected ratio	Observed (o)	Expected (e)
3/4	705	696.75
1/4	224	232.25

$$\chi^2 = 0.39$$

The *p* value in the table for 1 degree of freedom is still between 0.9 and 0.5; however; because the χ^2 value is larger in (b), we should say that the deviations from expectation are greater. The deviation in each case can be attributed to chance.

23. One must think of this problem as a dihybrid F_2 situation with the following expectations:

Expected ratio	Observed (o)	Expected (e)
9/16	315	312.75
3/16	108	104.25
3/16	101	104.25
1/16	32	34.75

$$\chi^2 = 0.47$$

Looking at the table in the text, one can see that this χ^2 value is associated with a probability greater than 0.90 for 3 degrees of freedom (because there are now four classes in the χ^2 test). The observed and expected values do not deviate significantly.

To deal with parts (b) and (c) it is easier to see the observed values for the monohybrid ratios if the phenotypes are listed:

smooth, yellow	315
smooth, green	108
wrinkled, yellow	101
wrinkled, green	32

For the smooth:wrinkled *monohybrid component*, the smooth types total 423 (315 + 108), while the wrinkled types total 133 (101 + 32).

Expected ratio	Observed (o)	Expected (e)
3/4	423	417
1/4	133	139

The χ^2 value is 0.35, and in examining the text for 1 degree of freedom, the *p* value is greater than 0.50 and less than 0.90. We fail to reject the null hypothesis and are confident that the observed values do not differ significantly from the expected values.

(c) For the yellow:green portion of the problem, see that there are 416 yellow plants (315 + 101) and 140 (108 + 32) green plants.

Expected ratio	Observed (o)	Expected (e)
3/4	416	417
1/4	140	139

The χ^2 value is 0.01 and in examining the text for 1 degree of freedom, the p value is greater than 0.90. We fail to reject the null hypothesis and are confident that the observed values do not differ significantly from the expected values.

24. It would be best to set up two tables based on the two hypotheses:

Expected ratio	Observed (o)	Expected (e)
3/4	250	300
1/4	150	100

Expected ratio	Observed (o)	Expected (e)
1/2	250	200
1/2	150	200

For the test of a 3:1 ratio, the χ^2 value is 33.3, with an associated p value of less than 0.01 for 1 degree of freedom. For the test of a 1:1 ratio, the χ^2 value is 25.0, again with an associated p value of less than 0.01 for 1 degree of freedom. Based on these probability values, both null hypotheses should be rejected.

25. Use of the $p = 0.10$ as the "critical" value for rejecting or failing to reject the null hypothesis instead of $p = 0.05$ would allow more null hypotheses to be rejected. Notice in the text that as the χ^2 values increase, there is a higher likelihood that the null hypothesis will be rejected because the higher values are more likely to be associated with a p value that is less than 0.05.

As the critical p value is increased, it takes a smaller χ^2 value to cause rejection of the null hypothesis. It would take less difference between the expected and observed values to reject the null hypothesis; therefore, the stringency of failing to reject the null hypothesis is increased.

26. Although many different inheritance patterns will be described later in the text (codominance, incomplete dominance, sex-linked inheritance, etc.), the range of solutions to this question is limited to the concepts developed in the first three chapters, namely, dominance or recessiveness.

If a gene is dominant, it will not skip generations; nor will it be passed to offspring unless the parents have the gene. On the other hand, genes that are recessive can skip generations and exist in a carrier state in parents. For example, notice that II-4 and II-5 produce a female child (III-4) with the affected phenotype. Based on these criteria alone, the gene must be viewed as being recessive. *Note:* If a gene is recessive and X-linked (to be discussed later), the pattern will often be from affected male to carrier female to affected male.

To provide genotypes for each individual, consider that if the box or circle is shaded, the *aa* genotype is to be assigned. If offspring are affected (shaded), a recessive gene must have come from both parents.

I-1 (*Aa*), I-2 (*aa*), I-3 (*Aa*), I-4(*Aa*)

II-1 (*aa*), II-2 (*Aa*), II-3 (*aa*), II-4 (*Aa*), II-5 (*Aa*), II-6 (*aa*), II-7 (*AA* or *Aa*), II-8 (*AA* or *Aa*)

III-1 (*AA* or *Aa*), III-2 (*AA* or *Aa*), III-3 (*AA* or *Aa*), III-4 (*aa*), III-5 (probably *AA*), III-6 (*aa*)

IV-1 through IV-7 all *Aa*.

27. Applying the same logic as in question 26, the gene is inherited as an autosomal recessive. Notice that two normal individuals II-3 and II-4 have produced a daughter (III-2) with myopia.

I-1 (*aa*), I-2 (*Aa* or *AA*), I-3 (*Aa*), I-4 (*Aa*)
II-1 (*Aa*), II-2 (*Aa*), II-3 (*Aa*), II-4 (*Aa*), II-5 (*aa*), II-6 (*AA* or *Aa*), II-7 (*AA* or *Aa*)
III-1 (*AA* or *Aa*), III-2 (*aa*), III-3 (*AA* or *Aa*)

28. Given the cross $AaBbCC \times AABbCc$, we can apply the product rule, which states that when two or more events occur independently but simultaneously, their combined probability is equal to the product of their individual probabilities.

The probability of getting *AA* from

$$Aa \times AA \text{ is } 1/2$$

The probability of getting *Bb* from

$$Bb \times Bb \text{ is } 1/2$$

The probability of getting *Cc* from

$$CC \times Cc \text{ is } 1/2$$

The *overall* probability then is

$$1/2 \times 1/2 \times 1/2 = 1/8$$

29. The probability of getting *aabbcc* from the *AaBbCC* × *AABbCc* mating is zero because of homozygosity for *AA* and *CC*.

30. Because all the offspring will show the dominant A and C phenotypes and 3/4 will show the B phenotype, the probability of an offspring showing all three dominant traits would be $1 \times 3/4 \times 1 = 3/4$.

31. (a) 1/6

(b) Apply the product law: $1/6 \times 1/6 = 1/36$

(c, d) Consider that there are two ways of coming up with the 3 and 6, and it doesn't matter in which way it is achieved: $(1/6 \times 1/6) + (1/6 \times 1/6) = 1/18$. Perhaps another way to think of it is the following: the probability is 1/3 that one die will come up a 3 or a 6, and 1/6 that the other die will come up with the appropriate number. Therefore, the answer is again $1/3 \times 1/6 = 1/18$.

(e) 1/3

32. Calculate each allelic pair separately and know that for each plant expressing the dominant phenotype, there is a 2/3 probability that it is heterozygous. Since the 2/3 probability applies to two independent loci, the product law is applied:

$$2/3 \times 2/3 = 4/9$$

33. (a) There are two possibilities. Either the trait is dominant, in which case I-1 is heterozygous as are II-2 and II-3, or the trait is recessive and I-1 is homozygous and I-2 is heterozygous. Under the condition of recessiveness, both II-1 and II-4 would be heterozygous; II-2 and II-3 are homozygous.

(b) recessive: parents *Aa, Aa*

(c) recessive: parents *Aa, Aa*

(d) recessive or dominant, not sex-linked; if recessive, parents *Aa, aa*

34. Assuming that both parents are heterozygous, the probability of being a carrier (for the male and female) is 2/3 for each. Since a child has a 1/4 chance of being homozygous recessive from carrier parents, the overall probability of the child having cystic fibrosis is:

$$2/3 \times 2/3 \times 1/4 = 1/9$$

35. (a) $P = [5!(1/2)^5(1/2)^0]/5!0! = 1/32$

(b) $P = [5!(1/2)^3(1/2)^2]/3!2! = 5/16$

(c) $P = [5!(1/2)^2(1/2)^3]/2!3! = 5/16$

(d) There are two ways of all being the same sex, all males or all females. Therefore the final probability is the sum of the two independent probabilities:

$$1/32 + 1/32 = 1/16$$

36. $P = [8!(3/4)^6(1/4)^2]/6!2!$

37. (a) By noting that traits passed unaltered from parental to subsequent generations, Mendel not only postulated the "unit" or "particulate" nature of hereditary elements, but he also described their behavior. Results of various crosses provided the basis for knowing that factors can remain hidden in some circumstances, thereby implying two participating elements, one dominating the other. Predictable ratios in crosses supported the hypothesis of two hereditary elements involved in the expression of a given trait.

(b) Typically, by conducting a testcross, one readily tests whether an organism is homozygous or heterozygous for a given trait.

(c) In general, a chi-square analysis is used to compare observed data with various genetic models.

(d) Pedigree analysis is often used to determine whether and how traits are inherited in humans. However, other methods are also used and are discussed in subsequent chapters.

38. (a) First consider that each parent is homozygous (true-breeding in the question) and since in the F_1 only round, axial, violet, and full phenotypes were expressed, they must each be dominant.

(b) Because all genes are on nonhomologous chromosomes, independent assortment will occur. Round, axial, violet and full would be the most frequent phenotypes:

$$3/4 \times 3/4 \times 3/4 \times 3/4$$

(c) Wrinkled, terminal, white, and constricted would be the least frequent phenotypes:

$$1/4 \times 1/4 \times 1/4 \times 1/4$$

(d) $3/4 \times 1/4 \times 3/4 \times 1/4$
$\quad + 1/4 \times 3/4 \times 1/4 \times 3/4 = 18/256$

(e) There would be 16 different phenotypes in the testcross offspring, just as there are 16 different phenotypes in the F_2 generation.

39. (a) The first task is to draw out an accurate pedigree (one of several possibilities):

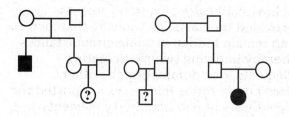

(b) The probability that the female (whose maternal uncle had TSD) is heterozygous is 1/3 because she is not TSD and her mother had a 2/3 chance of being heterozygous and she has a 1/2 chance of passing the TSD gene to her daughter ($2/3 \times 1/2 = 1/3$). The male (whose paternal first cousin had TSD)

has a 1/4 chance of being heterozygous, assuming that either (but not both, because the gene is said to be rare) his grandmother or grandfather was heterozygous. Therefore, the probability that both the male and female are heterozygous is:

$$1/3 \times 1/4 = 1/12$$

(c) The probability that neither is heterozygous is:

$$2/3 \times 3/4 = 6/12$$

(d) The probability that one is heterozygous is:

$$(1/3 \times 3/4) + (2/3 \times 1/4) = 5/12$$

Also, there are only three possibilities: both are heterozygous, neither is heterozygous, and at least one is heterozygous. You have already calculated the first two probabilities; the last is simply $1 - (1/12 + 6/12) = 5/12$.

40. (a) Ignoring flower color for the present, notice in the first cross that a 3:1 ratio exists for the spiny to smooth phenotypes in the first cross. Thus, we would predict that the *spiny* allele is dominant to *smooth*. Applying the same reasoning to the second cross, notice that there is a 3:1 ratio of purple to white. We would also predict that the *purple* allele is dominant to *white*.

(b) One could cross a homozygous purple, spiny plant to a homozygous white, smooth plant. The purple, spiny F_1 would support the hypothesis that *purple* is dominant to *white* and *spiny* is dominant to *smooth*. In the F_2, a 9:3:3:1 ratio would not only support the above hypothesis, but it would also indicate the independent inheritance and expression of the two traits.

41. (a) Notice in cross 1 that the ratio of straight wings to curled wings is 3:1 and that the ratio of short bristles to long bristles is also 3:1. This would indicate that straight is dominant to curled and short is dominant to long.

Possible symbols would be (using standard *Drosophila* symbolism):

straight wings = w^+ curled wings = w
short bristles = b^+ long bristles = b

(b)

Cross #1: w^+/w; b^+/b $\times$ w^+/w; b^+/b

Cross #2: w^+/w; b/b $\times$ w^+/w; b/b

Cross #3: w/w; b/b $\times$ w^+/w; b^+/b

Cross #4: w^+/w^+; $b^+/b \times w^+/w^+$; b^+/b
(one parent could be w^+/w)

Cross #5: w/w; b^+/b $\times$ w^+/w; b^+/b

42.

$$P = [5!(3/4)^3(1/4)^2]/3!2!$$
$$= 135/512$$

43. Because there are three possibilities within the group, it probably represents a case of incomplete dominance or codominance (see Chapter 4).

44. (a) First, consider that the data represent a 3:1 ratio based on the information given in the problem: $Ss \times Ss$. Compute the expected quantities for each class by multiplying the totals by 3/4 and 1/4.

Set I Expected Numbers:

Tall = 26.25   Short = 8.75

Set II Expected Numbers:

Tall = 262.5   Short = 87.5

For Set I the χ^2 value would be:

$(30 - 26.25)^2/26.25 + (5 - 8.75)^2/8.75 = 2.15$
with p being between 0.2 and 0.05

so one would accept the null hypothesis of no significant difference between the expected and observed values.

For Set II, the χ^2 value would be 21.43 and $p < 0.001$, and one would reject the null hypothesis and assume a significant difference between the observed and expected values.

(b) Clearly, with an increase in sample size, a different conclusion is reached. In fact, most statisticians recommend that the expected values in each class not be less than 10. In most cases, more confidence is gained as the sample size increases; however, depending on the organism or experiment, there are practical limits on sample size.

45. (a) Mendel postulated that each pair of hereditary elements separated independently from other pairs of hereditary elements during gamete formation. The work of Sutton and Carothers indicates that chromosomes also separate independently of each other.

(b) If Mendel's hereditary factors are on chromosomes as proposed by the chromosome theory of heredity, one could explain the independent assortment of genes on the basis of the independent assortment of chromosomes.

46. Given that dentinogenesis imperfecta is inherited as a dominant allele and that the man's mother had normal teeth, the man with six children must be heterozygous. Therefore, the probability that their first child will be a male with dentinogenesis imperfecta would be 1/2 (passage of the allele) $\times$ 1/2 (probability of child being male) = 1/4. The probability that three of their six children will have the disease is best determined by application of the following formula.

$$p = \frac{n!}{s!t!}a^s b^t$$

where:

n = total number of events (six in this case)

s = number of times outcome a happens (three in this case)

t = number of times outcome b happens (three in this case)

a = probability of being normal in this family (1/2)

b = probability of having the disease in this family (1/2)

$$p = \frac{6!}{3!3!}\, 1/2^3\, 1/2^3$$

The overall probability (p) would be 5/16 or about 0.31 (31%). All these types of questions are handled in the same manner.

Determine first the total number of events (n), and then how many times one outcome will occur (s). Determine how many times the alternative outcome will occur (t). Once you know the probability (a) of the "s" outcome and the probability (b) of outcome "t," you have all the components for the equation.

Chapter 4: Extensions of Mendelian Genetics

Concept Areas	Corresponding Problems
Function/Symbolism of Alleles (Genes)	31, 48
Incomplete Dominance, Codominance	1, 2, 5, 12, 13, 14, 23
Multiple Alleles	5, 6, 7, 8, 10, 11
Lethal Alleles	3, 4, 9, 41
Gene Interaction	8, 20, 22, 29, 38, 39, 43, 45, 47
Epistasis	16, 17, 18, 19, 21, 41
Novel Phenotypes	15
X-Linkage	24, 25, 26, 27, 28, 29, 30, 32, 35, 46
Sex-Limited/Sex-Influenced Inheritance	33, 34, 42, 44
Phenotypic Expression	36, 37, 47, 49
Genetic Anticipation and Imprinting	38

Vocabulary: Organization and Listing of Terms and Concepts

Structures and Substances

Wild type, mutations

  wild-type allele

  loss of function

  null

  gain of function

Native antigens

Antibodies

  glycoprotein

  isoagglutinogen

Ommatidia

  drosopterin

  xanthommatin

Hexosaminidase

Heterochromatin

Processes/Methods

Incomplete (partial) dominance
  pink flowers, 1:2:1

Codominance

  MN blood groups

Multiple allelism

  ABO blood types

  antigen-antibody reaction

    agglutination

    H substance

    galactose

    N-acetylglucosamine

    Bombay phenotype

  white eye in *Drosophila*

Lethal alleles

  recessive, dominant

    yellow coat color in mice

    Huntington disease

Gene interaction: discontinuous variation

  epigenesis

  epistasis

  homozygous recessive, 9:3:4

    coat color in mice

    Bombay phenotype

  dominant

    fruit color in squash, 12:3:1

  other

    white flowers in peas, 9:7

  novel phenotypes

    fruit shape in *Cucurbita*

    eye color in *Drosophila*

Complementation

  complementation group

X-linkage, Chromosome Theory

  hemizygous

    crisscross pattern

Sex-limited inheritance

  feathering in chickens

Sex-influenced inheritance

  pattern baldness

Penetrance

Expressivity

  genetic background

  position effect

  suppression

Pleiotropy

Conditional mutation

  temperature

  nutritional mutant

    auxotroph

    phenylketonuria

    galactosemia

  Marfan syndrome

  porphyria variegata

  Tay-Sachs

  Lesch-Nyhan

  Duchene muscular dystrophy (DMD)

  Huntington Disease

Genetic anticipation

Genomic (parental) imprinting

  Prader-Willi syndrome

  Angelman syndrome

Concepts

Gene interaction (F4.1)

Neo-Mendelian genetics

Allele (F4.2)

  wild type, mutation

    loss of wild-type function

    reduced or increased function

Symbolism (F4.2)

  recessive trait *(e, e$^+$)*

  dominant trait *(Wr, Wr$^+$)*

  no dominance *(R1, R2) (L^M, L^N)*

  leu–, leu+, dnaA, BRCA1

Modified ratios (T4.1), lethality

    3:1, 1:2:1, 9:3:3:1

    3:6:3:1:2:1

    9:3:4, 12:3:1, 9:7, 1:4:6:4:1

Complementation analysis

X-linked inheritance

Sex-limited inheritance

Sex-influenced inheritance

Phenotypic expression

    penetrance, expressivity

Genetic background

Environmental effects

T4.1 Examples of typical monohybrid and dihybrid ratios with several modifications.

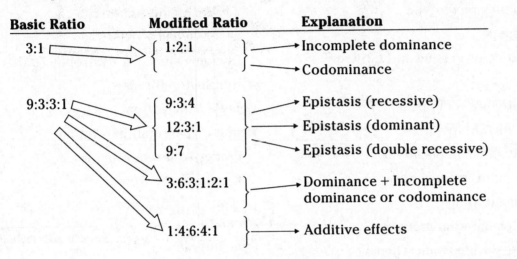

Basic Ratio	Modified Ratio	Explanation
3:1	1:2:1	Incomplete dominance
		Codominance
9:3:3:1	9:3:4	Epistasis (recessive)
	12:3:1	Epistasis (dominant)
	9:7	Epistasis (double recessive)
	3:6:3:1:2:1	Dominance + Incomplete dominance or codominance
	1:4:6:4:1	Additive effects

F4.1 Illustration of gene interaction where products from more than one gene pair influence one characteristic or phenotypic trait.

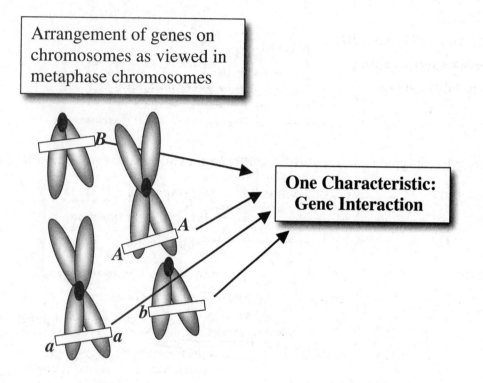

Arrangement of genes on chromosomes as viewed in metaphase chromosomes

One Characteristic: Gene Interaction

Example: Two gene pairs influencing the pigmentation pattern on the shark. Various gene products contribute in a variety of ways to generate a particular pigment pattern.

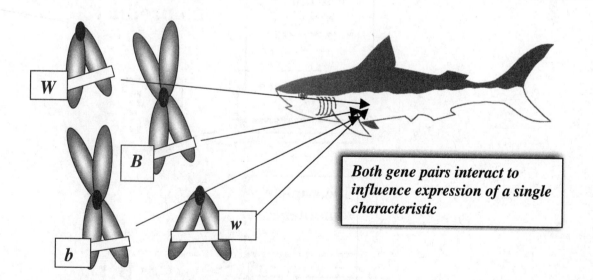

Both gene pairs interact to influence expression of a single characteristic

F4.2 Symbolism associated with the wild-type activity of a gene and several possible outcomes of the mutant state: **A.** wild type; **B.** too much product; **C.** too little product; **D.** no product; **E.** both products expressed; **F.** reduced product.

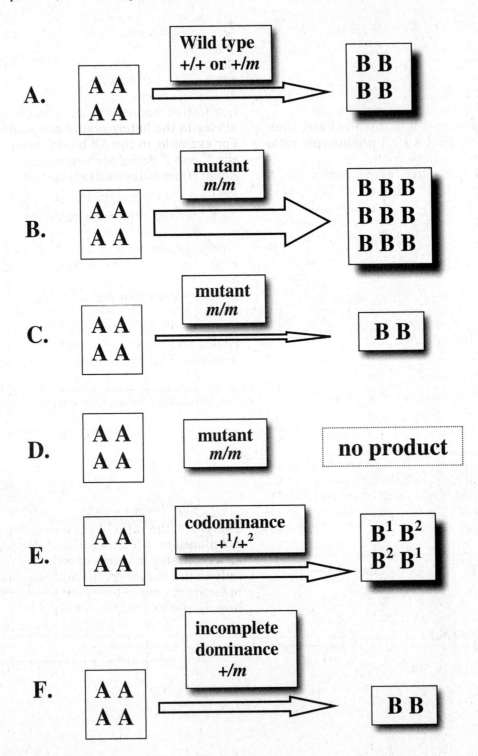

Solutions to Problems and Discussion Questions

1. In the first sentence of this problem, notice the mention of one characteristic (coat color) and three phenotypes: red, white, and roan. The fact that roan is intermediate between red and white suggests that this may be a case of incomplete dominance, with roan being the intermediate and, therefore, the heterozygous type. If that is the case, then we should suspect a 1:2:1 phenotypic ratio in crosses of "roan to roan."

Looking at the data given, notice that a cross of the "extremes" (red × white) gives roan, suggesting its heterozygous nature and the homozygous nature of the parents. Seeing the 1:2:1 ratio in the offspring of

roan   ×   roan

confirms the hypothesis of incomplete dominance as the mode of inheritance.

> Symbolism:
>
> *AA* = red
>
> *aa* = white
>
> *Aa* = roan

Crosses: It is important at this point that you not be fully dependent on writing out complete Punnett squares for each cross. Begin working these simple problems in your head.

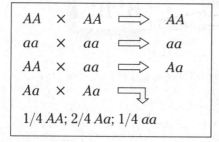

2. *Incomplete dominance* can be viewed primarily as a quantitative phenomenon where the heterozygote is intermediate (approximately) between the limits set by the homozygotes. Pink is intermediate between red and white.

Codominance can be viewed in a more qualitative manner where both of the alleles in the heterozygote are expressed. For example, in the AB blood group, both the I^A and I^B genes are expressed. There is no intermediate class that is part I^A and part I^B.

3. Notice that there is one typical (coat color) and one atypical (lethality) characteristic mentioned. Often under this condition of two characteristics, we must decide if the problem involves one or more than one gene pair. Because the genotypes are given here, it is obvious that lethality is associated with expression of the coat color alleles and therefore one gene pair is involved. This is a monohybrid condition.

> *Pp*   ×   *Pp*
>
> 1/4 *PP* (**lethal**)
>
> 2/4 *Pp* (platinum)
>
> 1/4 *pp* (silver)

Therefore, the ratio of surviving foxes is 2/3 platinum, 1/3 silver. The *P* allele behaves as a recessive in terms of lethality (seen only in the homozygote) but as a dominant in terms of coat color (seen in the homozygote).

4. In this problem it would be helpful first to diagram the phenotypes of the crosses so that you can get some idea of the inheritance pattern. From those phenotypic crosses, a suggestion as to the genotypes can be made and verified.

Cross 1:

short tail × normal long tail ⇨

approximately 1/2 short, 1/2 long

This tells you that one type is heterozygous and the other homozygous.

Cross 2:

short tail × short tail ⇨

6 short tail, 3 long tail (2/3 short, 1/3 long)

At this point, one would consider that the 2/3 *short* are heterozygotes and *long* is the homozygous class. Also, short is dominant to long. Since these ratios were repeated and verified, one can conclude that a 2:1 ratio is not a statistical artifact and that the following genotypic model would hold. Because long is the "normal" does not mean that it is dominant.

Symbolism:

S = short, s = long

Cross 1:

Ss × ss ⇨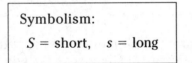

1/2 Ss (short), 1/2 ss (long)

Cross 2:

Ss × Ss ⇨

1/4 SS (lethal), 2/4 Ss (short), 1/4 ss (long)

---

5. The section on multiple alleles in the text presents a table that indicates all the genotypes requested.

Blood Group (phenotype)	Genotype(s)
A	$I^A I^A$, $I^A I^o$
B	$I^B I^B$, $I^B I^o$
AB	$I^A I^B$
O	$I^o I^o$

I^A and I^B are codominant (notice the AB blood group), while being dominant to I^o.

6. In this problem remember that individuals with blood type B can have the genotype $I^B I^B$ or $I^B I^o$ and that those with blood type A can have the genotype $I^A I^A$ or $I^A I^o$.

Male Parent: must be $I^B I^o$ because the mother is $I^o I^o$ and one inherits one homolog (therefore one allele) from each parent.

Female Parent: must be $I^A I^o$ because the father is $I^B I^o$ and one inherits one homolog (therefore one allele) from each parent. The father cannot be $I^B I^B$ and have a daughter of blood type A.

Offspring:

$$I^A I^o \times I^B I^o$$

	I^B	I^o
I^A	$I^A I^B$(AB)	$I^A I^o$(A)
I^o	$I^B I^o$(B)	$I^o I^o$(O)

The ratio would be

1(A):1(B):1(AB):1(O)

7. Given that a child is blood type O (genotype $I^o I^o$) and the mother blood type A (she must be $I^A I^o$ to have had a type O child), the father could have the following genotypes: $I^B I^o$, $I^A I^o$, or $I^o I^o$. In other words, the father must have been able to contribute I^o to the child. The only *blood type* that would exclude a male from being the father would be AB, because no I^o allele is present.

Because many individuals in a population could have genotypes with the I^O allele, one could not prove that a particular male was the father by this method.

8. Symbolism:

$$Se = \text{secretor} \quad se = \text{nonsecretor}$$

$$I^A I^B \, Sese \quad \times \quad I^O I^O \, Sese$$

(a)

	$I^O Se$	$I^O \, se$
$I^A \, Se$	A, secretor	A, secretor
$I^A \, se$	A, secretor	A, nonsecretor
$I^B \, Se$	B, secretor	B, secretor
$I^B \, se$	B, secretor	B, nonsecretor

Overall ratio: 3/8 A, secretor
 1/8 A, nonsecretor
 3/8 B, secretor
 1/8 B, nonsecretor

(b) 1/4 of all individuals will have blood type O.

9. Given that creepers never breed true and half of the offspring of a creeper crossed with a noncreeper are creepers, one would expect the creeper gene to be dominant and homozygous lethal. When creepers are interbred, two-thirds of the offspring are creepers (heterozygotes), while one-third are normal (homozygous recessive). The simplest explanation is that the homozygous creepers combination is lethal.

10. It is important to see that this problem involves multiple alleles, meaning that monohybrid type ratios are expected, and that there is an order of dominance that will allow certain alleles to be "hidden" in various heterozygotes. As with most genetics problems, one must look at the phenotypes of the offspring to assess the genotypes of the parents.

(a)

Phenotypes:

 Himalayan $\times$ Himalayan $\Longrightarrow$ albino

Genotypes: $c^h c^a$ $c^h c^a$ $c^a c^a$

Both Himalayan parents must be heterozygous to produce an albino offspring.

Phenotypes:

 full color $\times$ albino $\Longrightarrow$ chinchilla

Genotypes: Cc^{ch} $c^a c^a$ $c^{ch} c^a$

Because of the cc albino parent, the genotype of the chinchilla F_1 must be $c^{ch} c^a$. Also, in order to have a chinchilla offspring at all, the full color parent must be heterozygous for chinchilla.

Therefore, the cross of albino with chinchilla would be as follows:

$$c^a c^a \quad \times \quad c^{ch} c^a \quad \Longrightarrow$$

1/2 chinchilla; 1/2 albino

(b)

Phenotypes:

 albino $\times$ chinchilla $\Longrightarrow$ albino

Genotypes: $c^a c^a$ $c^{ch} c^a$ $c^a c^a$

Phenotypes:

 full color $\times$ albino $\Longrightarrow$ full color

Genotypes: $C\_$ $c^a c^a$ Cc^a

It is impossible to determine the complete genotype of the full color parent, but the full color offspring must be as indicated, Cc^a.

Therefore, the cross of the albino with full color would be as follows:

$$c^a c^a \times C c^a \Rightarrow$$
$$\text{1/2 full color; 1/2 albino}$$

(c)

Phenotypes:

chinchilla × albino ⟹ Himalayan

Genotypes: $c^{ch}c^h$ $c^a c^a$ $c^h c^a$

The chinchilla parent must be heterozygous for Himalayan because of the Himalayan offspring.

Phenotypes:

full color × albino ⟹ Himalayan

Genotypes: Cc^h $c^a c^a$ $c^h c^a$

Therefore, a cross between the two Himalayan types would produce the following offspring:

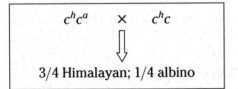

$$c^h c^a \quad \times \quad c^h c$$
$$\Downarrow$$
$$\text{3/4 Himalayan; 1/4 albino}$$

11. This problem involves multiple alleles, meaning that monohybrid type ratios are expected and that there is an order of dominance that will allow certain alleles to be "hidden" in various heterozygotes. As with most genetics problems, one must look at the phenotypes of the offspring to assess the genotypes of the parents.

(a)

Parents: sepia × cream

Because both guinea pigs had albino parents, both are heterozygous for the *ca* allele.

Cross:

$$c^k c^a \times c^d c^a \Rightarrow$$
$$\text{2/4 sepia; 1/4 cream; 1/4 albino}$$

Parents: sepia × cream

Because the sepia parent had an albino parent, it must be $c^k c^a$. Because the cream guinea pig had two sepia parents

$$(c^k c^d \times c^k c^d \text{ or } c^k c^d \times c^k c^a)$$

the cream parent could be $c^d c^d$ or $c^d c^a$.

Crosses:

$$c^k c^a \times c^d c^d \Rightarrow$$
$$\text{1/2 sepia; 1/2 cream*}$$
$$\text{*(if parents are assumed to be homozygous)}$$

$$\text{or } c^k c^a \times c^d c^a \Rightarrow$$
$$\text{1/2 sepia; 1/4 cream; 1/4 albino}$$

(b)

Parents: sepia × cream

Because the sepia guinea pig had two full color parents, which could be

$$Cc^k, Cc^d, \text{ or } Cc^a$$

(not *CC* because sepia could not be produced), its genotype could be

$$c^k c^k, c^k c^d, \text{ or } c^k c^a$$

Because the cream guinea pig had two sepia parents

$$(c^k c^d \times c^k c^d \quad \text{or} \quad c^k c^d \times c^k c^a)$$

the cream parent could be $c^d c^d$ or $c^d c^a$.

Crosses:

$c^k c^k$ × $c^d c^d$ ⟹ all sepia

$c^k c^k$ × $c^d c^a$ ⟹ all sepia

$c^k c^d$ × $c^d c^d$ ⟹ 1/2 sepia; 1/2 cream

$c^k c^d$ × $c^d c^a$ ⟹ 1/2 sepia; 1/2 cream

$c^k c^a$ × $c^d c^d$ ⟹ 1/2 sepia; 1/2 cream

$c^k c^a$ × $c^d c^a$ ⟹

1/2 sepia; 1/4 cream; 1/4 albino

(c)

Parents: sepia × cream

Because the sepia parent had a full color parent and an albino parent (Cc^k × $c^a c^a$), it must be $c^k c^a$. The cream parent had two full color parents, which could be Cc^d or Cc^a. Therefore, it could be $c^d c^d$ or $c^d c^a$.

Crosses:

$c^k c^a$ × $c^d c^d$ ⟹ 1/2 sepia; 1/2 cream

$c^k c^a$ × $c^d c^a$ ⟹

1/2 sepia; 1/4 cream; 1/4 albino

12. Three independently assorting characteristics are being dealt with: flower color (incomplete dominance), flower shape (dominant/recessive), and plant height (dominant/recessive). Establish appropriate gene symbols:

Flower color:

RR = red; Rr = pink; rr = white

Flower shape:

P = personate; p = peloric

Plant height:

D = tall; d = dwarf

(a)

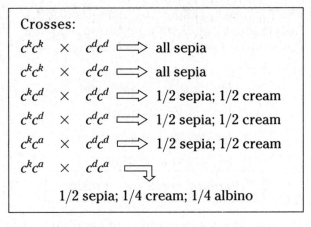

$RRPPDD$ × $rrppdd$

$RrPpDd$ (pink, personate, tall)

(b) Use *components* of the forked-line method as follows:

2/4 pink × 3/4 personate × 3/4 tall

$= \dfrac{18}{64}$

13. There are two characteristics: flower color and flower shape. Because pink results from a cross of red and white, one would conclude that flower color is "monohybrid" with incomplete dominance.

In addition, because personate is seen in the F_1 when personate and peloric are crossed, personate must be dominant to peloric. Results from crosses (c) and (d) verify these conclusions. The appropriate symbols would be as follows:

Flower color:

RR = red; Rr = pink; rr = white

Flower shape:

P = personate; p = peloric

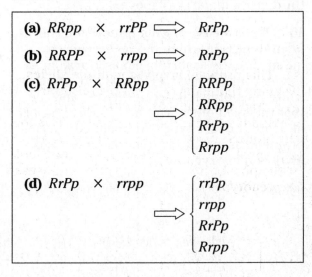

(a) $RRpp$ × $rrPP$ ⟹ $RrPp$

(b) $RRPP$ × $rrpp$ ⟹ $RrPp$

(c) $RrPp$ × $RRpp$ ⟹ $\begin{cases} RRPp \\ RRpp \\ RrPp \\ Rrpp \end{cases}$

(d) $RrPp$ × $rrpp$ ⟹ $\begin{cases} rrPp \\ rrpp \\ RrPp \\ Rrpp \end{cases}$

In the cross of the F_1 of (a) to the F_1 of (b), both of which are double heterozygotes, one would expect the following:

$$RrPp \times RrPp$$

1/4 red
- 3/4 personate → 3/16 red, personate
- 1/4 peloric → 1/16 red, peloric

2/4 pink
- 3/4 personate → 6/16 pink, personate
- 1/4 peloric → 2/16 pink, peloric

1/4 white
- 3/4 personate → 3/16 white, personate
- 1/4 peloric → 1/16 white, peloric

14. (a) This is a case of incomplete dominance in which, as shown in the third cross, the heterozygote (palomino) produces a typical 1:2:1 ratio. Therefore, one can set the following symbols:

$C^{ch}C^{ch}$ = chestnut

C^cC^c = cremello

$C^{ch}C^c$ = palomino

(b) The F_1 resulting from matings between cremello and chestnut horses would be expected to be all palomino. The F_2 would be expected to fall in a 1:2:1 ratio as in the third cross in part (a) above.

15. This is a case of gene interaction (novel phenotypes) in which the recessive, independently assorting genes *brown* and *scarlet* (both recessive) interact to give the white phenotype. Refer to the text and see that the symbolism uses a "+" superscript to indicate the wild type. For simplicity in this problem, assume that all parental crosses involve homozygotes.

(a) $bw^+/bw^+; st^+/st^+ \times bw/bw; st/st$

⇓

$bw^+/bw; st^+/st$ (wild)

The F_2 would produce the expected 9:3:3:1 ratio except that gene interaction will give the white phenotype in the 1/16 class.

$bw^+/\_; st^+/\_$	= wild type
$bw^+/\_; st/st$	= scarlet
$bw/bw; st^+/\_$	= brown
$bw/bw; st/st$	= white

(b)

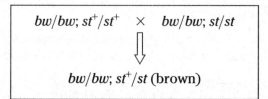

$$bw^+/bw^+; st^+/st^+ \times bw^+/bw^+; st/st$$
⇓
$$bw^+/bw^+; st^+/st \text{ (wild)}$$

The F_2, resulting from a cross of

$$bw^+/bw^+; st^+/st \times bw^+/bw^+; st^+/st$$

would produce a 3:1 ratio of wild to scarlet.

(c)

$$bw/bw; st^+/st^+ \times bw/bw; st/st$$
⇓
$$bw/bw; st^+/st \text{ (brown)}$$

The F_2, resulting from a cross of

$$bw/bw; st^+/st \times bw/bw; st^+/st$$

would produce a 3:1 ratio of brown to white. Notice that in the F_2 crosses in parts (b) and (c) one of the parents in each is homozygous; therefore, the crosses will give monohybrid types of ratios.

16. This is a case in which epistasis (from cc) results in a "masking" of genes at the *A* locus. In this case, there will be modifications of typical 9:3:3:1 and 1:1:1:1 ratios because of gene interactions.

(a) In a cross of

$$AACC \quad \times \quad aacc$$

the offpsring are all *AaCc* (agouti) because the *C* allele allows pigment to be deposited in the hair and when it is, it will be agouti. F_2 offspring would have the following "simplified" genotypes with the corresponding phenotypes:

A_C_ = 9/16 (agouti)

A_cc = 3/16

(colorless because *cc* is epistatic to *A*)

aaC_ = 3/16 (black)

aacc = 1/16

(colorless because *cc* is epistatic to *aa*)

The two colorless classes are phenotypically indistinguishable; therefore, the final ratio is 9:3:4.

(b) Results of crosses of female agouti

$$(A\_C\_) \quad \times \quad aacc \text{ (males)}$$

are given in three groups:

(1) To produce an even number of agouti and colorless offspring, the female parent must have been *AACc* so that half of the offspring are able to deposit pigment because of *C*. When they do, they are all agouti (having received only *A* from the female parent).

(2) To produce an even number of agouti and black offspring, the mother must have been *Aa* and so that no colorless offspring were produced, the female must have been *CC*. Her genotype must have been *AaCC*.

(3) Notice that half of the offspring are colorless; therefore, the female must have been *Cc*. Half of the pigmented offspring are black and half are agouti; therefore, the female must have been *Aa*. Overall, the *AaCc* genotype seems appropriate.

17. Notice that the distribution of observed offspring fits a 9:3:4 ratio quite well. This suggests that two independently assorting gene pairs with epistasis are involved. Assign gene symbols in the usual manner:

> *A* = pigment; *a* = pigmentless (colorless)
> *B* = purple; *b* = red

> AaBb × AaBb
> ⇓
> A_B_ = purple
> A_bb = red
> aaB_ = colorless
> aabb = colorless

One may see this occurring in the following manner:

precursor —+→ cyanidin —+→ purple pigment

> (colorless) *aa*   (red) *bb*

18. This is a case of gene interaction (novel phenotypes) where the yellow and black types (double mutants) interact to give the cream phenotype and epistasis where the *cc* genotype produces albino.

(a) *AaBbCc* ⟹ gray (*C* allows pigment)

(b) *A_B_Cc* ⟹ gray (*C* allows pigment)

(c) Use the forked-line method for this portion.

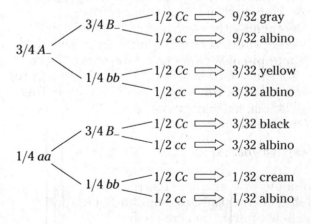

Combining the phenotypes gives (always count the proportions to see that they add up to 1.0):

16/32   albino

9/32   gray

3/32   yellow

3/32   black

1/32   cream

(d) Use the forked-line method for this portion.

$$3/4\ A\_ \Longrightarrow \begin{array}{l} 1/1\ BB - 1/4\ cc \Longrightarrow 3/16\ (albino) \\ \nearrow 3/4\ C\_ \Longrightarrow 9/16\ (gray) \end{array}$$

3/4 A_ $\Longrightarrow$ 1/1 *BB* − 1/4 *cc* $\Longrightarrow$ 3/16 (albino)

1/4 aa $\Longrightarrow$ 1/1 *BB* − 3/4 *C*_ $\Longrightarrow$ 3/16 (black)

1/4 *cc* $\Longrightarrow$ 1/16 (albino)

Combining the phenotypes gives (always count the proportions to see that they add up to 1.0):

9/16   (gray)

3/16   (black)

4/16   (albino)

(e) Use the forked-line method for this portion.

1/1 *AA*

3/4 *B*_ ── 1/2 *Cc* $\Longrightarrow$ 3/8 (gray)

1/2 *cc* $\Longrightarrow$ 3/8 (albino)

1/4 *bb* ── 1/2 *Cc* $\Longrightarrow$ 1/8 (yellow)

1/2 *cc* $\Longrightarrow$ 1/8 (albino)

The final ratio would be

3/8   (gray)

1/8   (yellow)

4/8   (albino)

19. Treat each cross as a series of monohybrid crosses, remembering that albino is epistatic to color and black and yellow interact to give cream.

(a) Since this is a 9:3:3:1 ratio with no albino phenotypes, the parents must each have been double heterozygotes and incapable of producing the *cc* genotype.

Genotypes:

    AaBbCC × *AaBbCC*

        or

    AaBbCC × *AaBbCc*

Phenotypes:

    gray × gray

(b) Since there are no black offspring, no combination in the parents can produce *aa*. The 4/16 proportion indicates that the *C* locus is heterozygous in both parents.

If the parents are

    AABbCc × *AaBbCc*

        or

    AABbCc × *AABbCc*

then the results would follow the pattern given.

Phenotypes: gray × gray

(c) First, notice that 16/64 or 1/4 of the offspring are albino; therefore, both parents are heterozygous at the *C* locus. Second, notice that without considering the *C* locus, there is a 27:9:9:3 ratio that reduces to a 9:3:3:1 ratio. Given this information, the genotypes must be

    AaBbCc × *AaBbCc*

Phenotypes: gray × gray

(d) Notice that 2/8 or 1/4 of the offspring are albino, which indicates that both parents are *Cc*. Also notice that the ratio of black to cream is 1:1, suggesting that the parents are *Bb* and *bb*. Because there are no gray or yellow offspring, there can be no *A* alleles.

Genotypes:

$$aaBbCc \times aabbCc$$

Phenotypes: black × cream

(e) Notice that half of the offspring are albino indicating that, for the *C* locus, the genotypes are *Cc* and *cc*. There is a 3:1 ratio of black to cream indicating heterozygosity for the *B* locus in each parent. Because there are no gray or yellow offspring, there can be no *A* alleles.

Genotypes:

$$aaBbCc \times aaBbcc$$

Phenotypes: black × albino

---

20. After reading the problem, glance at the kinds of F_1 and F_2 ratios. Notice that the first two, (A) and (B), appear as monohybrid ratios and that (C) is clearly dihybrid. You need to see this combination of crosses as being solved with one set of gene symbols. The fact that cross (c) yields a 9:3:3:1 ratio gives you a start.

(a) Going back to the basics, set up the relationship that you know holds for a 9:3:3:1 ratio as follows:

$$A\_B\_ = 9/16$$
$$A\_bb = 3/16$$
$$aaB\_ = 3/16$$
$$aabb = 1/16$$

Then assign the phenotypes from cross (C) as indicated:

$$A\_B\_ = 9/16 \text{ (green)}$$
$$A\_bb = 3/16 \text{ (brown)}$$
$$aaB\_ = 3/16 \text{ (gray)}$$
$$aabb = 1/16 \text{ (blue)}$$

Now it should become clear that blue results from interaction of the *aa* and *bb* genotypes and brown and gray result from homozygosity of either of the two genes as shown above. From this model, see if crosses (a), (b), and (c) and the resulting progeny make sense.

Cross A:

P_1:	$AABB \times aaBB$
F_1:	$AaBB$
F_2:	3/4 *A_BB*: 1/4 *aaBB*

Cross B:

P_1:	$AABB \times AAbb$
F_1:	$AABb$
F_2:	3/4 *AAB_*: 1/4 *AAbb*

Cross C:

P_1:	$aaBB \times AAbb$
F_1:	$AaBb$
F_2:	9/16 *A_B_*: 3/16 *A_bb*:
	3/16 *aaB_*: 1/16 *aabb*

(b) This question is exactly the same as that in cross C. The genotype of the unknown P_1 individual would be *AAbb* (brown), while the F_1 would be *AaBb* (green).

21. First, see in this problem that a 9:7 ratio is involved, which implies a dihybrid condition with epistasis. Going back to a basic 9:3:3:1 ratio, one can see that if the 3:3:1 groups were lumped together, the 9:7 ratio would result. Assign tall to any plant with both *A* and *B* and to any dwarf plant that is homozygous for either or both of the recessive alleles. The initial cross must have been

$$AABB \times aabb$$

There are two gene pairs involved.

(a)

$$A\_B\_ = 9/16 \text{ (tall)}$$
$$A\_bb = 3/16 \text{ (dwarf)}$$
$$aaB\_ = 3/16 \text{ (dwarf)}$$
$$aabb = 1/16 \text{ (dwarf)}$$

(b) There are three different classes of dwarf plants. Within each of the 3/16 classes there are two types:

$$A\_bb = 3/16 \text{ (dwarf)}$$
$$= 1/3 \; AAbb \text{ and } 2/3 \; Aabb$$

and

$$aaB\_ = 3/16 \text{ (dwarf)}$$
$$= 1/3 \; aaBB \text{ and } 2/3 \; aaBb$$

Therefore, the true-breeding dwarf plants would be the following:

$$AAbb, \; aaBB, \text{ and } aabb$$

and they would constitute 3/7 of the dwarf group.

22. Problems of this type often pose difficulties for students. It is important for students to go back to basic patterns of inheritance when getting started. First, see that a 9:3:3:1 ratio is involved as indicated below:

$$A\_B\_ = 9/16$$
$$A\_bb = 3/16$$
$$aaB\_ = 3/16$$
$$aabb = 1/16$$

(a) Assign the phenotypes as given; then see if patterns emerge.

$$A\_B\_ = 9/16 \text{ (yellow)}$$
$$A\_bb = 3/16 \text{ (blue)}$$
$$aaB\_ = 3/16 \text{ (red)}$$
$$aabb = 1/16 \text{ (mauve)}$$

From this information, the genotypes for the various phenotypes and the solution to the problem become clear. As stated in the problem all colors *may* be true-breeding. See that each type can exist as a full homozygote. If plants with blue flowers (homozygotes) are crossed to red-flowered homozygotes, the F_1 plants will have yellow flowers. Also as stated in the problem, if yellow-flowered plants are crossed with mauve-flowered plants, the F_1 plants are yellow and the F_2 will occur in a 9:3:3:1 ratio. All of the observations fit the model as proposed.

(b) If one crosses a true-breeding red plant (*aaBB*) with a mauve plant (*aabb*), the F_1 should be red (*aaBb*). The F_2 would be as follows:

---

aaBb $\times$ *aaBb* →

3/4 *aaB_* (red); 1/4 *aabb* (mauve)

---

23. First, make certain that you understand the genetics of all the gene pairs being described in the problem. The ABO system involves multiple alleles, codominance, and dominance. The MN system is codominant. The easiest way to approach these types of problems is to consider those gene pairs that produce a low number of options in the offspring. Notice in cross #1 that there are two options in the offspring for the ABO system (types A and O), but only one option for the MN system (type MN). By looking at the most restrictive classes, one can see that option (c) is the only one that is both MN and O. The remainder of the combinations can be determined using the same logic.

Cross #1 = (c)

Cross #2 = (d)

Cross #3 = (b)

Cross #4 = (e)

Cross #5 = (a)

Given that each parental/offspring grouping can only be used once, there are no other combinations.

24. In order to solve this problem, one must first see the possible genotypes of the parents and the grandfathers. Since the gene is X-linked, the cross will be symbolized with the X chromosomes.

RG = normal vision; rg = color-blind

Mother's father: X^{rg}/Y

Father's father: X^{rg}/Y

Mother: $X^{RG}X^{rg}$

Father: X^{RG}/Y

Notice that the mother must be heterozygous for the rg allele (being normal-visioned and having inherited an X^{rg} from her father) and the father, because he has normal vision, must be X^{RG}. The fact that the father's father is color-blind does not mean that the father will be color-blind. On the contrary, the father will inherit his X chromosome from his mother.

$$X^{RG}X^{rg} \times X^{RG}/Y$$

$X^{RG}X^{RG}$ = 1/4 daughter normal

$X^{RG}X^{rg}$ = 1/4 daughter normal

X^{RG}/Y = 1/4 son normal

X^{rg}/Y = 1/4 son color-blind

Looking at the distribution of offspring:

(a) 1/4

(b) 1/2

(c) 1/4

(d) zero

25. The mating is $X^{RG}X^{rg}; I^A I^O \times X^{RG}Y; I^A I^O$

Based on the son who is color-blind and blood type O, the mother must have been heterozygous for the RG locus and both parents must have had one copy of the I^O

gene. The probability of having a female child is 1/2, that she has normal vision is 1 (because the father's X is normal), and that she has type O blood is 1/4. The final product of the independent probabilities is

$$1/2 \ \times \ 1 \ \times \ 1/4 \ = \ 1/8$$

26. Symbolism: Normal wing margins = sd^+; scalloped = sd

(a)

P_1: $X^{sd}X^{sd} \times X^+/Y$

F_1: 1/2 X^+X^{sd} (female, normal)

1/2 X^{sd}/Y (male, scalloped)

F_2: 1/4 X^+X^{sd} (female, normal)

1/4 $X^{sd}X^{sd}$ (female, scalloped)

1/4 X^+/Y (male, normal)

1/4 X^{sd}/Y (male, scalloped)

(b)

P_1: $X^+/X^+ \times X^{sd}/Y$

F_1: 1/2 X^+X^{sd} (female, normal)

1/2 X^+/Y (male, normal)

F_2: 1/4 X^+X^+ (female, normal)

1/4 X^+X^{sd} (female, normal)

1/4 X^+/Y (male, normal)

1/4 X^{sd}/Y (male, scalloped)

If the *scalloped* gene were not X-linked, then all of the F_1 offspring would be wild (phenotypically) and a 3:1 ratio of normal to scalloped would occur in the F_2.

27. Assuming that the parents are homozygous, the crosses would be as follows. Notice that the X symbol may remain to remind us that the *sd* gene is on the X chromosome. It is extremely important that one account for both the mutant genes and each of their wild-type alleles.

P$_1$: $X^{sd}X^{sd}$; e^+/e^+ × X^+/Y; e/e

F$_1$:

       1/2 X^+X^{sd}; e^+/e (female, normal)

       1/2 X^{sd}/Y; e^+/e (male, scalloped)

F$_2$:

	X^+e^+	X^+e	$X^{sd}e^+$	$X^{sd}e$
$X^{sd}e^+$				
$X^{sd}e$	Fill in box on your own.			
Ye^+				
Ye				

Phenotypes:

    3/16 normal females

    3/16 normal males

    1/16 ebony females

    1/16 ebony males

    3/16 scalloped females

    3/16 scalloped males

    1/16 scalloped, ebony females

    1/16 scalloped, ebony males

Forked-line method:

P$_1$: $X^{sd}X^{sd}$; e^+/e^+ × X^+/Y; e/e

F$_1$:   1/2 X^+X^{sd}; e^+/e (female, normal)

          1/2 X^{sd}/Y; e^+/e (male, scalloped)

F$_2$:

	Wings	Color	
1/4	females, normal	3/4 normal	3/16
		1/4 ebony	1/16
1/4	females, scalloped	3/4 normal	3/16
		1/4 ebony	1/16
1/4	males, normal	3/4 normal	3/16
		1/4 ebony	1/16
1/4	males, scalloped	3/4 normal	3/16
		1/4 ebony	1/16

28. Set up the symbolism and the cross in the following manner:

P$_1$: X^+X^+; *su-v/su-v*   × X^v/Y; *su-v$^+$/su-v$^+$*

F$_1$:   1/2 X^+X^v; *su-v$^+$/su-v* (female, normal)

      1/2 X^+/Y; *su-v$^+$/su-v* (male, normal)

F$_2$:   2/4   females, $X^+/_-$ 3/4 $su - v^+/_-$

                          1/4 $su - v/su - v$

        1/4   males, X^+/Y 3/4 $su - v^+/_-$

                          1/4 $su - v/su - v$

        1/4   males, X^v/Y 3/4 $su - v^+/_-$

                          1/4 $su - v/su - v$

8/16 are wild-type females (none of the females are homozygous for the *vermilion* gene).

5/16 are wild-type males (4/16 because they have no *vermilion* gene and 1/16 because the X-linked, hemizygous *vermilion* gene is suppressed by *su-v/su-v*).

3/16 are vermilion males (no suppression of the *vermilion* gene).

29. It is extremely important that one account for both the mutant genes and each of their wild-type alleles.

(a)

P₁: $X^vX^v; +/+ \times X^+/Y; b^r/b^r$

F₁:
  1/2 $X^+X^v; +/b^r$ (female, normal)
  1/2 $X^v/Y; +/b^r$ (male, vermilion)

F₂:

Eye color (X)	Eye color (autosomal)	
1/4 females, normal	3/4 normal	3/16
	1/4 brown	1/16
1/4 females, vermilion	3/4 normal	3/16
	1/4 brown	1/16
1/4 males, normal	3/4 normal	3/16
	1/4 brown	1/16
1/4 males, vermilion	3/4 normal	3/16
	1/4 brown	1/16

3/16 = females, normal
1/16 = females, brown eyes
3/16 = females, vermilion eyes
1/16 = females, white eyes
3/16 = males, normal
1/16 = males, brown eyes
3/16 = males, vermilion eyes
1/16 = males, white eyes

(b)

P₁: $X^+X^+; b^r/b^r \times X^v/Y; +/+$

F₁:
  1/2 $X^+X^v; +/b^r$ (female, normal)
  1/2 $X^+/Y; +/b^r$ (male, normal)

F₂:

Eye color (X)	Eye color (autosomal)
2/4 females, normal	3/4 normal
	1/4 brown
1/4 males, normal	3/4 normal
	1/4 brown
1/4 males, vermilion	3/4 normal
	1/4 brown

6/16 = females, normal
2/16 = females, brown eyes
3/16 = males, normal
1/16 = males, brown eyes
3/16 = males, vermilion eyes
1/16 = males, white eyes

(c)

P₁: $X^vX^v; b^r/b^r \times X^+/Y; +/+$

F₁: 1/2 $X^+X^v; +/b^r$ (female, normal)
    1/2 $X^v/Y; +/b^r$ (male, vermilion)

F₂:

Eye color (X)	Eye color (autosomal)
1/4 females, normal	3/4 normal
	1/4 brown
1/4 females, vermilion	3/4 normal
	1/4 brown
1/4 males, normal	3/4 normal
	1/4 brown
1/4 males, vermilion	3/4 normal
	1/4 brown

3/16 = females, normal
1/16 = females, brown eyes
3/16 = females, vermilion eyes
1/16 = females, white eyes
3/16 = males, normal
1/16 = males, brown eyes
3/16 = males, vermilion eyes
1/16 = males, white eyes

30. (a)

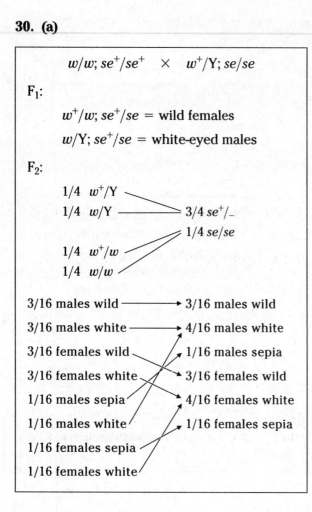

$$w/w; se^+/se^+ \quad \times \quad w^+/Y; se/se$$

F₁:

$w^+/w; se^+/se$ = wild females

$w/Y; se^+/se$ = white-eyed males

F₂:

1/4 w^+/Y

1/4 w/Y ——→ 3/4 $se^+/_-$

1/4 se/se

1/4 w^+/w

1/4 w/w

3/16 males wild ——————→ 3/16 males wild

3/16 males white ————→ 4/16 males white

3/16 females wild → 1/16 males sepia

3/16 females white → 3/16 females wild

1/16 males sepia → 4/16 females white

1/16 males white → 1/16 females sepia

1/16 females sepia

1/16 females white

(b)

$$w^+/w^+; se/se \quad \times \quad w/Y; se^+/se^+$$

⇓

F₁: $w^+/w; se^+/se$ = wild females

$w^+/Y; se^+/se$ = wild males

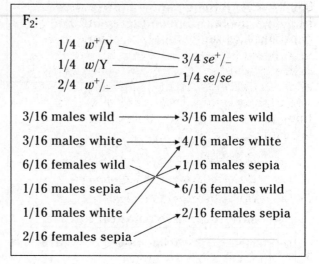

F₂:

1/4 w^+/Y

1/4 w/Y ——→ 3/4 $se^+/_-$

2/4 $w^+/_-$ ——→ 1/4 se/se

3/16 males wild ——————→ 3/16 males wild

3/16 males white ————→ 4/16 males white

6/16 females wild → 1/16 males sepia

1/16 males sepia → 6/16 females wild

1/16 males white → 2/16 females sepia

2/16 females sepia

31. (a,b) In looking at the pedigrees, one can see that the condition cannot be dominant because it appears in the offspring (II-3 and II-4) and not the parents in the first two cases. The condition is therefore *recessive*. In the second cross, note that the father is not shaded, yet the daughter (II-4) is. If the condition is recessive, then it must also be *autosomal*.

(c)   II-1 = *AA* or *Aa*

II-6 = *AA* or *Aa*

II-9 = *Aa*

32. For all three pedigrees, let *a* represent the mutant gene and *A* represent its normal allele.

(a) This pedigree is consistent with an X-linked recessive trait because the male would contribute an X chromosome, carrying the *a* mutation to the *aa* daughter. The mother would have to be heterozygous *Aa*.

(b) This pedigree is consistent with an X-linked recessive trait because the mother could be *Aa* and transmit her *a* allele to her one son (*a*/Y) and her *A* allele to her other son.

(c) This pedigree is not consistent with an X-linked mode of inheritance because the *aa* mother has an *A*/Y son.

56

33. In view of the different distribution between males and females, one might consider sex-influenced inheritance as a model and have males more likely to express bearded and females more likely to express beardless in the heterozygote. This situation is similar to pattern baldness in humans. Consider two alleles that are autosomal and let

> BB = beardless in both sexes
> Bb = beardless in females
> Bb = bearded in males
> bb = bearded in both sexes

P_1:

female: bb (bearded) × male: BB (beardless)

F_1:

Bb = females beardless; males bearded

Because half of the offspring are males and half are females, one could, for clarity, rewrite the F_2 as:

	1/2 females	*1/2 males*
1/4 *BB*	1/8 beardless	1/8 beardless
2/4 *Bb*	2/8 beardless	2/8 bearded
1/4 *bb*	1/8 bearded	1/8 bearded

One could test the above model by crossing F_1 (heterozygous) beardless females with bearded (homozygous) males. Comparing these results with the reciprocal cross would support the model if the distributions of sexes with phenotypes were the same in both crosses.

34. In looking at the information provided in the text, notice that the only genotype that gives cock-feathering in males is *hh*, while three genotypes give hen-feathering in females,

> *HH, Hh,* and *hh*

Remember that these genes are sex-limited and autosomal.

P_1:   female: *HH* × male: *hh*

F_1:

   all hen-feathering

F_2:

	1/2 females	*1/2 males*
1/4 *HH*	hen-feathering	hen-feathering
2/4 *Hh*	hen-feathering	hen-feathering
1/4 *hh*	hen-feathering	cock-feathering

All of the offspring would be hen-feathered except for 1/8 of the males, which are cock-feathered.

35. Passage of X-linked genes typically occurs from carrier mother to affected son. The fact that the father in couple #2 has hemophilia would not predispose his son to hemophilia. The #1 couple has no valid claim.

36. Phenotypic expression is dependent on the genome of the organism, the immediate molecular and cellular environment of the genome, and numerous interactions between a genome, the organism, and the environment.

37. *Penetrance* refers to the percentage of individuals that expresses the mutant phenotype, while *expressivity* refers to the range of expression of a given phenotype.

38. *Anticipation* occurs when a heritable disorder exhibits a progressively earlier age of onset and an increased severity in successive generations. *Imprinting* occurs when phenotypic expression is influenced by the parental origin of the chromosome carrying a particular gene.

39. (a) In general, they observed results of crosses that did not produce offspring in typical Mendelian ratios.

(b) Modifications of dihybrid and higher-level ratios indicated that loci were not expressed independently. A 9:3:4 ratio illustrates such a dihybrid modification. The number of gene pairs involved is often determined by the sum of the components of each ratio. For example, a 1:2:1 or 3:1 ratio adds to 4, indicating a monohybrid cross. A 9:3:4 or 15:1 ratio adds to 16, indicating a dihybrid ratio.

(c) Morgan and his colleagues observed that the sex of the parent carrying a mutant allele influenced the results of crosses when compared to a reciprocal cross. When correlated with the sex chromosome differences between males and females, a model placing a gene on the X chromosome was supported.

(d) When a gene is X-linked, ratios from crosses are influenced by which parent contributes a particular allele. When sex-limited or sex-influenced inheritance occurs, the parental source of the allele is irrelevant.

40. First, look for familiar ratios that will inform you as to the general mode of inheritance. Notice that the last cross (h) gives a 9:4:3 ratio, which is typical of epistasis. From this information one can develop a model to account for the results given.

Symbolism:

$$A\_B\_ = \text{black}$$
$$A\_bb = \text{golden}$$
$$aabb = \text{golden}$$
$$aaB\_ = \text{brown}$$

The combination of *bb* is epistatic to the *A* locus.

(a) *AAB_* × *aaBB* (other configurations possible, but each must give all offspring with *A* and *B* dominant alleles)

(b) *AaB_* × *aaBB* (other configurations are possible but no types can be produced)

(c) *AABb* × *aaBb*

(d) *AABB* × *aabb*

(e) *AaBb* × *Aabb*

(f) *AaBb* × *aabb*

(g) *aaBb* × *aaBb*

(h) *AaBb* × *AaBb*

Those genotypes that will breed true will be as follows:

$$\text{black} = AABB$$
$$\text{golden} = \text{all genotypes that are } bb$$
$$\text{brown} = aaBB$$

41. A first glance would seem to favor a 9:7 ratio; however, the phenotypes would have to be reversed for such a result to fit. Therefore, one must consider an alternative explanation. A 27:9:9:9:3:3:3:1 ratio fits very well with *A_B_C_* being purple and any homozygous recessive combination giving white. Thus, a 27 (purple):37 (white) ratio fits well. To test this hypothesis, one might take the purple F$_1$'s and cross them to the pure breeding (*aabbcc*) white type. Such a cross should give a 1 (purple):7 (white) ratio.

42. The clue to the solution comes from the description of the Dexters as not true-breeding and of low fertility. This indicates that Dexters are heterozygous and that the Kerry breed is homozygous recessive. The homozygous dominant type is lethal. Polled is caused by an independently assorting dominant allele, whereas horned is caused by the recessive allele to polled.

43. (a) Because the denominator in the ratios is 64, one would begin to consider that there are three independently assorting gene pairs operating in this problem. There are only two characteristics (eye color and croaking), but one might hypothesize that two gene pairs are involved in the inheritance of one trait, while one gene pair is involved in the other.

(b) Notice that there is a 48:16 (or 3:1) ratio of rib-it to knee-deep and a 36:16:12 (or 9:4:3) ratio of blue to green to purple eye color. Because of these relationships, one would conclude that croaking is due to one (dominant/recessive) gene pair, while eye color is due to two gene pairs. Because there is a (9:4:3) ratio regarding eye color, some gene interaction (epistasis) is indicated.

(c,d) Symbolism:

Croaking: $R\_$ = rib-it; rr = knee-deep

Eye color:

Since the most frequent phenotype is blue eye, let $A\_B\_$ represent the genotypes. For the purple class, "a 3/16 group" uses the A_bb genotypes. The "4/16" class (green) would be the $aaB\_$ and the $aabb$ groups.

(e) The cross involving a blue-eyed, knee-deep frog and a purple-eyed, rib-it frog would have the genotypes:

$$AABBrr \times AAbbRR$$

which would produce an F_1 of $AABbRr$ that would be blue-eyed and rib-it. The F_2 will follow a pattern of a 9:3:3:1 ratio because of homozygosity for the A locus and heterozygosity for both the B and R loci.

9/16 $AAB\_R\_$ = blue-eyed, rib-it

3/16 AAB_rr = blue-eyed, knee-deep

3/16 $AAbbR\_$ = purple-eyed, rib-it

1/16 $AAbbrr$ = purple-eyed, knee-deep

(f) The different results can arise because of the genetic variety possible in producing the green-eyed frogs. Since there is no dependence on the B locus, the following genotypes can define the green phenotype:

$$aaBB, aaBb, aabb$$

(g) In doing these types of problems, take each characteristic individually, then build the complete genotypes. Notice that the ratio of purple-eyed to green-eyed frogs is 3:1; therefore, expect the parents to be heterozygous for the A locus. Because the ratio of rib-it to knee-deep is also 3:1 expect both parents to be heterozygous at the R locus.

The B locus would have the bb genotype because both parents are purple-eyed as given in the problem. Both parents would therefore be $AabbRr$.

44. In looking at the pedigree, one can see that the typical carrier mother-to-son X-linked pattern is not present. One cannot default to a Y-linked pattern because of sons (II-1, IV-1) not having precocious puberty. We might then consider a sex-limited form of inheritance where the gene(s) is(are) autosomal, but expression is limited to one sex, male in this case. Because of the relatively high frequency of occurrence of precocious puberty in the pedigree, one might consider a dominant gene to be involved. Indeed, there is no skipping of generations typical of recessive traits.

Notice, however, that there is an apparent skipping of generations in giving rise to the IV-5 son. This is because females are not capable of expressing the gene. Given the degree of outcrossing, that the gene is probably quite rare and therefore heterozygotes are uncommon, and that the frequency of transmission is high, it is likely that this form of male precious puberty is caused by an autosomal dominant, sex-limited gene.

45. Given that both parents are true-breeding and that the sort of gene interaction described is occurring, one can come up with the following symbols:

(a) P_1: $YYBB \times yWbb$

F_1: $YyBb$ and $YWBb$

Crossing these F_1's gives the observed ratios in the F_2.

(b) Given a blue male with the genotype $yyBb$ and a green female with the genotype $YWBb$, the offspring are as given in part **(b)** of the question.

46. The reduced ratio is 12 white, 3 orange, and 1 brown, and in a dihybrid cross (*AaBb* × *AaBb*) the following would occur:

12 white	*A_B_* or *aaB_*
3 orange	*A_bb*
1 brown	*aabb*

47. Given the following genotypes of the parents:

$$aabb = \text{crimson}$$
$$AABB = \text{white}$$

the F$_1$ consist of *AaBb* genotypes with a rose phenotype.

In the F$_2$, the following genotypes correspond to the given phenotypes:

*AAB_*	= white	4/16
AaBB	= magenta	2/16
AaBb	= rose	4/16
Aabb	= orange	2/16
aaBB	= yellow	1/16
aaBb	= pale yellow	2/16
aabb	= crimson	1/16

Notice that different phenotypes result from heterozygous vs. homozygous dominant states. *AaBB* gives magenta, while *AaBb* gives rose. However, in the presence of *AA*, the same phenotype is found regardless of *Bb* or *BB* genotypes. Gene interaction is occurring along with the absence of complete dominance.

48. Since proto oncogenes stimulate a cell to progress through a cell cycle, loss of function of such genes should inhibit such cellular progress. In this case, the gene would likely function as a recessive. However, if overproduction of a proto oncogene should occur, then the cell would be stimulated to undergo more rapid cycles (perhaps), which would lead to an expressed phenotype such as a tumor or cancer. Under this condition (gain of function), the gene would behave as a dominant. If the regulatory region of a proto oncogene is mutated such that loss of control occurs and the proto oncogene is overexpressed, then it would "gain function" and be dominant. If the proto oncogene product is defective, there would be a loss of function and it would more than likely behave as a recessive.

49. (a) The term *pleiotropy* is used when there are multiple phenotypic manifestations of a single gene.

(b) Each phenotypic response is a result of the inability of the red blood cells to adequately supply tissues. Sickle-cell hemoglobin fails to adequately carry oxygen, and the sickle shape of the red blood cells blocks their passage to various tissues. As a result of a vaso-occlusive (blockage) crisis, tissue necrosis occurs, and a variety of health problems result.

(c) The molecular basis of sickle-cell anemia is a substitution of valine for glutamic acid at the sixth position of the β chain.

Chapter 5: Chromosome Mapping in Eukaryotes

Concept Areas	Corresponding Problems
Linkage vs. Independent Assortment	1, 26, 34, 38, 40
Chromosome Mapping	3, 4, 5, 6, 7, 8, 9, 10, 11, 12, 13, 20, 24, 25, 26, 27, 28, 29, 30, 31, 32, 33, 35, 36, 37, 38, 39
Multiple Crossovers and Three-Point Mapping	5, 14, 15, 16, 17, 18, 19
Determining Gene Sequence	15, 16, 17, 20
Interference and Coefficient of Coincidence	6, 15, 16, 41
Crossing Over in the Four-Strand Stage	2
Mechanism of Crossing Over	2, 18, 23
Mitotic Recombination	21, 22
Somatic Cell Hybridization and Human Maps	34

Vocabulary: Organization and Listing of Terms and Concepts

Structures and Substances

Chromosome map

  interlocus distance

  linkage group

  isogamete

  tetrad

  parental ditype

  nonparental ditype

  tetratype

Heterokaryon

Synkaryon

Ascospores

Ascus (pl. asci)

Rh antigen

Elliptocytosis

Cystic fibrosis

Bromodeoxyuridine (BUdR)

DNA helicase

DNA markers

  microsatellite

  minisatellite

  restriction fragment length polymorphism (RFLP)

    cystic fibrosis

physical map

single nucleotide polymorphism (SNP)

Processes/Methods

Linkage

  crossing over

  crossover gametes (recombinant)

  recombination

    reciprocal classes

  parental (noncrossover gametes)

  incomplete

Linkage (continued)

    chiasmata (chiasma)

    three-point mapping

    product rule (multiple crossovers)

        noncrossovers (NCO)

        single crossovers (SCO)

        double crossovers (DCO)

Linkage ratio

Determining gene sequence

    correct heterozygous arrangement

    correct sequence of genes

        method I

        method II

Poisson distribution

    2-strand double

    3-strand double

    4-strand double

        mapping function

Cytological evidence (crossing over)

Mechanism of crossing over

Human chromosome maps

    lod score

Somatic cell hybridization

    random loss of human chromosomes

    synteny testing

    translocation

Haploid organisms

    tetrad analysis

Mapping to the centromere

    first-division segregation

    second-division segregation

Gene conversion

Mitotic recombination

    synapsis

    genetic exchange

    twin spots

Sister chromatid exchange

    bromodeoxyuridine (BUdR)

    Bloom syndrome

Chromosome walking

Chromosome jumping

Mendel and linkage

    independent assortment

Concepts

Linked genes (linkage groups)

    arrangement (gene sequence) (F5.1)

Chromosome Theory of Inheritance

Chromosome maps

    map unit (% recombination)

    50% maximum

Interference

    coefficient of coincidence

    expected frequency of DCO

    observed frequency of DCO

        positive

        negative

    lod score

Synteny testing

Generation of variation

Mitotic recombination

Use of molecular genetic markers

F5.1 Illustration of critical arrangements of linked genes. Notice that there are two possible arrangements for an *AaBb* double heterozygote. In order to do linkage problems correctly, such arrangements must be understood.

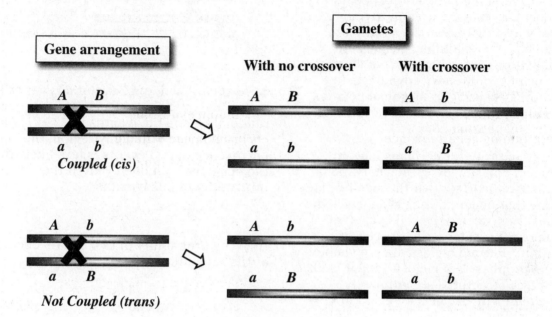

Solutions to Problems and Discussion Questions

1. The biological significance of genetic exchange and recombination appears to be to generate genetic variation in gametes, thereby leading to genetic variation in organisms. By reshuffling genes, new combinations are generated, which may then be of evolutionary advantage. In addition, because chromosomal position can influence gene function, variation is created by *position effect*.

2. First, in order for chromosomes to engage in crossing over, they must be in proximity. It is likely that the side-by-side pairing that occurs during synapsis is the earliest time during the cell cycle that chromosomes achieve that necessary proximity. Second, chiasmata are visible during prophase I of meiosis, and it is likely that these structures are intimately associated with the genetic event of crossing over.

3. With some qualification, especially around the centromeres and telomeres, one can say that crossing over is somewhat randomly distributed over the length of the chromosome. Two loci that are far apart are more likely to have a crossover between them than two loci that are close together.

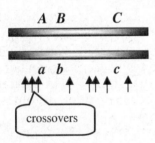

4. Because crossing over occurs at the four-strand stage of the cell cycle (that is, after the S phase) notice that each single crossover involves only two of the four chromatids.

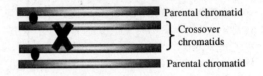

5. As mentioned in an earlier answer (#3), with some qualifications, crossovers occur randomly along the lengths of chromosomes. Within any region, the occurrence of two events is less likely than the occurrence of one event. If the probability of one event is

$$1/X$$

then the probability of two events occurring at the same time will be

$$1/X^2$$

6. Positive interference occurs when a crossover in one region of a chromosome interferes with crossovers in nearby regions. Such interference ranges from zero (no interference) to 1.0 (complete interference). Interference is often explained by a physical rigidity of chromatids such that they are unlikely to make sufficiently sharp bends to allow crossovers to be close together.

7. Each cross must be set up in such a way as to reveal crossovers because it is on the basis of crossover frequency that genetic maps are developed. It is necessary that genetic heterogeneity exist so that different arrangements of genes, generated by crossing over, can be distinguished.

The organism that is heterozygous must be the sex in which crossing over occurs. In other words, it would be useless to map genes in *Drosophila* if the male parent is the heterozygote since crossing over is not typical in *Drosophila* males.

Lastly, the cross must be set up so that the phenotypes of the offspring readily reveal their genotypes. The best arrangement is one where a fully heterozygous organism is crossed with an organism that is fully recessive for the genes being mapped.

8. Since the distance between *dp* and *ap* is greatest, they must be on the "outside" and *cl* must be in the middle. The genetic map would be as follows:

$$dp\cdots cl\cdots\cdots\cdots\cdots\cdots\cdots ap$$
$$\underbrace{\qquad}_{3\ mu}\underbrace{\qquad\qquad\qquad\qquad}_{39\ mu}$$

9. The initial cross for this problem would be

$$AaBb \quad \times \quad aabb$$

(a) If the two loci are on different chromosomes, independent assortment would occur and the following distribution (1:1:1:1) is expected:

1/4	*AaBb*
1/4	*Aabb*
1/4	*aaBb*
1/4	*aabb*

(b) Even though the two loci are linked and on the same chromosome, the frequency of crossing over is so high that crossovers always occur. Under that condition, independent assortment would occur and the following distribution (1:1:1:1) is expected:

1/4	*AaBb*
1/4	*Aabb*
1/4	*aaBb*
1/4	*aabb*

(c) If crossovers never occur, then all of the gametes from the heterozygous parent are *parental*. If the arrangement is

$$AB/ab \quad \times \quad ab/ab$$

then the two types of offspring will be

1/2	*AB/ab*
1/2	*ab/ab*

Under this condition *AB* are *coupled*. If, however, *A* and *B* are not coupled then the symbolism would be

$$Ab/aB \times aabb$$

The offspring would occur as follows:

1/2	*Ab/ab*
1/2	*aB/ab*

(d) If the loci are linked with 10 map units between them, then the two recombinant classes must add up to 10 percent of the total. Assuming that *A* and *B* are coupled, the following distribution would occur:

45%	*AaBb*	(parental)
5%	*Aabb*	(crossover)
5%	*aaBb*	(crossover)
45%	*aabb*	(parental)

10. In looking at this problem, one can immediately conclude that the two loci (kernel color and plant color) are linked because the testcross progeny occur in a ratio other than 1:1:1:1 (and epistasis does not appear because all phenotypes expected are present).

The question is whether the arrangement in the parents is *coupled*

$$RY/ry \quad \times \quad ry/ry$$

or *not coupled*

$$Ry/rY \quad \times \quad ry/ry$$

Notice that the most frequent phenotypes in the offspring, the parentals, are colored, green (88) and colorless, yellow (92). This indicates that the heterozygous parent in the testcross is coupled

$$RY/ry \quad \times \quad ry/ry$$

with the two dominant genes on one chromosome and the two recessives on the homolog (F5.1). Seeing that there are 20 crossover progeny among the 200, or 20/200, the map distance would be 10 map units (20/200 × 100 to convert to percentages) between the *R* and *Y* loci.

11. Start this problem by working through the expected offspring under two models: one with no crossing over and the second with 30 percent crossing over in the female.

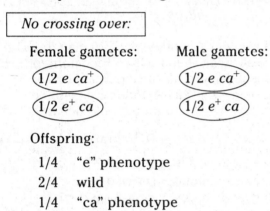

No crossing over:

Female gametes: Male gametes:

1/2 *e ca*⁺   1/2 *e ca*⁺

1/2 *e*⁺ *ca*   1/2 *e*⁺ *ca*

Offspring:

1/4   "e" phenotype

2/4   wild

1/4   "ca" phenotype

With 30% crossing over:

Female gametes: Male gametes:

35% *e ca*⁺   1/2 *e ca*⁺

35% *e*⁺ *ca*   1/2 *e*⁺ *ca*

15% *e*⁺ *ca*⁺

15% *e ca*

Offspring: (obtained by combining gametes and phenotypes)

"e" phenotype = 17.5% + 7.5% = **25%**

wild phenotype =

17.5% + 7.5% + 17.5% + 7.5% = **50%**

"ca" phenotype = 17.5% + 7.5% = **25%**

Notice that the distribution of phenotypes is the same, regardless of the contribution of the crossover classes.

12. Since there is no indication as to the configuration of the *P* and *Z* genes (*coupled or not coupled*) in the parent, one must look at the percentages in the offspring. Notice that the most frequent classes are *PZ* and *pz*. These classes represent the parental (noncrossover) groups, which indicate that the original parental arrangement in the testcross was

$$PZ/pz \quad \times \quad pz/pz$$

Adding the crossover percentages together (6.9 + 7.1) gives 14 percent, which would be the map distance between the two genes.

13. This problem can be approached by looking for the most distant loci (*adp* and *b*) and then filling in the intermediate loci. In this case the map for parts **(a)** and **(b)** is the following:

| *d* · · · · · *b* · · · · · *pr* · · · · · *vg* · · · · · *c* · · · · · *adp* |
| 31   48   54   67   75   83 |
| **Map Units** |

The expected map units between *d* and *c* would be 44, *d* and *vg* would be 36, and *d* and *adp* 52. However, because there is a theoretical maximum of 50 map units possible between two loci in any one cross, that distance would be below the 52 determined by simple subtraction.

14.

	female A:	female B:	Frequency:
NCO	3, 4	7, 8	first
SCO	1, 2	3, 4	second
SCO	7, 8	5, 6	third
DCO	5, 6	1, 2	fourth

The single-crossover classes that represent crossovers between the genes that are closer together (*d-b*) would occur less frequently than the classes of crossovers between more distant genes (*b-c*).

15. For two reasons, it is clear that the genes are in the *coupled* configuration in the F_1 female. First, a completely homozygous female was mated to a wild-type male, and second, the phenotypes of the offspring indicate the following parental classes:

$$sc\ s\ v \text{ and } +++$$

(a)

P_1: $sc\ s\ v/sc\ s\ v$ $\times$ $+++/Y$

F_1: $+++/sc\ s\ v$ $\times$ $sc\ s\ v/Y$

(b) Using method I or II for determining the sequence of genes, examine the parental classes and compare the arrangement with the double-crossover (least frequent) classes. Notice that the v gene "switches places" between the two groups (parentals and double crossovers). The gene that switches places is in the middle.

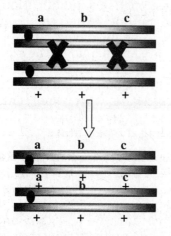

The map distances are determined by first writing the proper arrangement and sequence of genes, and then computing the distances between each set of genes.

$$\frac{sc\ v\ s}{+++}$$

$$sc - v = \frac{150 + 156 + 10 + 14}{1000} \times 100$$

$$= 33\% \text{ (map units)}$$

$$v - s = \frac{46 + 30 + 10 + 14}{1000} \times 100$$

$$= 10\% \text{ (map units)}$$

Double crossovers are always added into each crossover group because they represent a crossover in each region.

$$sc \cdots\cdots v \cdots\cdots s$$
$$\underbrace{\hspace{1.5cm}}_{33} \underbrace{\hspace{1.5cm}}_{10}$$

(c,d) The coefficient of coincidence =

$$\frac{\text{observed freq. double C/O}}{\text{expected freq. double C/O}}$$

$$= \frac{(14+10)/1000}{0.33 \times .1}$$

$$= \frac{0.024}{0.033}$$

$$= 0.727$$

which indicates that there were fewer double crossovers than expected; therefore, positive chromosomal interference is present.

16. This setup involves an F_1 in which the fully heterozygous female has the genes y and w in *coupled* and ct *not coupled*. The arrangement for the cross is therefore:

(a) $y\ w+/++ct$ $\times$ $y\ w+/Y$

It is important at this point to determine the gene sequence. Using method I or II, examine the parental classes and compare the arrangement with the double-crossover (least frequent) classes. Notice that the w gene "switches places" between the two groups (parentals and double crossovers). The gene that switches places is in the middle.

Therefore, the arrangement as written above is correct.

(b)

$$y - w = \frac{9 + 6 + 0 + 0}{1000} \times 100$$

$$= 1.5 \text{ map units}$$

$$w - ct = \frac{90 + 95 + 0 + 0}{1000} \times 100$$

$$= 18.5 \text{ map units}$$

$$y \cdots\cdots\cdots w \cdots\cdots\cdots ct$$
$$0.0 \qquad\qquad 1.5 \qquad\qquad\qquad 20.0$$

(c) There were

$$0.185 \times 0.015 \times 1000 = 2.775$$
double crossovers expected.

(d) Because the cross to the F_1 males included the normal (wild-type) gene for *cut wings,* it would not be possible to unequivocally determine the genotypes from the F_2 phenotypes for all classes.

17. (a) The cross will be as follows. Represent the *Dichete* gene as an upper-case letter because it is dominant.

P_1:	$D + +/+ + +$	$\times$	$+ e\,p/+ e\,p$
F_1:	$D + +/+ e\,p$	$\times$	$+ e\,p/+ e\,p$
F_2:	$D + + /+e\,p$	Dichete	
	$+e\,p/+e\,p$	ebony, pink	
	$D\,e+/+e\,p$	Dichete, ebony	
	$+ + p/+e\,p$	pink	
	$D + p/+e\,p$	Dichete, pink	
	$+e + /+e\,p$	ebony	
	$D\,e\,p/+e\,p$	Dichete, ebony, pink	
	$+ + +/+e\,p$	wild type	

(b) Determine which gene is in the middle by comparing the parental classes with the double-crossover classes. Notice that the *pink* gene "switches places" between the two groups (parentals and double crossovers). The gene that switches places is in the middle. So, rewriting the sequence of genes with the correct arrangement gives the following:

F_1:
$$D+ +/+p\,e \quad \times \quad + p\,e/+p\,e$$

Distances: Remember to add in the double-crossover classes.

$$D - p = \frac{12 + 13 + 2 + 3}{1000} \times 100$$
$$= 3.0 \text{ map units}$$

$$p - e = \frac{84 + 96 + 2 + 3}{1000} \times 100$$
$$= 18.5 \text{ map units}$$

18. The fact that two of the genes are linked and are 20 map units apart on the third chromosome, and that one is on the second chromosome, the problem is a combination of linkage and independent assortment. First, provide the genotypes of the parents in the original cross and the reciprocal. Use a semicolon to indicate that two different chromosome pairs are involved.

P_1:
$$\text{females:} \quad +/+; \quad p\,e/p\,e$$
$$\times$$
$$\text{males:} \quad dp/dp; \quad + +/+ +$$

F_1:
$$\text{females:} \quad +/dp; \quad + +/p\,e$$
$$\times$$
$$\text{males:} \quad dp/dp; \quad p\,e/p\,e$$

Female gametes: Use a modification of the forked-line method to determine the types of gametes to be produced. The *dumpy* locus will give $0.5 +$ and $0.5\ dp$ to the gametes because of independent assortment (on a different chromosome), and the other two loci will segregate, with 20 percent (map units) being the recombinants and 80 percent being the parentals.

	0.4 +	+ (parental)	= 0.20 + + +
0.5 +	0.1 +	e (crossover)	= 0.05 + + e
	0.1 p	+ (crossover)	= 0.05 + p +
	0.4 p	e (parental)	= 0.20 + p e
	0.4 +	+ (parental)	= 0.20 dp + +
	0.1 +	e (crossover)	= 0.05 dp + e
0.5 dp	0.1 p	+ (crossover)	= 0.05 dp p +
	0.4 p	e (parental)	= 0.20 dp p e

Crossing with $dp\ p\ e$ from the male gives the following offspring:

0.20 wild type
0.05 ebony
0.05 pink
0.20 pink, ebony
0.20 dumpy
0.05 dumpy, ebony
0.05 dumpy, pink
0.20 dumpy, pink, ebony

For the reciprocal cross:

> F$_1$:
>
> males: $+/dp$; $++/p\,e$
>
> $\times$
>
> females: dp/dp; $p\,e/p\,e$

there would be no crossover classes.

$$0.5+ \diagup \begin{array}{l} 0.5+ \quad +\text{(parental)} = 0.25 + + + \end{array}$$
$0.5+ \!\!-\!\! 0.5\,p \quad e\ \text{(parental)} = 0.25 + p\,e$
$$0.5\,dp \diagup \begin{array}{l} 0.5+ \quad +\text{(parental)} = 0.25\,dp + + \end{array}$$
$0.5\,dp \!\!-\!\! 0.5\,p \quad e\ \text{(parental)} = 0.25\,dp\,p\,e$

Crossing with $dp\,p\,e$ from the female gives the following offspring:

0.25 wild type

0.25 pink, ebony

0.25 dumpy

0.25 dumpy, pink, ebony

The results would change because of no crossing over in males.

19. Since *stubble* is a dominant mutation (and homozygous lethal), one can determine whether it is heterozygous ($Sb/+$) or homozygous wild type ($+/+$). One would use the typical testcross arrangement with the *curled* gene so the arrangement would be

$$+\,cu/+\,cu$$

20. In typical trihybrid crosses, one expects eight kinds of offspring. In this example, only six are listed, and one can assume that since the double-crossover class is the least frequent, it is the double crossovers that are not listed.

To work this type of problem, examine the list to see which types are not present. In this case, the double-crossover classes are the following:

$$+ + c \quad \text{and} \quad a\,b +$$

(a,b) Notice that if you compare the parental classes (most frequent) with the double-crossover classes (zero in this case) you can, by using the logic of the methods described in the text, determine that the gene *b* is in the middle and the arrangement is as follows. *Note:* For consistency the zeros (double crossovers) are included in the calculations.

$$+\,b\,c/a + +$$

$$a - b = \frac{32 + 38 + 0 + 0}{1000} \times 100$$
$$= 7 \text{ map units}$$

$$b - c = \frac{11 + 9 + 0 + 0}{1000} \times 100$$
$$= 2 \text{ map units}$$

(c) The progeny phenotypes that are missing are $+ + c$ and $a\,b +$, which, of 1000 offspring, 1.4 ($0.07 \times 0.02 \times 1000$) would be expected. Perhaps by chance or some other unknown selective factor, they were not observed.

21. You will notice that it would take two crossovers to "isolate" the *singed* gene for a spot, and one exchange for a twin spot. Therefore, the likelihood of a twin spot is greater than the likelihood of a singed spot. The arrangement of the "marker" being discussed in the second part of this question is as follows:

$$\cdots\cdot t \cdots\cdots\cdots f \cdots\cdots c \cdots\cdot$$
$$\quad 27.5 \qquad\qquad 56.7 \qquad 66$$

Because the distance between *forked* and *tan* loci is relatively great, crossovers in this region would be most frequent (and produce a tan spot). The region between the centromere and *forked* is approximately nine map units; therefore, one would expect crossovers to occur in this region at the next highest frequency, thereby yielding twin spots. The least frequent event would probably be forked spots because it would take two crossovers to "isolate" the *forked* gene.

22. Because sister chromatids are genetically identical (with the exception of rare new mutations), crossing over between sisters provides no increase in genetic variability. Individual genetic variability could be generated by somatic crossing over because certain patches on the individual would be genetically different from other regions. This variability would in all likelihood be of only minor consequence. Somatic crossing over would have no influence on the offspring produced.

23. These observations, as well as the results of other experiments, indicate that the synaptonemal complex is required for crossing over.

24. (a) There would be $2^n = 8$ genotypic and phenotypic classes, and they would occur in a 1:1:1:1:1:1:1:1 ratio.

(b) There would be two classes, and they would occur in a 1:1 ratio.

(c) There are 20 map units between the *A* and *B* loci, and locus *C* assorts independently from both *A* and *B* loci.

25. Since the genetic map is more accurate when relatively small distances are covered and when large numbers of offspring are scored, this map would probably not be too accurate with such a small sample size.

26. Assign the following symbols, for example:

    R = Red   *r* = yellow
    O = Oval   *o* = long

  Progeny A: *Ro/rO* × *rroo* = 10 map units
  Progeny B: *RO/ro* × *rroo* = 10 map units

27. The easiest way to approach this problem is to set up fractions representing the proportions of gametes, with the frequency of the recombinant gametes adding up to 25 percent. For each, the gamete proportions would be the following:

    3/8 *Ab*; 3/8 *aB*; 1/8 *AB*; 1/8 *ab*

Now, combine the gametes from each parent (they are the same) and arrive at the following frequency:

  *A_B_* 33/64; *A_bb* 15/64; *aaB_* 15/64; *aabb* 1/64

28. The map distance of a gene to the centromere in *Neurospora* is determined by dividing the percentage of second-division asci (tetrads) by two. Patterns other than *BBbb* or *bbBB* are "second division" as discussed in the text and represent a crossover between the gene in question and the centromere. In the data given, the percentage of second-division segregation is 20/100 or 20 percent. Dividing by two (because only two of the four chromatids are involved in any single-crossover event) gives 10 map units.

29. Because the two types of tetrads occurred at equal frequency, one could say that the gene loci are not linked. Also, looking at the individual loci, notice that gene *a* segregates just as often with gene *b* as it does with its allele +. Because there are no arrangements characteristic of second-division segregation (*a+a+*, or *b++b*, for example), the two genes must be very close to their centromeres.

30. The general formula for determining map distances is as follows:

$$\text{Map distance} = \frac{NP + 1/2(T)}{\text{Total \# Tetrads}} \times 100$$

    NP = Nonparental ditypes

    T = Tetratypes

For Cross 1:

$$\frac{36 + 14}{100} \times 100 = 50 \text{ map units}$$

Because there are 50 map units between genes *a* and *b*, they are not linked.

For Cross 2:

$$\frac{3 + 9}{100} \times 100 = 12 \text{ map units}$$

Because genes *a* and *b* are not linked, they could be on nonhomologous chromosomes or far apart (50 map units or more) on the same chromosome. Because genes *c* and *b* are linked and therefore on the same chromosome, it is also possible that genes *a* and *c* are on different chromosome pairs. Under that condition, the NP and P (parental ditypes) would be equal; however, there is a possibility that the following arrangement occurs and that genes *a* and *c* are linked.

$$\underbrace{a \cdots\cdots\cdots \overset{<50}{c} \cdots\cdots \overset{12}{b}}_{>50}$$

31.

(a)

Tetrad	Category
1	parental ditype
2	parental ditype
3	nonparental ditype
4	tetratype
5	tetratype
6	tetratype

(b) If a single crossover occurs between the centromere and the two linked genes, then the arrangement in tetrad 2 will occur.

(c)

$$Map\ distance = \frac{NP + 1/2(T)}{Total\ \#\ Tetrads} \times 100$$

NP = Nonparental ditypes

T = Tetratypes

$$= \frac{6 + 11}{71} \times 100 = about\ 24\ map\ units$$

32. (a) One can see the various arrangements and crossover events that are labeled as parental ditype (P), nonparental ditype (NP), and tetratype (T). From that information, the following can be listed:

Tetrad in Problem	Class
1	NP
2	T
3	P
4	NP
5	T
6	P
7	T

(b) The easiest way to determine whether the *c* and *d* genes are linked is to compare the frequencies of the parental ditype (P)

and nonparental ditype (NP) classes. If P > NP, then the genes are linked. If P = NP, they are independently assorting. In the problem given here, P = 44 and NP = 2. Therefore, the genes are linked.

(c) The gene to centromere distances are computed by dividing the percent second-division segregation by two.

For the centromere to *c* distance:

$$\frac{1 + 5 + 3 + 1}{69} \times 100 = 14.5$$

now divide by 2 = 7.2 map units

For the centromere to *d* distance:

$$\frac{17 + 1 + 3 + 1}{69} \times 100 = 31.9$$

now divide by 2 = 15.9 map units

The map would be, according to these figures:

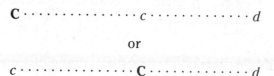

$$\text{C} \cdots\cdots\cdots\cdots\cdots c \cdots\cdots\cdots\cdots d$$

or

$$c \cdots\cdots\cdots\cdots \text{C} \cdots\cdots\cdots\cdots d$$

By mapping the genes to the centromeres, one can come up with two configurations. Either the genes are on the same side of the centromere, or they are on opposite sides. To decide which configuration is occurring, one should see what types of crossovers are required in each case. The two tetrad arrangements that are critical in dealing with the above configurations are #4 and #5.

Notice that, for tetrad arrangement #4, it takes three crossovers if genes *c* and *d* are on the same side of the centromere, while it takes two crossovers if they are on opposite sides. For tetrad arrangement #5, it takes two crossovers if genes *c* and *d* are on the same side of the centromere, while it takes three crossovers if they are on opposite sides.

Notice that the frequency of tetrad arrangement #5 (5) is much greater than tetrad arrangement #4 (1). This would make sense if the genes were on the same side of the centromere because the highest number of tetrads (5) is in tetrad arrangement #5 where the lowest number of crossovers is required.

If the two genes were on opposite sides of the centromere, the highest number of tetrad arrangements (5 in #5) would be associated with three crossover events. Since the likelihood of multiple crossovers decreases as the number of crossovers increases, it would seem reasonable that the genes are on the same side of the centromere.

Tetrad class #4

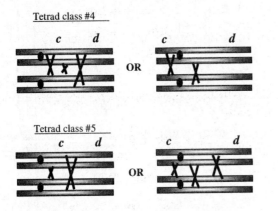

Tetrad class #5

(d) The formula for calculating the distance between the two loci is as follows:

$$Map\ distance = \frac{NP + 1/2(T)}{Total\ \#\ Tetrads} \times 100$$

NP = Nonparental ditypes

T = Tetratypes

$$= \frac{2 + 12}{69} = 20\ map\ units$$

(e)

$$C \cdots\cdots\cdots c \cdots\cdots\cdots d$$
$$\underbrace{}_{7.9} \underbrace{}_{16.4}$$

The discrepancy between the two mapping systems is caused by the manner in which first- and second-division segregation products are scored. For instance, in tetrad arrangement #1 there are actually two crossovers between the *d* gene and the centromere, but it is still scored as a

first-division segregation. In tetrad arrangement #4, three crossovers occur between the *d* gene and the centromere, but they are scored as one. If one draws out all the crossovers needed to produce the tetrad arrangements in this problem, it becomes clear that there are many crossovers between the *d* gene and the centromere that go undetected in the scoring of the arrangements of the *d* gene itself. This will cause one to underestimate the distance and give the discrepancy noted. One could account for these additional crossover classes to make the map more accurate.

(f)

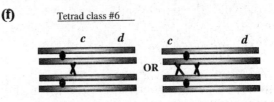

Tetrad class #6

33. (a)

10 *AB, Ab, aB, ab* (tetratype)

102 *Ab, aB, Ab, aB* (nonparental ditype)

99 *AB, AB, ab, ab* (parental ditype)

(b) Since the parental ditype class is approximately equal to the nonparental ditype class, one would conclude that there is no linkage.

(c) Since there is no linkage, one would conclude that the two loci are either on nonhomologous chromosomes or far apart on homologous chromosomes.

34. (a) Morgan and his students, especially Alfred Sturtevant, correlated chiasma frequency with the distance between linked genes. The farther apart the two genes, the higher the chiasma and, therefore, crossover frequency. The most important hint was that recombination frequency between gene *a* and *c* could equal to recombination frequency between *a* and *b*, plus recombination frequency between *b* and *c*.

(b) The discovery of linkage, genes segregating together during gamete formation, indicated a physical association among genes.

(c) Two experimental lines, one using maize (Creighton and McClintock) and the other using *Drosophila* (Stern), showed that each time a crossover occurred, an actual physical exchange of chromosomes also occurred. Each experiment demonstrated a switch in chromosomal markers when genetic markers exchanged.

(d) Even when sister chromatid exchanges do not produce new allelic combinations, they can be demonstrated using molecular markers such as bromodeoxyuridine.

(e) Linkage analysis in humans was historically accomplished by Lod score analysis, somatic cell hybridization (synteny testing), and pedigree analysis. Modern methods combine these historical approaches, with database analyses often employing a variety of physical markers (microsatellites, minisatellites, RFLPs, and SNPs).

35. Look for overlap between chromosome number in given clones and genes expressed. Note that *ENO1* is expressed in clones B, D, and E; chromosomes 1 and 5 are common to these clones. However, since *ENO1* is not expressed in clone C, which is missing chromosome 1 (and has chromosome 5), *ENO1* must be on chromosome 1.

    MDH1:   chromosome 2

    PEPS: chromosome 4

    PMG1:   chromosome 1

36. First make a drawing with the genes placed on the homologous chromosomes as follows:

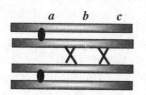

Realize that there are four chromatids in each tetrad and that a single crossover involves only two of the four chromatids.

Noninvolved chromatids must be added to the noncrossover classes. Do all the crossover classes first; then add up the noncrossover chromatids. For example, in the first crossover class (20 between *a* and *b*), notice that there will be 40 chromatids that were not involved in the crossover. These 40 must be added to the *abc* and +++ classes.

$$
\begin{aligned}
a\,b\,c\ &=\ 168 \\
+\ +\ +\ &=\ 168 \\
a\ +\ +\ &=\ 20 \\
+\ b\,c\ &=\ 20 \\
+\ +\ c\ &=\ 10 \\
a\,b\ +\ &=\ 10 \\
+\ b\ +\ &=\ 2 \\
a\ +\ c\ &=\ 2
\end{aligned}
$$

The map distances would be computed as follows:

$$
a - b = \frac{20 + 20 + 2 + 2}{400} \times 100
$$

$$
= 11 \text{ map units}
$$

$$
b - c = \frac{10 + 10 + 2 + 2}{400} \times 100
$$

$$
= 6 \text{ map units}
$$

37. There is no crossing over in males, and if two genes are on the same chromosome, there will be complete linkage of the genes in the male gametes. In females, crossing over will produce parental and crossover gametes. What you will have is the following gametes from the females (left) and males (right):

$bw^{+}\,st^{+}$	1/4		$bw^{+}\,st^{+}$	1/2
$bw^{+}\,st$	1/4		$bw\,st$	1/2
$bw\,st^{+}$	1/4			
$bw\,st$	1/4			

Combining these gametes will give the ratio presented in the table of results.

38. (a) There are several ways to think through this problem. Remember that there is no crossing over in *Drosophila* males.

Therefore, any gene on the same chromosome will be completely linked to any other gene on the same chromosome. Since you can get *pink* by itself, *short* cannot be completely linked to it. This leaves linkage to *black* on the second chromosome, the 4th chromosome, or the X chromosome. Since the distribution of phenotypes in males and females is essentially the same, the gene cannot be X-linked. In addition, the F_1 males were wild and if the *short* gene is on the X, the F_1 males would be short.

It is also reasonable to state that the gene cannot be on the 4th chromosome because there would be eight phenotypic classes (independent assortment of three genes) instead of the four observed. Through these insights, one could conclude that the *short* gene is on chromosome 2 with the *black* gene.

Another way to approach this problem is to make three chromosomal configurations possible in the F_1 male. By producing gametes from this male, the answer becomes obvious.

Case A	*Case B*	*Case C*
p b sh	p sh b	b sh p
+ + +	+ + +	+ + +

Develop the gametes from Case C and cross them out to the completely recessive triple mutant. You will get the results in the table.

(b) The parental cross is now the following:

Females: b sh   p   ×   *Males: b sh   p*
+ +   +   b sh p

The new gametes resulting from crossing over in the female would be *b +* and *+ sh*. Since the gene *p* is assorting independently, it is not important in this discussion. Because 15 percent of the offspring now contain these recombinant chromatids, the map distance between the two genes must be 15.

39. Notice that in the description of the genotype of the female, no mention is made of the *cis-trans* (coupling-repulsion) arrangement of the genes. The data will supply that information. Begin with a set of symbols as follows:

B^+ = wild eye shape

B = Bar eye shape

m^+ = wild wings

m = miniature wings

e^+ = wild body color

e = ebony body color

Superficially, the cross would be as follows:

$B^+B \ m^+m \ e^+e$ X B^+? *m*? *e*? (The *?* is used at this point to indicate that we have no information allowing us to decide whether any of the alleles in the male are X-linked.)

Notice from the data that there are approximately as many ebony offspring (282) as those with wild body color (283). Therefore, we can conclude that the *ebony* locus is not linked to *B* or *m*. Notice, too, that the most frequent offspring regarding eye shape and wing size are wild-miniature and Bar-wild. This suggests that the arrangement is "trans" or "repulsion" as indicated below:

$$B \ m^+/B^+m; \ e^+/e$$

Observe that a semicolon is used to indicate that the *ebony* locus is on a different chromosome.

At this point and without prior knowledge, we still do not know whether any of the genes are X-linked; however, it is of no consequence to the solution of the problem. (In actuality, both *B* and *m* loci are X-linked.)

To determine the map distances (again, *ebony* is out of the mapping picture at this point because it is not linked to either *B* or *m*):

111 + 115 = 226   = wild miniature
                                  = parental

117 + 101 = 218   = Bar wild
                                  = parental

26 + 31 = 57   = Bar miniature
                                  = crossover

29 + 35 = 64   = wild wild
                                  = crossover

Mapping the distance between B and m would be as follows:

$(57 + 64)/(226 + 218 + 57 + 64) \times 100 =$

$$121/565 \times 100 = 21.4 \text{ map units.}$$

We would conclude that the *ebony* locus is either far away from B and m (50 map units or more) or that it is on a different chromosome. In fact, *ebony* is on a different chromosome.

40. Once the pedigree is established as requested in part (a), one can address part (b) by detailing the genotypes of each daughter and her husband. To symbolize the two alleles at the *EMWX* locus, a "+" superscript is used for the normal allele, and a "−" superscript is used for the mutant allele.

Daughter 1:

$$EMWX^+ \, Xg^+/EMWX^- \, Xg^- \times Xg^+/Y$$

Daughter 2:

$$EMWX^+ \, Xg^+/EMWX^- \, Xg^- \times Xg^-/Y$$

Daughter 3:

$$EMWX^+ \, Xg^+/EMWX^- \, Xg^- \times Xg^-/Y$$

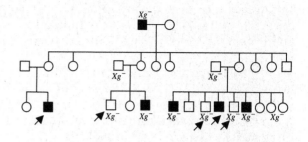

By examining the chromosomal configurations in the three daughters along with their husbands, one can determine, at least for the male offspring, whether a crossover was required to produce the given phenotypes. Crossover offspring are noted by an arrow.

41. (a) A number of studies have suggested a relationship between maternal chromosome nondisjunction and crossover frequency and/or chromosomal location of crossovers. Data presented in this table show an inverse correlation between recombination frequency and live-born children having various trisomies. As the frequency of crossing over decreases, the frequency of trisomy increases. While these data indicate a correlation, other factors such as intrauterine survival are also likely to play a role in determining trisomy live-born frequencies.

(b) If positive interference does spread out crossovers among and within chromosomes, then ensuring that crossovers are distributed among all the chromosomes (and all portions of chromosomes) may reduce nondisjunction and therefore be of selective advantage. This model assumes that the total number of crossovers per oocyte is limiting.

Chapter 6: Genetic Analysis and Mapping in Bacteria and Bacteriophages

Concept Areas	Corresponding Problems
Growth Characteristics	17, 28
Genetic Recombination in Bacteria	1, 23
Conjugation	2, 3, 4, 5, 6, 22, 31, 32
Chromosome Mapping	4, 2, 27
Transformation	7, 8, 9, 26, 29, 30
Bacteriophages	11, 15, 16
Transduction	10, 11, 12, 13
Mutation and Recombination in Viruses	14, 33
Intragenic Recombination in Phages	18, 19, 20, 21, 24, 25

Vocabulary: Organization and Listing of Terms and Concepts

Structures and Substances

Bacteria

Bacteriophage

Spontaneous mutations

Growth conditions

  minimal medium

  liquid culture

  prototroph

  auxotroph

Donor strain

  E. coli K12

  F sex pilus

  fertility factor, F factor

  RecA, RecBCD proteins

  rec genes

  lysozyme

  Hfr, circular chromosome

F′, merozygotes

  partial diploid

Plasmids

  F factors

  R plasmids

    resistance transfer factor (RTF)

    r-determinants

    antibiotic resistance

Col plasmids

ColE1

  colicins

  colicinogenic

Protein capsid

Lysozyme

Plaque

Episome

Prophage P22

Cistron

Hot spot

Processes/Methods

Sensitive

Resistant

  lag, log, stationary phases

Bacterial recombination

  conjugation

    F^+, F^-

    physical contact

    unidirectional

  donor, "male"

  recipient, "female"

  high-frequency recombination, Hfr

    oriented transfer

    interrupted mating technique

    circular map

F' state

  merozygotes

Transformation

  competence

  heteroduplex

  single-strand displacement

  linkage

  cotransformation

Transduction

  phage life cycle

    plaque (plaque assay)

    lysis

    lysogenized bacteria

    temperate phage

    U-tube experiment

    filterable agent (FA)

    prophage P22

  generalized transduction (F6.1)

  specialized transduction

    abortive transduction

    complete transduction

  cotransduction

    mapping

    specialized transduction

    intragenic exchanges

    fine structure analysis

    *r*II, T4

    E. coli B, K12

  complementation

  deletion testing

    hot spots

  mixed infection experiments

Mutations (viral)

  rapid lysis, host range

Concepts

Dilution

Bacterial recombination—all forms

Relationship to *rec* genes

Fine structure analysis

  complementation

  cistron

  recombinational analysis

  deletion testing

F6.1 Simple illustration comparing abortive and complete transduction.

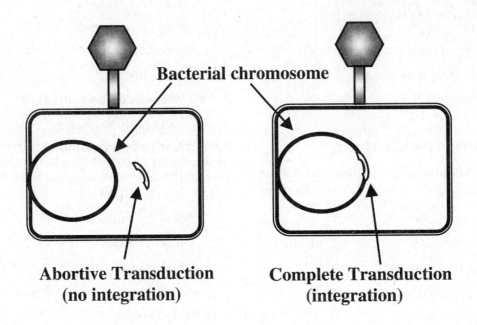

Bacterial chromosome

Abortive Transduction
(no integration)

Complete Transduction
(integration)

Solutions to Problems and Discussion Questions

1. Three modes of recombination in bacteria are *conjugation, transformation,* and *transduction.* Conjugation is dependent on the F factor, which, by a variety of mechanisms, can direct genetic exchange between two bacterial cells. Transformation is the uptake of exogenous DNA by cells. Transduction is the exchange of genetic material using a bacteriophage.

2. (a) The requirement for physical contact between bacterial cells during conjugation was established by placing a filter in a U-tube such that the medium can be exchanged, but the bacteria cannot come in contact. Under this condition, conjugation does not occur.

(b) By treating cells with streptomycin, an antibiotic, it was shown that recombination would not occur if one of the two bacterial strains was inactivated. However, if the other was similarly treated, recombination would occur. Thus, directionality was suggested, with one strain being a donor strain and the other being the recipient.

(c) An F$^+$ bacterium contains a circular, double-stranded, structurally independent DNA molecule that can direct recombination.

3. (a) In an F$^+$ × F$^-$ cross, the transfer of the F factor produces a recipient bacterium, which is F$^+$. Any gene may be transferred on an F′, and the frequency of transfer is relatively low. Crosses that are Hfr × F$^-$ produce recombinants at a higher frequency than the F$^+$ × F$^-$ cross. The transfer is oriented (nonrandom), and the recipient cell remains F$^-$.

(b) Bacteria that are F$^+$ possess the F factor, while those that are F$^-$ lack the F factor. In Hfr cells the F factor is integrated into the bacterial chromosome, and in F′ bacteria, the F factor is free of the bacterial chromosome, yet it possesses a piece of the bacterial chromosome.

4. Mapping the chromosome in an Hfr × F$^-$ cross takes advantage of the oriented transfer of the bacterial chromosome through the conjugation tube. For each F type, the point of insertion and the direction of transfer are fixed; therefore, breaking the conjugation tube at different times produces partial diploids, with corresponding portions of the donor chromosome being transferred. The length of the chromosome being transferred is contingent on the duration of conjugation; thus, mapping of genes is based on time.

5. In an Hfr × F$^-$ cross, the F factor is directing the transfer of the donor chromosome. It takes approximately 90 minutes to transfer the entire chromosome. Because the major portion of the F factor is the last element to be transferred and the conjugation tube is fragile, the likelihood for complete transfer is low.

6. As shown in the text, the F$^+$ element can enter the host bacterial chromosome, and upon returning to its independent state, it may pick up a piece of a bacterial chromosome. When combined with a bacterium with a complete chromosome, a partial diploid, or merozygote, is formed.

7. Transformation requires *competence* on the part of the recipient bacterium, meaning that only under certain conditions are bacterial cells capable of being transformed. Transforming DNA must be *double stranded* to begin with, yet it is converted to a single-stranded structure upon insertion into the host cell. The most efficient length of the transforming DNA is about 1/200 of the size of the host chromosome. Transformation is an energy-requiring process, and the number of sites on the bacterial cell surface is limited.

8. In the first dataset, the transformation of each locus, a^+ or b^+, occurs at a frequency of 0.031 and 0.012, respectively. To determine if there is linkage, one would determine whether the frequency of double transformants a^+b^+ is greater than that expected by a multiplication of the two independent events. Multiplying 0.031 × 0.012 gives 0.00037 or approximately 0.04 percent. From this information, one would consider no linkage between these two loci. Notice that this frequency is approximately the same as the frequency in the second experiment, where the loci are transformed independently.

9. Notice that the incorporation of loci a^+ and b^+ occurs much more frequently than the incorporation of b^+ and c^+ together (210 to 1), and the incorporation of all three genes $a^+b^+c^+$ occurs relatively infrequently. If a and b loci are close together and both are far from locus c, then fewer crossovers would be required to incorporate the two linked loci compared to all three loci (see diagram). If all three loci were close together, then the frequency of incorporation of all three would be similar to the frequency of incorporation of any two contiguous loci, which is not the case.

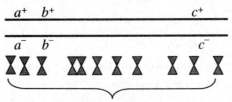

Sites of crossing over

10. In their experiment, a filter was placed between the two auxotrophic strains; this would not allow contact. F-mediated conjugation requires contact; without that contact, such conjugation cannot occur. The treatment with DNase showed that the filterable agent was not naked DNA.

11. A *plaque* results when bacteria in a "lawn" are infected by a phage and the progeny of the phage destroy (lyse) the bacteria. A somewhat clear region called a plaque is produced.

Lysogeny is a complex process whereby certain temperate phages can enter a bacterial cell and, instead of following a lytic developmental path, integrate their DNA into the bacterial chromosome. In doing so, the bacterial cell becomes lysogenic. The latent, integrated phage chromosome is called a *prophage*.

12. In *generalized transduction,* virtually any genetic element from a host strain may be included in the phage coat and thereby be transduced. In *specialized (restricted) transduction,* only those genetic elements of the host that are closely linked to the insertion point of the phage can be transduced. Specialized transduction involves the process of lysogeny.

Because only certain genetic elements are involved in specialized transduction, it is not useful in determining linkage relationships. Cotransduction of genes in generalized transduction allows linkage relationships to be determined.

13. The first problem to be solved is the gene order. Clearly, the parental types are

$$a^+b^+c^+ \text{ and } a^-b^-c^-$$

because they are the most frequent. The double-crossover types are the least frequent:

$$a^-b^-c^+ \text{ and } a^+b^+c^-$$

Because it is the gene in the middle that switches places when one compares the parental and double-crossover classes, the c gene must be in the middle. The map distances are as follows:

a to c = (740 + 670 + 90 + 110)/10,000

$\quad\quad$ = 16.1 map units

c to b = (160 + 140 + 90 + 110)/10,000

$\quad\quad$ = 5 map units

To determine the type of interference, first determine the *expected* frequency of double crossovers ($0.161 \times 0.05 = 0.000805$), which when multiplied by 10,000 gives approximately 80. The *observed* number of double crossovers is $90 + 110$, or 200. Since many more double crossovers are observed than expected, negative interference is occurring.

14. Phage recombination occurs when there is a sufficiently high number of infecting viruses, so that there is a high likelihood that more than one type of phage will infect a given bacterium. Under this condition, phage chromosomes can recombine by crossing over.

15. The translation machinery of the infected bacterium provides the necessary materials for protein synthesis.

16. Starting with a single bacteriophage, one lytic cycle produces 200 progeny phages; three more lytic cycles would produce $(200)^4$ or 1,600,000,000 phages.

17. (a) The concentration of phage is greater than 10^4.

(b) The concentration of phage is around 1.4×10^6.

(c) The concentration of phage is less than 10^6.

18. The approach for determining the complementation groupings and the results of the missing data are to recall that if a "+" is registered, different complementation groups (genes) exist. If a "−" results, then the two mutations are in the same complementation group. For Group A, *d* and *f* are in the same complementation group (gene), while *e* is in a different one. Therefore,

$$e \times f = +$$

For Group B, all three mutations are in the same gene, hence

$$h \times i = -$$

In Group C, *j* and *k* are in different complementation groups, as are *j* and *l*. It would be impossible to determine whether *l* and *k* are in the same or different complementation group if the *r*II region had more than two cistrons. However, because only two complementation regions exist, and both are not in the same one as *j*, *k* and *l* must both be in the other.

19. Because there are only two complementation groups in the *r*II region, one would have the following groupings:

   Group A: 1,4,5   *Group* B: 2,3

(a) Therefore, the result of testing is

   2×3 = no lysis
   2×4 = lysis
   3×4 = lysis

(b) Because mutant 5 failed to complement with mutations in either cistron, it probably represents a major alteration in the gene such that both cistrons are altered. A deletion that overlaps both cistrons could cause such a major alteration.

20. The recombination frequency is given by the following formula. Recall that only one of the two recombinant types is recovered in this type of experiment where the assay of growth on *E. coli* B is used. Remember to include the dilution factor in the setting of the observed values.

General formula:

$$\frac{2(\text{number of recombinant types})}{\text{total number of progeny}}$$

$$= 2(5 \times 10^1)/(2 \times 10^5) = 5 \times 10^{-4}$$

21. Because mutant 6 complemented mutations 2 and 3, it is likely to be in the cistron with mutants 1, 4, and 5. A lack of recombinants with mutant 4 indicates that mutant 6 is a deletion that overlaps mutation 4. Recombinants with 1 and 5 indicate that the deletion does not overlap these mutations.

22. One can approach this problem by lining up the data from the various crosses in the following order:

Hfr Strain	*Order*
1	T C H R O
2	H R O M B
3	<<C H R O M
4	M B A K T>>
5	<<B A K T C>

Overall: $\boxed{\text{T C H R O M B A K}}$

Notice that all of the genes can be linked together to give a consistent map and that the ends overlap, indicating that the map is circular. The order is reversed in two of the crosses, indicating that the orientation of transfer is reversed.

23. (a) Genetic variants of bacteria were discovered by their resistance to infection by bacteriophage and their dependence on certain media. Mutant strains could be established that provided the raw material for the discovery of a variety of recombinant strategies. Mutant bacteriophages were discovered by variations in their plaque morphology and host range.

(b) A variety of experiments involving transformation, conjugation, and transduction showed that genetic elements from one bacterial strain can be transferred to another strain. Historically, transformation set the stage for the discovery that DNA is the genetic material in bacteria.

(c) The general strategy for determining the dependence of cell-to-cell contact in one form of bacterial recombination involved a Davis U-tube and a filter. When the filter separated two auxotrophic strains, no genetic recombination occurred.

(d) A filterable agent was discovered such that when two auxotrophic strains were placed on opposite sides of a Davis U-tube apparatus, there was a one-way passage of genetic material. The filterable agent was insensitive to DNase treatment and was therefore not naked DNA.

(e) Intergenic recombination in bacteria was demonstrated by mixed infections that yielded recombinants. Such recombinants can be used in the mapping of genes.

(f) Early experiments by Benzer showed that in certain pair-wise combinations of rII mutant strains, wild-type function could be restored. Such complementation experiments demonstrated the presence of functional domains (cistrons) within certain complex genes.

24. (a)

Combination	*Complementation*
1, 2	−
1, 3	+
2, 4	+
4, 5	−

25. (a) Because mutants can lyse *E. coli* B but not K12, one can determine the total number of plaque-forming units (phages) as 4×10^7. The number of recombinants (those that grow on K12) would be 8×10^2. The recombination frequency would therefore be

$$2(8 \times 10^2/4 \times 10^7) = 4 \times 10^{-5}$$

(b) The dilution would be 10^{-3}, and the colony number would be 8×10^3.

(c) Mutant 7 might well be a deletion spanning parts of both A and B cistrons.

26. Because the frequency of double transformants is quite high (compare the *trp⁺tyr⁺* transformants in A and B experiments), one may conclude that the genes are quite closely linked together. Part B in the experiment gives one the frequencies of transformations of the individual genes and the frequency of transformants receiving two pieces of DNA (2 in the data table). One must know these numbers in order to estimate the actual number of *trp⁺tyr⁺* cotransformations.

27. **(a)** Rifampicin eliminates the donor strain which is *rif* ˢ.

(b) <u>*b a*   *c*   </u> F

(c) To determine the location of the *rif* gene, one could use a donor strain, which was *rif* ʳ but sensitive to another antibiotic (ampicillin, for example). The interrupted mating experiment is conducted as usual on an ampicillin-containing medium, but the recombinants must be replated on a rifampicin medium to determine which ones are sensitive.

28. Because 1/10 ml of a 10^{-6} dilution is used to add to the bacterial suspension, the concentration of the original phage suspension would be:

$$10 \times 10^6 \times 17 = 1.7 \times 10^8$$

plaque-forming units per ml or pfu/ml.

29. The basis for answering this question rests in the fact that it is easier to transform two genes that are close together (that is, cotransform) than if the same two genes are far apart. If two genes are cotransforming at a relatively high rate, they are said to be "linked" in a sense that they are closer together than two genes that do not cotransform. The data indicate that *a* and *d* are linked, *b* and *c* are linked, and since *f* cotransforms with *b*, *b*, *c*, and *f* are likely to be linked. However, if the arrangement is *c b f*, or the reverse, there is a possibility that whereas both *c* and *f* are "linked" to *b*, *c* and *f* may not be strongly linked enough to cotransform. Gene *e* does not cotransform with any gene, so it must be independent of the other linkage groups.

30. Since *g* cotransforms with *f*, it is likely to be in the *c b f* "linkage group" and would be expected to cotransform with each. One would not expect transformation with *a*, *d* or *e*.

31. **(a)** Some strains, *E. fergusonii,* for example, undergo relatively low transfer as a donor strain, while others, *E. chrysanthemi*, undergo relatively frequent transfer as a donor strain. Within-species transfer is not necessarily more frequent than between-species transfer. The direction of transfer (which is the donor and recipient strain) in some cases influences the frequency of transfer; for example, notice the frequencies of transfer when *E. chrysanthemi* is the donor and *E. coli* is the recipient (−1.7), compared with when *E. coli* is the donor and *E. chrysanthemi* is the recipient (−3.7).

(b) The answers are: *E. chrysanthemi,* (−2.4); *Ecoli-E. chrysanthem* (−1.7).

(c) Conjugative plasmids can share genes when bacteria are in proximity, and since such plasmids may contain either pathological genes or genes that compromise the use of antibiotics, any harmful variant that develops in one species may be spread to others. While a particular gene may be harmless in one bacterium, it may confer pathogenicity or drug resistance to a different species.

32. **(a)** No, all functional groups do not impact similarly on conjugative transfer of R27. Regions 1, 2, and 4 appear to be least influenced by mutation because transfer is at 100 percent.

(b) Regions 3, 5, 6, 8, 9, 10, 12, 13, and 14 appear to have the most impact on conjugation because, when mutant, conjugation is abolished.

(c) Regions 7 and 11, when mutant, only partially abolish conjugation; therefore, they probably have less impact on conjugation than those listed in part **(b)**.

(d) The data in this problem provide some insight into the complexity of the genetic processes involved in bacterial conjugation. The regions that have the most impact on conjugation fall into three different functional groups. In addition, notice that regions 1, 2, 4, 7, and 11, those that appear to have little, if any, impact on conjugation, are functionally related, as indicated by their shading.

33. (a) Each process, mutation, recombination, and reassortment provides genetic diversity upon which sustained infectivity is dependent. As host defenses adapt, viral diversity provides for viral survival.

(b) Because of its relatively volatile genome, the influenza virus is able to present a variety of unique surface elements that are foreign to the human immune system. As the immune system responds to viral uniqueness, new variants are generated that again evade the immune system.

(c) A successful vaccine is one that stimulates a response in the immune system to a specific antigen or array of antigens presented by a pathogen or toxin. Since the influenza virus alters its surface antigens at a relatively rapid pace, by the time a vaccine is developed, new strains have evolved. Recently, researchers have become more successful at developing useful short-term vaccines for variants of influenza viruses that evolve relatively rapidly.

Chapter 7: Sex Determination and Sex Chromosomes

Concept Areas	Corresponding Problems
Sex Chromosomes	1, 3, 9, 10, 13, 14, 17, 28, 32
Life Cycles	2
Sex Determination	4, 5, 6, 7, 9, 12, 15, 16, 17, 22, 27, 33, 37, 38
Sexual Differentiation	8, 3, 4, 11, 24, 25, 26, 27
Dosage Compensation	7, 17, 18, 19, 20, 21, 22, 23, 31, 34, 35, 36

Vocabulary: Organization and Listing of Terms and Concepts

Structures and Substances

Heteromorphic sex chromosomes

isogamete

zoospore

gametophyte

sporophyte

stamen (tassels)

microgametophyte

pistil

endosperm nuclei

oocyte nucleus

synergids

antipodal nuclei

heterochromosome

Y chromosome

heterogametic sex

homogametic sex

aromatase

Testis-determining factor (TDF)

MSY region of the Y

X-transposed region

Xq21

X-degenerative region

pseudogenes

ampliconic region

amplicon

glucose-6-phosphate dehydrogenase deficiency (*G-6-PD*)

clone

X-inactivation center (*XIC*)

X-inactive specific transcript (*XIST*)

Xic, Xist (mouse)

open reading frame (ORF)

transformer gene (*tra*)

sex-lethal (*Sxl*)

double-sex (*dsx*)

maleless (*mle*)

Processes/Methods

Sexual differentiation

primary, secondary

unisexual

dioecious

gonochoric

bisexual

monoecious

hermaphroditic

intersex

Chlamydomonas

isogametes

Zea mays

    double fertilization

    C. elegans

    XX/XO *Protenor* mode

    XX/XY *Lygaeus* mode

    ZZ/ZW

Sex determination (humans)

    XX = female, XY = male

       intersexuality

    Klinefelter syndrome 47, XXY

    48, XXXY

    48, XXYY, etc.

    Turner syndrome 45, X

    mosaics 45X/46XY, 45X/46XX

    47, XXX; 48, XXXX

    49, XXXXX

    47, XYY

sexual differentiation

    gonadal primordia

    cortex, medulla

    human Y chromosome

       pseudoautosomal regions (PARS)

       NRY

    testis-determining factor (TDF)

    sex-determining region (SRY)

       XX males

       XY females

       transgenic mice

       SOX9, WT1, SF1

Sex ratio (humans)

    primary

    secondary

Dosage compensation

    sex chromatin body (Barr body)

    N-1 rule

    Lyon hypothesis, Lyonization

       G-6-PD

       red-green color blindness

       anhidrotic ectodermal

    dysplasia

    X-inactivating center (*XIC*)

    X-inactive specific transcript (*XIST*)

    open reading frame (ORF)

    epigenetic event

Sex determination (*Drosophila*)

    nondisjunction

       XO = sterile male

       XXY = normal female

    ratio (number of X chromosomes to number of haploid sets of autosomes)

       superfemale (metafemale)

       metamale

       intersex

    RNA splicing, alternative splicing

    dosage compensation

    mosaics, bilateral

    gynandromorph

Concepts

Sex determination (humans, *Drosophila*)

Sex differentiation

Dosage compensation

Solutions to Problems and Discussion Questions

1. The term *homomorphic* refers to the situation in which the sex chromosomes have the same form. The term *heteromorphic* refers to the condition in many organisms in which there are two different forms (morphs) of chromosomes such as X and Y. In *isogamous* species, there is little visible difference between the haploid vegetative cells that reproduce asexually and the haploid gametes that are involved in sexual reproduction. The two gametes that fuse during mating are morphologically indistinguishable and are called *isogametes*. An organism that is *heterogamous* is one in which there are two morphologically distinct gametes.

2. Maize (*Zea mays*) is a monoecious seed plant in which the sporophyte phase predominates during the life cycle. Both male and female structures are present on the adult plant. The stamens produce diploid microspore mother cells, which undergo meiosis to produce four haploid microspores. Each haploid microspore develops into a microgametophyte that contains two sperm nuclei. Female diploid cells, megaspore mother cells, are located in the pistil of the sporophyte. Following meiosis, only one of the four haploid megaspores survives and divides mitotically three times, producing a total of eight haploid nuclei. Two of these nuclei unite to become the endosperm nuclei. At the end of the sac where the sperm enters, three nuclei remain: the oocyte nucleus and two synergids. The other three antipodal nuclei cluster at the opposite end of the embryo sac.

When pollen grains make contact with the stigma and successfully develop, two sperm nuclei enter the embryo sac: one sperm nucleus unites with the haploid oocyte nucleus, and the other sperm nucleus unites with two endosperm nuclei.

In *Caenorhabditis elegans*, there are two sexual phenotypes: males, which have only testes, and hermaphrodites, which contain both testes and ovaries. While in the larval stage of development of hermaphrodites, testes produce sperm, which is stored. Oogenesis does not occur until the adult stage is reached. The eggs are fertilized (self-fertilized) by the stored sperm. The majority of the offspring are hermaphrodites, while less than 1 percent of the offspring is male. As adults, males can mate with hermaphrodites, producing about half male and half hermaphrodite offspring.

3. The life cycle of the green alga *Chlamydomonas* exhibits occasional sexual reproduction. Spending most of their life cycle as haploids, they asexually produce daughter cells by mitosis. In unfavorable nutrient conditions, some daughter cells function as gametes, forming a diploid zygote after fertilization. When conditions become acceptable, meiosis ensues and haploid vegetative cells are again produced. *Zea mays*, like many plants, alternate between the haploid gametophyte stage and the diploid sporophyte stage, which are linked together by meiosis and fertilization. It is a monoecious seed plant in which the sporophyte phase predominates the life cycle. Both male and female structures are present in the adult plant. The stamens produce diploid mother cells that undergo meiosis to produce four haploid microspores. Each microspore develops into a mature microgametophyte that contains two sperm nuclei. Similar female diploid cells, megaspore mother cells, occur in the pistil and following meiosis produce one of the four haploid megaspores, which divides mitotically three times, thus producing a total of eight haploid nuclei. Two of these nuclei unite becoming the endosperm nuclei.

Double fertilization results in a diploid zygotic nucleus and the triploid endosperm nucleus. Each ear of corn contains as many as 1000 fertilization products, and each kernel may germinate and give rise to a new plant (sporophyte).

The roundworm *Caenorhabditis elegans* consists of only about 1000 cells found in two sexual phenotypes: males, having testes, and hermaphrodites, which have both testes and ovaries. Early in the development of a hermaphrodite, testes form and produce sperm, which is then stored. Ovaries are produced too, but oogenesis occurs in the adult stage. Eggs may be fertilized by the stored sperm from self-fertilization.

Most of the offspring are hermaphrodites, and less than 1 percent of the offspring is male.

Genes located on both the X chromosome and autosomes determine the development of males or hermaphrodites. Hermaphrodites have two X chromosomes, whereas males have only one X chromosome and no Y chromosome is present. As in *Drosophila*, the ratio of X chromosomes to the number of sets of autosomes determines the sex of these worms.

4. Sexual differentiation is the response of cells, tissues, and organs to signals provided by the genetic mechanisms of sex determination. In other words, genes are present that signal developmental pathways whereby the sexes are generated. Sexual differentiation is the complex set of responses to those genetic signals.

5. The *Protenor* form of sex determination involves the XX/XO condition, while the *Lygaeus* mode involves the XX/XY condition.

6. Calvin Bridges (1916) studied nondisjunctional *Drosophila*, which had a variety of sex-chromosome complements. He noted that XO produced sterile males, while XXY produced fertile females. Other investigators have determined that the Y chromosome is male determining in humans. Individuals with the 47, XXY complement are males, while those with 45, XO are females.

In *Drosophila* it is the balance between the number of X chromosomes and the number of haploid sets of autosomes that

determines sex. In humans a small region on the Y chromosome determines maleness.

7. Mammals possess a system of X chromosome inactivation whereby one of the two X chromosomes in females becomes a chromatin body or Barr body. If one of the two X chromosomes is randomly inactivated, the dosage of genetic information is more or less equivalent in males (XY) and females (XX).

8. While a specific region on the Y chromosome specifies the eventual cellular fate as male in humans, sexual differentiation of the genital ridge does not occur until around the seventh week of development. In the absence of the Y chromosome, no male development occurs, and the cortex of the genital ridge forms ovarian tissue.

9. The Y chromosome is male determining in humans. It is a particular region of the Y chromosome that causes maleness, the sex-determining region (SRY). SRY encodes a product called the testis-determining factor (TDF), which causes the undifferentiated gonadal tissue to form testes. Individuals with the 47, XXY complement are males, while those with 45, XO are females. In *Drosophila* it is the balance between the number of X chromosomes and the number of haploid sets of autosomes that determines sex. In contrast to humans, XO *Drosophila* are males, and the XXY complement is female.

10. In *primary* nondisjunction, half of the gametes contain two X chromosomes, while the complementary gametes contain no X chromosomes. In secondary nondisjunction you get two normal gametes: one with two X chromosomes and one with no X. Fertilization, by a Y-bearing sperm cell, of those female gametes with two X chromosomes would produce the XXY Klinefelter syndrome. Fertilization of the "no-X" female gamete with a normal X-bearing sperm will produce Turner syndrome.

11. (a) female $X^{rw}Y$ $\times$ male X^+X^+

F_1: females: X^+Y (normal)
        males: $X^{rw}X^+$ (normal)

F_2: females: X^+Y (normal)
                  $X^{rw}Y$ (reduced wing)
        males: $X^{rw}X^+$ (normal)
                  X^+X^+ (normal)

(b) female $X^{rw}X^{rw}$ $\times$ male X^+Y

F_1: females: $X^{rw}X^+$ (normal)
        males: $X^{rw}Y$ (reduced wing)

F_2: females: $X^{rw}X^+$ (normal)
                  $X^{rw}X^{rw}$ (reduced wing)
        males: X^+Y (normal)
                  $X^{rw}Y$ (reduced wing)

12. No, since the Y chromosome cannot be detected in these crosses, there is no way to distinguish the two modes of sex determination.

13. Males and females share a common placenta and, therefore, hormonal factors carried in blood. Hormones and other molecular species (transcription factors perhaps) triggered by the presence of a Y chromosome lead to a cascade of developmental events, which both suppress female organ development and enhance masculinization. Other mammals also exhibit a variety of similar effects depending on the sex of their uterine neighbors during development.

14. Because attached-X chromosomes have a mother-to-daughter inheritance and the father's X is transferred to the son, one would see daughters with the white-eye phenotype and sons with the miniature wing phenotype.

15. If the offspring were typical (that is, if there were no attached-X chromosome to begin with), one would strongly suspect that the X chromosome had become unattached. Specifically, if the male offspring had white eyes and the female offspring were wild type, one might suspect that the attached-X had become unattached. All "expected" offspring would require that the detachment had occurred well before meiosis—early in germ-line formation. If it occurs *during* meiosis in some meiotic mother cells, we would see irregular numbers of the normal genotypes.

16. Because synapsis of chromosomes in meiotic tissue is often accompanied by crossing over, it would be detrimental to sex-determining mechanisms to have sex-determining loci on the Y chromosome transferred, through crossing over, to the X chromosome.

17. A *Barr body* is a differentially staining chromosome seen in some interphase nuclei of mammals with two X chromosomes. There will be one less Barr body than number of X chromosomes. The Barr body is an X chromosome that is considered to be genetically inactive.

18. There is a simple formula for determining the number of Barr bodies in a given cell: N-1, where N is the number of X chromosomes.

Klinefelter syndrome (XXY)	= 1
Turner syndrome (XO)	= 0
47, XYY	= 0
47, XXX	= 2
48, XXXX	= 3

19. The *Lyon hypothesis* states that the inactivation of the X chromosome occurs at random early in embryonic development. Such X chromosomes are in some way "marked," such that all clonally related cells have the same X chromosome inactivated.

20. Unless other markers, cytological or molecular, are available, one cannot test the Lyon hypothesis with homozygous X-linked genes. The test requires identification of allelic alternatives to see differences in X chromosome activity.

21. Females will display mosaic retinas with patches of defective color perception. Under these conditions, their color vision may be influenced.

22. Refer to the text and notice that the phenotypic mosaicism is dependent on the heterozygous condition of genes on the two X chromosomes. Dosage compensation and the formation of Barr bodies occur only when there are two or more X chromosomes. Males normally have only one X chromosome; therefore, such mosaicism cannot occur. Females normally have two X chromosomes. There are cases of male calico cats that are XXY.

23. Many organisms have evolved over millions of years under the fine balance of numerous gene products. Many genes required for normal cellular and organismic function in *both* males and females are located on the X chromosome. These gene products have nothing to do with sex determination or sex differentiation.

24. In mammals, the scheme of sex determination is dependent on the presence of a piece of the Y chromosome. If present, a male is produced. In *Bonellia viridis*, the female proboscis produces some substance that triggers a morphological, physiological, and behavioral developmental pattern that produces males. To elucidate the mechanism, one could attempt to isolate and characterize the active substance by testing different chemical fractions of the proboscis. Second, mutant analysis usually provides critical approaches into developmental processes. Depending on characteristics of the organism, one could attempt to isolate mutants that lead to changes in male or female development. Third, by using micro-tissue transplantations, one could attempt to determine which anatomical "centers" of the embryo respond to the chemical cues of the female.

25. In general, information about the primary sex ratio in humans is obtained from abortions and miscarriages.

In addition, some studies (Barczyk 2001) using "hamster oocyte–human sperm" have been successful in determining some of the causal factors involved in determining the primary sex ratio.

26. Several possibilities are discussed in the text. One could account for the significant departures from a 1:1 ratio of males to females by suggesting that at anaphase I of meiosis, the Y chromosome more often goes to the pole that produces the more viable sperm cells. One could also speculate that the Y-bearing sperm has a higher likelihood of surviving in the female reproductive tract, or that the egg surface is more receptive to Y-bearing sperm. At this time the mechanism is unclear.

As Pergament et al. (2002) explain:

A number of environmental, physiological and genetic factors have been observed to impact on the primary sex ratio: sexual behaviour, variation in hormonal concentrations, natural disasters, environmental pollutants and timing of conception. Nevertheless, no biological mechanism or interaction of factors has suitably explained this phenomenon, or that of the prenatal vulnerability of the male, the suspected higher sex ratio in spontaneous abortion and the male excesses in adult diseases related to the intrauterine environment.

27. Since there is a region of synapsis close to the SRY-containing section on the Y chromosome, crossing over in this region would generate XY translocations, which would lead to the condition described.

28. Because of the homology between the *red* and *green* genes, there exists the possibility for an irregular synapsis (see the figure below), which, following crossing over, would give a chromosome with only one (*green*) of the duplicated genes. When this X chromosome combines with the normal Y chromosome, the son's phenotype can be explained.

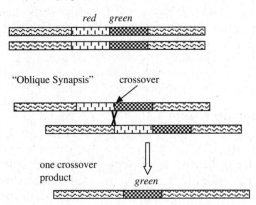

"Normal Synapsis"

red   green

"Oblique Synapsis"   crossover

one crossover
product   green

29. **(a)** Mutations such as *tassel seed (ts)*, *silkless (sk)*, and *barren stalk (ba)* have provided insight into sex determination in a monoecious plant such as *Zea mays*. Studies on such mutations indicate that many genes are responsible for sex differentiation in maize.

(b) The Y chromosome has been shown to play a crucial role in sex determination in mammals and some insects because its presence or absence determines sex. In others, such as *Drosophila*, the presence of certain X chromosome complements, such as a ratio to the autosomes, determines sex.

(c) Supported by the discovery of sex-chromosome aneuploids (e.g., XO, XXY) the presence or absence of a Y chromosome has been shown to be fundamental in sex determination in humans.

(d) Based on consensus data on the sex of embryos and fetuses recovered from miscarriages and abortions, showing that fetal mortality is higher in males than females, it is estimated that the primary sex ratio favors males.

(e) The most direct evidence in support of random inactivation of either X chromosome in an XX cell came from experiments using electrophoretic variants of the G6PD locus. Such studies, coupled with mosaic coat patterns in cats, support the random inactivation hypothesis.

(f) Calvin Bridges studied a number of chromosomal compositions in *Drosophila* and determined that the critical factor in sex determination is the ratio of X chromosomes to the number of haploid sets of autosomes. Given two haploid sets, XO is male and XXY is female.

30. The presence of the Y chromosome provides a factor (or factors) that leads to the initial specification of maleness. Subsequent expression of secondary sex characteristics must be dependent on the interaction of the normal X-linked *Tfm* allele with testosterone. Without such interaction, differentiation takes the female path.

31. **(a)** Something is missing from the male-determining system of sex determination either at the level of the genes, gene products, or receptors, and so on.

(b) The *SOX9* gene, or its product, is probably involved in male development. Perhaps it is activated by *SRY*.

(c) There is probably some evolutionary relationship between the *SOX9* gene and *SRY*. There is considerable evidence that many other genes and pseudogenes are also homologous to *SRY*.

(d) Normal female sexual development does not require the *SOX9* gene or gene product(s).

32. Since all haploids are male and half of the eggs are unfertilized, 50 percent of the offspring would be male at the start; adding the X_a/X_a types gives 25 percent more male; the remainder X_a/X_b would be female. Overall, 75 percent of the offspring would be male, while 25 percent would be female.

33. In snapping turtles, sex determination is strongly influenced by temperature such that males are favored in the 26–34°C range. Lizards, on the other hand, appear to have their sex determined by factors other than temperature in the 20–40°C range.

34. Different cells manage X chromosome inactivation in different ways. The absence of orange patches is due to the fact that in gonadal tissue, while oogonia have a single active X chromosome, the inactive X chromosome is reactivated at, or more likely, shortly before, entry into meiotic prophase (Kratzer and Chapman 1981). Thus, X chromosome inactivation does not remain in certain ovarian cells as in somatic tissue. However, since the timing of reactivation is variable in different cell lines, there is some uncertainty as to which cell is in which state of inactivation. The actual result was a kitten (CC) with black spots on a white background. With *black* being expressed in the presence of orange, only black shows through in the Carbon Copy's coat. However, if one assumes that the somatic ovarian cell was engaging in X chromosome inactivation, the ovarian somatic cell that Rainbow donated to create CC contained an activated black gene and an inactivated orange gene (from X-inactivation). This would mean that as CC developed, her cells did not change that inactivation pattern. Therefore, unlike Rainbow, CC developed without any cells that specified orange coat color. The result is CC's black and white tiger-tabby coat.

35. The white patches of CC are due to an autosomal gene *S* for white spotting that prevents pigment formation in the cell lineages in which it is expressed. Homozygous *SS* cats have more white than heterozygous *Ss* cats, and there is no absolute pattern of patches due to the *S* allele. So the distribution of white patches would be expected to be different from Rainbow. In addition, since X chromosome inactivation is random, CC would have a different patch pattern from her genetic mother on the random X inactivation basis alone.

36. If one assumes that the somatic ovarian cell engaged in X chromosome inactivation, the ovarian somatic cell that Rainbow donated to create CC contained an activated black gene and an inactivated orange gene (from X-inactivation). This would mean that as CC developed, her cells did not change that inactivation pattern. Therefore, unlike Rainbow, CC developed without any cells that specified orange coat color. The result is CC's black and white tiger-tabby coat.

37. (a) *Bonellia viridis*: Environmental influence of female proboscis (see Problem 24). *Bracon hebetor*: Genotypic and parthenogenetic (see Problem 32). *Homo sapiens*: Region on the Y chromosome is male-determining. *Drosophila melanogaster*: Balance between number of X chromosomes and number of haploid sets of autosomes. *Caenorhabditis elegans*: Balance between number of X chromosomes and sets of autosomes. *Protenor*: XX/XO system where XX gives female and XO gives male. *Lygaeus*: XX/XY system where XX gives female and XY gives male. Birds, moths, butterflies: ZZ/ZW where ZZ gives male and ZW gives female. Lizards: Some XX/XY, some ZZ/ZW, and some, temperature of egg incubation. Crocodiles, most turtles: temperature of egg incubation.

Organism	*Group**
Bonellia viridis	Other
Bracon hebetor	CSD, GSD
Homo sapiens	CSD, GSD
Drosophila melanogaster	CSD, GSD
Caenorhabditis elegans	CSD, GSD
Protenor	CSD
Lygaeus	CSD
Birds, moths, butterflies	CSD, GSD
Lizards	CSD, TSD
Crocodiles	TSD
Turtles	TSD

*In many cases it is difficult to distinguish between CSD and GSD because, while there are clearly chromosomal differences between the two sexes, there are likely major genetic determinants on such chromosomes that play a major role in sex determination.

(b) Since temperature variation is common in determining sex in reptiles and can sometimes override other schemes in amphibians, it has been suggested that parthenogenetic, CSD, and GSD systems are more recent adaptations among amphibians. The ancestral system of sex determination in amphibians is perhaps TSD, though tempered and modified in some species.

(c) The variety of sex-determination mechanisms suggests that there is no real standard for determining sex. Rather, various species have evolved different but sometimes overlapping strategies. It is likely that remnants of ancestral systems are carried in the genome but are masked by more recently evolved systems. Since endotherms have evolved to withstand only a narrow internal temperature range, it would be difficult to test TSD systems in endotherms. However, if the genetic underpinnings for TSD can be determined, they may also be identified in other taxa like birds and mammals. Such information would therefore be useful in answering this question.

38. (a) The figures below depict only those chromosomes relevant to the *Mm* and *Dd* genotypes. With the *MmDd* genotype, both dyads separate intact to the secondary spermatocytes and are potentially capable of fertilizing the egg. (Only one configuration of the *MmDd* genotype is presented here.)

Primary Spermatocyte

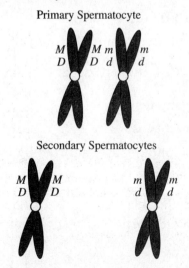

Secondary Spermatocytes

Below is the *Mm dd* genotype that leads to fragmentation of the *m*-bearing chromosome. Thus, only the *M*-bearing chromosome is available for fertilization.

Primary Spermatocyte

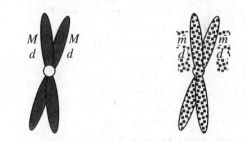

Secondary Spermatocytes

(b) Many attempts have been made to control pest species by hampering the production or fertility of one sex. In this case, if a sex ratio distorter could be successfully integrated into a large enough pool of males, then female numbers could drop. Whether one could successfully manage a pest population with such a method remains to be tested.

Chapter 8: Chromosome Mutations: Variation in Chromosome Number and Arrangement

Concept Areas	Corresponding Problems
Variation in Chromosome Number	1, 2, 3, 4, 5, 6, 13, 14, 15, 17, 18, 19, 20, 22, 26, 27, 29, 31, 32, 33
Deletions	7
Duplications	7, 10, 11, 32
Inversions	8, 9, 12, 16, 21, 23
Translocations	12, 25, 28, 30

Vocabulary: Organization and Listing of Terms and Concepts

Structures and Substances

Colchicine

Protoplast

rDNA

Nucleolar organizer (NOR)

Micronucleoli

Trinucleotide repeat

G-quartets

Knockout mice

Processes/ Methods

Chromosome mutations (aberrations)

  aneuploidy (F8.1)

Nondisjunction

  monosomy, trisomy, tetrasomy, pentasomy

  Klinefelter syndrome

  Turner syndrome

  haplo-VI (*Drosophila*)

  partial monosomy

    segmental deletions

    cri-du-chat syndrome

46,5p-

trisomy

  XXX (*Drosophila*, humans)

  Datura

pairing configurations

  trivalent

Down syndrome (G group)

  trisomy 21 (47, +21)

  amniocentesis

  chorionic villus sampling (CVS)

  familial Down syndrome

Patau syndrome (D group)

  trisomy 13 (47, +13)

Edwards syndrome (E group)

  trisomy 18 (47, +18) reduced viability

    gametes

    embryos

    spontaneously aborted fetuses

euploidy (F8.1)

  monoploid (*n*)

  diploid (2*n*)

polyploid
  triploid (3*n*)
  tetraploid (4*n*)
  pentaploid (5*n*)
autopolyploidy
autotriploids (3*n*)
complete nondisjunction
dispermic fertilization
  tetraploid × diploid
autotetraploids (4*n*)
cold or heat shock
allopolyploidy
  hybridization
allotetraploid (amphidiploid)
(cotton, *Triticale*)
Raphanus × *Brassica*
  somatic cell hybrids
  (protoplasts)
endopolyploidy
  endomitosis
Chromosome structure
  deletions (deficiency)
    terminal, intercalary
    loop (deficiency, compensation)
    pseudodominance
  duplications
  gene redundancy
    rDNA
      bobbed
  gene amplification
  nucleolar organizer (NOR)
    micronucleoli
  Bar eye in *Drosophila*
    semidominant

position effect
evolutionary aspects
  gene families
  rearrangements
inversions
  paracentric
  pericentric
    arm ratio
  heterozygotes
  inversion loops
  dicentric chromatids
  acentric chromatids
    dicentric bridges
  "suppression of crossing over"
  position effect
  evolutionary aspects
translocations
  reciprocal
  unorthodox synapsis
  semisterility
  familial Down syndrome
  centric fusion
  Robertsonian fusion
    14/21 or D/G
  fragile sites
    X chromosome
    Martin-Bell syndrome (MBS)
  genetic anticipation
  cancer
    recombinogenic
    tumor-suppressor gene
    apoptosis

Concepts

Significance of variation in chromosomes

    genomic balance

    sex chromosome balance

    evolution

Gene duplication (evolutionary aspects)

    sequence homology

        nucleic acids

        amino acids

Inversions

    "suppression of crossing over"

        evolutionary consequences

Translocations

Fragile sites

F8.1 Illustration of the chromosomal configurations of euploid and aneuploid genomes of *Drosophila melanogaster*.

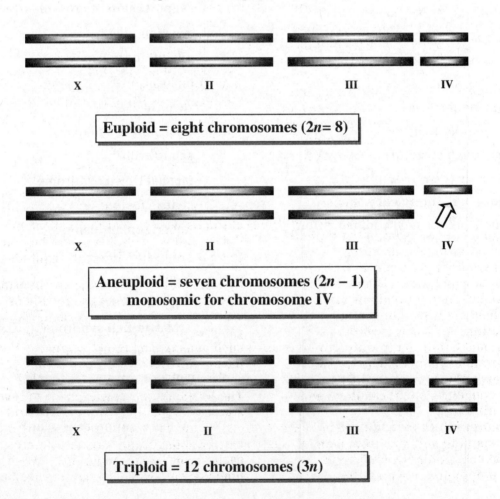

Drosophila melanogaster female

Euploid = eight chromosomes (2*n* = 8)

Aneuploid = seven chromosomes (2*n* − 1) monosomic for chromosome IV

Triploid = 12 chromosomes (3*n*)

Solutions to Problems and Discussion Questions

1. With a diploid chromosome number of 18 ($2n$), a haploid (n) would have 9 chromosomes, a triploid ($3n$) would have 27 chromosomes, and a tetraploid ($4n$) would have 36 chromosomes. A trisomic would have one extra chromosome (19), and a monosomic would have one less than the diploid (17).

2. With frequent exceptions, especially in plants, organisms typically inherit one chromosome complement (*haploid* = n = one representative of each chromosome) from each parent. Such organisms are *diploid*, or $2n$. When an organism contains complete multiples of the n complement ($3n$, $4n$, $5n$, etc.), it is said to be *euploid* in contrast with aneuploid in which complete haploid sets do not occur. An example of an aneuploid is *trisomic* where a chromosome is added to the $2n$ complement. In humans, trisomy 21 would be symbolized as $2n + 1$ or 47, +21.

Monosomy is an aneuploid condition in which one member of a chromosome pair is missing, thus producing the chromosomal formula of $2n - 1$. Haplo-IV is an example of monosomy in *Drosophila*. *Trisomy* is the chromosomal condition of $2n + 1$ where an extra chromosome is present. Down syndrome is an example in humans (47, +21). See the text and notice that all the chromosomes are present in the diploid state except chromosome #21.

Patau syndrome is a chromosomal condition in which there is an extra D group chromosome. Such individuals are 47, +13 and have multiple congenital malformations. *Edwards syndrome* is a chromosomal condition in which there is an extra E group chromosome (47, +18). Individuals with Edwards syndrome have multiple congenital malformations and reduced life expectancy.

Polyploidy refers to instances of more than two haploid sets of chromosomes in an individual cell. *Autopolyploidy* refers to cases of polyploidy in which the chromosomes in the individual originate from the same species. *Allopolyploidy* involves instances where the chromosomes originate from the hybridization of two different species, usually closely related. *Autotetraploids* arise within a species, while *amphidiploids* arise from two taxa followed by chromosome doubling.

Paracentric inversions require breakpoints that do not flank the centromere, while *pericentric* inversions do.

3. Individuals with Down syndrome, while suffering congenital defects with tendencies toward respiratory disease and leukemia, can live well into adulthood. Individuals with Patau or Edwards syndrome live less than four months on the average. Comparing the different sizes of the involved chromosomes (21, 13, and 18, respectively) in the text, for example, suggests that the larger the chromosome, the lower the likelihood of lengthy survival. In addition, it would be expected that certain chromosomes, because of their genetic content, may have different influences on development.

4. Because an allotetraploid has a possibility of producing bivalents at meiosis I, it would be considered the most fertile of the three. Having an even number of chromosomes to match up at the metaphase I plate, autotetraploids would be considered to be more fertile than autotriploids.

5. The sterility of interspecific hybrids is often caused by a high proportion of univalents in meiosis I. As such, viable gametes are rare, and the likelihood of two such gametes "meeting" is remote. Even if partial homology of chromosomes allows some pairing, sterility is usually the rule. The horticulturist may attempt to reverse the sterility by treating the sterile hybrid with colchicine. Such a treatment, if successful, may double the chromosome number, and each chromosome would then have a homolog with which to pair during meiosis.

6. American cultivated cotton has 26 pairs of chromosomes: 13 large and 13 small. Old world cotton has 13 pairs of large chromosomes, and American wild cotton has 13 pairs of small chromosomes. It is likely that an interspecific hybridization occurred, followed by chromosome doubling. These events probably produced a fertile amphidiploid (allotetraploid). Experiments have been conducted to reconstruct the origin of American cultivated cotton.

7. Basically, the synaptic configurations produced by chromosomes bearing a deletion or duplication (on one homolog) are very similar. There will be point-for-point pairing in all sections that are capable of pairing. The section that has no homolog will "loop out" as in the text.

8. While crossing over appears to be suppressed in inversion "heterozygotes," the phenomenon extends from the fact that the crossover chromatids end up being abnormal in genetic content. As such, they fail to produce viable (or competitive) gametes or lead to zygotic or embryonic death. Notice in the text that the crossover chromatids end up genetically unbalanced.

9. Examine the text and notice that in a paracentric inversion there are two genetically balanced chromatids (normal and inverted) and two chromatids resulting from a single crossover in the inversion loop, which are genetically unbalanced and abnormal (dicentric and acentric). The dicentric chromatid will often break, thereby producing highly abnormal fragments, whereas the acentric fragment is often lost in the meiotic process. In a pericentric inversion, all the chromatids have centromeres, but the two chromatids involved in the crossover are genetically unbalanced. The balanced chromatids are of normal or inverted sequence.

10. The mutant *Notch* in *Drosophila* produces flies with abnormal wings. It is a sex-linked dominant gene (a deletion) that also behaves as a recessive lethal. A deficiency (compensation) loop indicates that bands 3C2 through 3C11 are involved. Loci near *Notch* display pseudodominance. The *Bar* gene, on the other hand, results from a duplication of a sex-linked region (16A) and produces abnormal eye shape.

Females:	N^+/N	$\times$	males: B/Y
1/4	N^+/B	females; Bar	
1/4	N/B	females; Notch, Bar	
1/4	N^+/Y	males; wild	
1/4	N/Y	**lethal**	

The final phenotypic ratio would be 1:1:1 for the phenotypes shown above.

If a gene exists in a duplicated state and if that gene's product is required for survival, then mutation in either (but not both) the original gene or its duplicate will not ordinarily threaten the survival of the organism. Duplication of a gene provides a buffer to mutation.

11. In a work entitled *Evolution by Gene Duplication*, Ohno suggests that gene duplication has been essential in the origin of new genes. If gene products serve essential functions, mutation, and therefore evolution, would not be possible unless these gene products could be compensated for by products of duplicated, normal genes. The duplicated genes, or the original genes themselves, would be able to undergo mutational "experimentation" without necessarily threatening the survival of the organism.

12. It is likely that when certain combinations of genes are of selective advantage in a specific and stable environment, it would be beneficial to the organism to protect that gene combination from disruption through crossing over. By having the genes in an inversion, crossover chromatids are not recovered and, therefore, are not passed on to future generations.

Translocations offer an opportunity for new gene combinations by associations of genes from nonhomologous chromosomes. Under certain conditions, such new combinations may be of selective advantage. Meiotic conditions have evolved so that segregation of translocated chromosomes yields a relatively uniform set of gametes.

13. A Turner syndrome female has the sex chromosome composition of XO. If the father had hemophilia, it is likely that the Turner syndrome individual inherited the X chromosome from the father and no sex chromosome from the mother. If nondisjunction occurred in the mother, either during meiosis I or meiosis II, an egg with no X chromosome could be the result. (See the text for a diagram of primary and secondary nondisjunction.)

14. The primrose, *Primula kewensis*, with its 36 chromosomes, is likely to have formed from the hybridization and subsequent chromosome doubling of a cross between the two other species, each with 18 chromosomes. An example of this type of allotetraploidy (amphidiploidy) is seen in the text.

15. Given the basic chromosome set of nine unique chromosomes (a haploid complement), other forms with the "n multiples" are forms of autopolyploidy. In the illustration below, the n basic set is multiplied to various levels, as is the autotetraploid in the example.

Basic set of nine unique chromosomes (n)

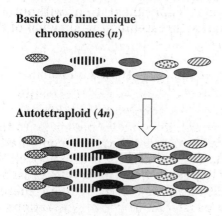

Autotetraploid ($4n$)

Individual organisms with 27 chromosomes ($3n$) are more likely to be sterile because there are trivalents at meiosis I, which cause a relatively high number of unbalanced gametes to be formed.

16. The rare double crossovers within the boundaries of a paracentric or pericentric inversion produce only minor departures from the standard chromosomal arrangement as long as the crossovers involve the same two chromatids. With two-strand double crossovers, the second crossover negates the first. However, three-strand and four-strand double crossovers have consequences that lead to anaphase bridges as well as a high degree of genetically unbalanced gametes.

17. Set up the cross in the usual manner, realizing that recessive genes in the Haplo-IV individual will be expressed.

Let b = bent bristles; b^+ = normal bristles.

(a) _/b × b^+/b^+ ⟶

F_1:   _/b^+ = normal bristles

          b/b^+ = normal bristles

F_2:   _/b^+ × b/b^+ ⟶

          _/b^+ = normal bristles

          _/b = bent bristles

          b^+/b^+ = normal bristles

          b/b^+ = normal bristles

(b) _/b^+ × b/b ⟶

F_1:   _/b = bent bristles

          b/b^+ = normal bristles

F_2:   _/b × b/b^+ ⟶

          _/b^+ = normal bristles

          _/b = bent bristles

          b^+/b = normal bristles

          b/b = bent bristles

18. In the trisomic, segregation will be "2 × 1" as illustrated below:

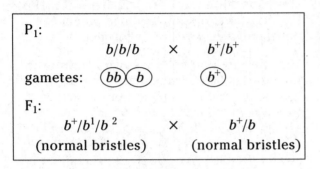

P$_1$:

$$b/b/b \quad \times \quad b^+/b^+$$

gametes: (bb)(b)   (b$^+$)

F$_1$:

$$b^+/b^1/b^2 \quad \times \quad b^+/b$$

(normal bristles)   (normal bristles)

Notice that the trivalent at anaphase I creates several segregation patterns.

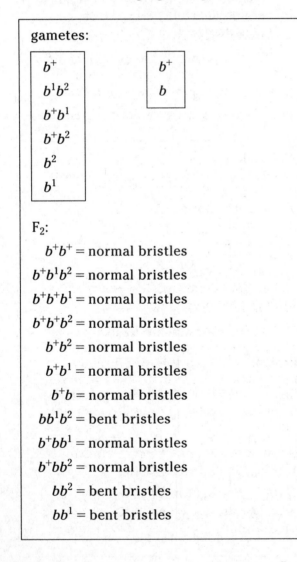

gametes:

b^+	b^+
b^1b^2	b
b^+b^1	
b^+b^2	
b^2	
b^1	

F$_2$:

b^+b^+ = normal bristles

$b^+b^1b^2$ = normal bristles

$b^+b^+b^1$ = normal bristles

$b^+b^+b^2$ = normal bristles

b^+b^2 = normal bristles

b^+b^1 = normal bristles

b^+b = normal bristles

bb^1b^2 = bent bristles

b^+bb^1 = normal bristles

b^+bb^2 = normal bristles

bb^2 = bent bristles

bb^1 = bent bristles

19. The cross would be as follows:

$$WWWW \quad \times \quad wwww$$

(assuming that chromosomes pair as bivalents at meiosis)

F$_1$: *WWww*

F$_2$:

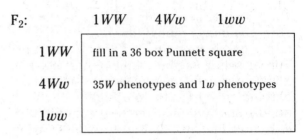

| | 1 *WW* | 4 *Ww* | 1 *ww* |

1 *WW*	fill in a 36 box Punnett square		
4 *Ww*	35 *W* phenotypes and 1 *w* phenotypes		
1 *ww*			

20. Given some of the information in Problem 19, the expression would be as follows:

$(35/36W:1/36w)(35/36A:1/36a)$

$(35/36)^2$	$W–A–$
$35/(36)^2$	$W–aaaa$
$35/(36)^2$	$wwwwA–$
$1/(36)^2$	$wwwwaaaa$

21. (a) In all probability, crossing over in the inversion loop of an inversion (in the heterozygous state) had produced defective, unbalanced chromatids, thus leading to stillbirths and/or malformed children.

(b) It is probable that a significant proportion (perhaps 50 percent) of the children of the man will be similarly influenced by the inversion.

(c) Since the karyotypic abnormality is observable, it may be possible to detect some of the abnormal chromosomes of the fetus by amniocentesis or CVS. However, depending on the type of inversion and the ability to detect minor changes in banding patterns, not all abnormal chromosomes may be detected.

22. (a) Before the advent of polymorphic markers, maternal involvement in trisomy 21 was strongly suspected because of the striking influence of maternal age on incidence.

(b) Karyotype analysis of spontaneously aborted fetuses has shown that a significant percentage of abortuses are trisomic and that every chromosome can be involved. Other forms of aneuploidy (monosomy, nullisomy) are less represented.

(c) A variety of studies, many tracing to early work with specialized (polytene) chromosomes in *Drosophila* and aneuploidy in other organisms, demonstrated that as chromosome structures or numbers are altered, phenotypic consequences are likely.

(d) By examining the polytene chromosomes of *Drosophila*, Bridges and Muller determined that the Bar-eye phenotype was caused by a chromosomal duplication of the 16A region on the X chromosome. In addition, unequal crossing over that resulted in reduced or increased numbers of 16A regions reverted or enhanced the Bar-eye phenotype, respectively.

(e) Ohno suggested that duplications provide a "reservoir" for new genes by buffering mutations, thus allowing a duplicated gene to evolve with little or no consequence. This model is supported by findings that many genes have a substantial amount of their DNA sequence in common. Gene families also support the model of gene origin by duplication.

23. Considering that there are at least three map units between each of the loci, and that only four phenotypes are observed, it is likely that genes *a b c d* are included in an inversion, and crossovers that do occur among these genes are not recovered because of their genetically unbalanced nature. In a sense, the minimum distance between loci *d* and *e* can be estimated as 10 map units

$$(48 + 52/1000)$$

However, this is actually the distance from the *e* locus to the breakpoint that includes the inversion.

The "map" is therefore drawn as:

$$\cdots \cdot / \cdot a \cdots b \cdots c \cdots d \cdots / \cdots e \cdots$$

$$\underbrace{\qquad\qquad\qquad\qquad}_{\textbf{Inversion}} \qquad \textbf{10}$$

24. (a) Reciprocal translocation

(b)

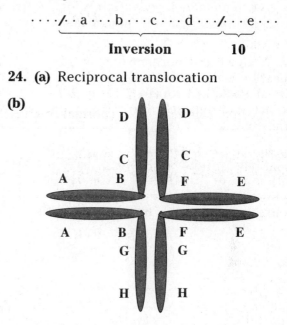

(c) Notice that all chromosomal segments are present and that there is no apparent loss of chromosomal material. However, if the breakpoints for the translocation occurred within genes, then an abnormal phenotype may be the result. In addition, a gene's function is sometimes influenced by its position (its neighbors, in other words). If such "position effects" occur, then a different phenotype may result.

25. The translocation is the likely cause of the miscarriages. Segregation of the chromosomal elements will produce approximately half unbalanced gametes. The chance of a normal child is approximately one in two; however, half of the normal children will be translocation carriers.

26. (a) The father must have contributed the abnormal X-linked gene.

(b) Since the son is XXY and heterozygous for anhidrotic dysplasia, he must have received both the defective gene and the Y chromosome from his father. Thus, nondisjunction must have occurred during meiosis I.

(c) This son's mosaic phenotype is caused by X chromosome inactivation, a form of dosage compensation in mammals.

27. Notice that a chromosome in this question is defined as having two sisters joined at the centromere. This is the expected chromosome structure at the end of meiosis I.

(a) In light of this information, meiosis I must have produced the abnormal oocytes with more or less than 24 chromosomes, indicating multiple conditions of nondisjunction. More likely, the oocytes

consisted of "22 $\frac{1}{2}$" chromosomes—those 22 normal dyads and a single monad.

(b) The result will be a monosomic and a normal zygote, assuming that the half chromosome (monad) migrates, intact, to one pole or the other.

(c) In all likelihood, premature division of the centromere (at meiosis I) probably causes the single (nonduplicated) chromosome at meiosis II.

(d) We generally consider nondisjunction occurring at meiosis I to consist of intact chromosomes, two sister chromatids, failing to separate appropriately. These data indicate that some forms of aneuploidy result from premature division of the centromere at meiosis I as in the figure below.

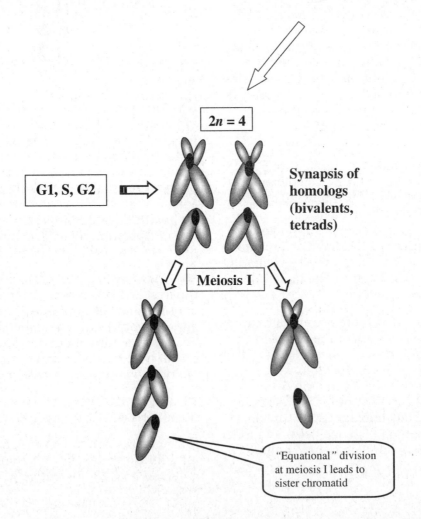

$2n = 4$

G1, S, G2

Synapsis of homologs (bivalents, tetrads)

Meiosis I

"Equational" division at meiosis I leads to sister chromatid

28. First, consider what is meant by a Robertsonian translocation: breaks at the short arms of two nonhomologous acrocentric chromosomes where the small acentric fragments are lost and the larger chromosomal segments fuse at or near the centromeric region, producing a compound, larger submetacentric or metacentric chromosome. Below is a description of breakage/reunion events that illustrate such a translocation in relatively small, similarly sized chromosomes 19 (metacentric) and 20 (metacentric/submetacentric). The case described here is shown occurring before S phase duplication. The same phenomenon is shown in the text as occurring after S phase. Since the likelihood of such a translocation is fairly small in a general population, inbreeding played a significant role in allowing the translocation to "meet itself."

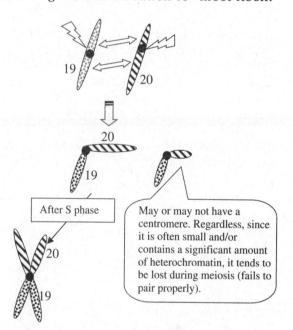

29. Mitotic nondisjunction likely contributed to the mosaic condition. If one of the X chromosomes failed to be included in a daughter mitotic cleavage cell, then a substantial proportion of the child's cells would be XO. Expression of Turner syndrome characteristics would depend on the percentage and location of the XO cell population.

30. This female will produce meiotic products of the following types:

normal: 18 + 21

translocated: 18/21

translocated plus 21: 18/21 + 21

deficient: 18 only

Note: The 18/21 + 18 gamete is not formed because it would require separation of primarily homologous chromosomes at anaphase I.

Fertilization with a normal 18 + 21 sperm cell will produce the following offspring:

normal: 46 chromosomes

translocation carrier: 45 chromosomes 18/21 + 18 + 21

trisomy 21: 46 chromosomes 18/21 + 21 + 21

monosomic: 45 chromosomes 18 + 18 + 21, lethal

31. Since the CF gene is on chromosome 7, which is a fairly large chromosome, we will assume that all chromosomes are present in the diploid state since a cell with only one copy of chromosome 7 is likely to be lethal. Several explanations may account for a CF child with only one parent who is a carrier of CF. First, a deletion or a new mutation could occur in the normal allele, thus exposing the mutant CF gene. Second, another interesting phenomenon, once thought to be rare, may explain the child's genetic state. Uniparental disomy is an occurrence in which both chromosomes of a pair (in this case, chromosome 7) originate from one parent. While there are many explanations for uniparental disomy, also called isodisomy, monosomic conception with subsequent chromosome gain or trisomic conception followed by chromosome loss are likely possibilities.

32. (a,b) Polyploidization provides an opportunity for novel combinations of relatively diverse genomes. However, because meiosis is often complicated by polyploidy, diploidization is often an evolutionary advantage. Since diploidization is apparently a gradual and relatively haphazard process, some genomic regions may become diploid while others may not. Such differential diploidization may lead to advantageous genomic combinations and serve as genetic reservoirs that may be tested by selection.

(c) Generally, diploidization is accomplished by deletions directly as well as chromosomal rearrangements, such as inversions and translocations, that lead to deletions.

33. *Trisomic rescue* is a condition in which an original trisomic zygote occurs, but a particular chromosome is lost. In the following diagram, two chromosomes originally came from the father (solid) and one came from the mother (striped). The one from the mother was eliminated during mitosis, leaving the two chromosomes from the father.

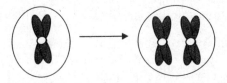

Monosomic rescue occurs when a chromosome is originally present in a zygote, and usually through mitotic nondisjunction, a duplicate of that chromosome occupies the cell.

Gamete complementation occurs when a cell without either homolog of a given chromosome is fertilized by a gamete with two copies of that homolog. The resulting zygote contains two homologous chromosome pairs from one parent.

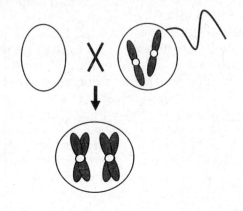

Isochromosome formation occurs when a chromosome contains two copies of one arm and has lost the homolog. Such a homolog loss can originate in mitosis or meiosis. The isochromosome compensates for the nullisomic condition. Effectively, the chromosome is "uniparental" because most of the chromosomal material of a given homolog is from one parent.

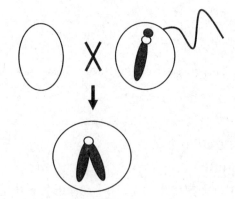

Chapter 9: Extranuclear Inheritance

Concept Areas	Corresponding Problems
Extranuclear Inheritance	1, 17, 18, 22, 23
Maternal Effect	9, 10, 11, 12, 15, 16, 19, 20, 24
Organelle Heredity	2, 3, 4, 5, 6, 13, 14, 15, 16, 25
Infectious Heredity	7, 8, 21

Vocabulary: Organization and Listing of Terms and Concepts

Structures and Substances

Chloroplast DNA

Mitochondrial DNA

Heterokaryon

Conidia

Kappa

Paramecin

Sigma

Kynurenine

Tryptophan

Processes/Methods

Organelle heredity (cytoplasmic inheritance)

    chloroplast DNA (cpDNA)

        coding products

            rRNA, tRNA

            ribosomal proteins, *etc.*

    Mirabilis jalapa

    RuBP (ribulose-1-5-bisphosphate carboxylase)

    Chlamydomonas reinhardi

      mt^+, mt^-

    mitochondrial DNA (mtDNA)

coding products

    rRNA, tRNA, proteins

    Neurospora crassa (*poky*)

      mi-1

      suppressive mutations

    Saccharomyces cerevisiae (*petite*)

      segregational

      neutral

      suppressive

    endosymbiotic hypothesis

humans

    heteroplasmy

    myoclonic epilepsy (MERRF)

Paramecium aurelia

    killers, paramecin

    kappa

    conjugation

    autogamy

    Drosophila

    CO_2 sensitivity

      D. bifasciata, D. willistoni

    sex ratio

maternal effect (influence)

Ephestia kuhniella (A, a)

Limnaea peregra (D, d)

Leber's hereditary optic

neuropathy (LHON)

Kearns-Sayre syndrome

Infectious heredity

dextral, sinistral

first cleavage division

spindle orientation

injection experiments

molecular gradients

bicoid

Concepts

Extranuclear inheritance (F9.1)

Products of cpDNA and mtDNA

Non-Mendelian patterns (F9.1)

maternal, infectious, organelle

Heteroplasmy

F9.1 Illustration of the common pattern seen in many cases of extranuclear inheritance. The condition of the female (egg) parent has a stronger influence on the phenotype of the offspring than the male (sperm/pollen) parent. Reciprocal crosses give different results in offspring.

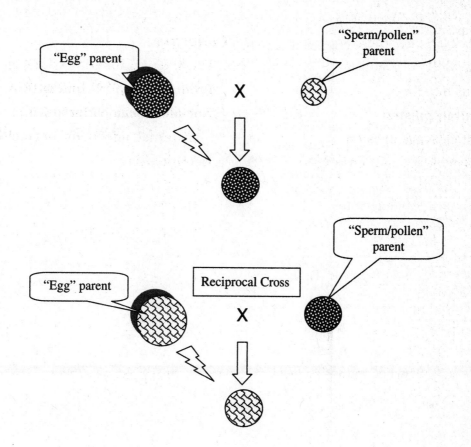

Solutions to Problems and Discussion Questions

1. In cases of extranuclear inheritance, the phenotype is determined by the nuclear (maternal effect) or cytoplasmic (organelle or infectious) condition of the parent that contributes the bulk of the cytoplasm to the offspring. In most cases, the maternal parent provides the basis for the cytoplasmic inheritance.

    The pattern of inheritance is more often from one parent to the offspring. One does not see both parents contributing to the characteristics of the offspring as is the case with Mendelian (chromosomal) forms of inheritance. Standard Mendelian ratios (3:1) are usually not present. In general, the results of reciprocal crosses differ. (See F9.1.)

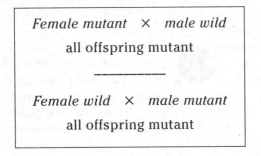

> *Female mutant* × *male wild*
>
>   all offspring mutant
>
> ------------
>
> *Female wild* × *male mutant*
>
>   all offspring mutant

    In sex-linked inheritance, the pattern is often from grandfather through carrier mother to son. Patterns of extranuclear inheritance are often not influenced by the sex of the individual.

2. The mt^+ strain (resistant for the nuclear and chloroplast genes) contributes the "cytoplasmic" component of streptomycin resistance, which would negate any contribution from the mt^- strain. Therefore, all the offspring will have the streptomycin resistance phenotype. In the reciprocal cross, with the mt^+ strain being streptomycin sensitive, all the offspring will be sensitive.

3. Because the ovule source furnishes the cytoplasm to the embryo and thus the chloroplasts, the offspring will have the same phenotype as the plant providing the ovule.

(a) green

(b) white

(c) white, variegated, or green (as illustrated below)

(d) green

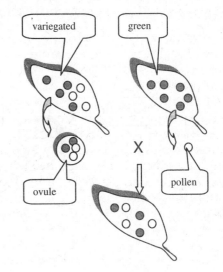

4. See the text for a comparison of results involving various petite strains.

(a) neutral

(b) segregational (nuclear mutations)

(c) suppressive

5. As with any description of dominance, one looks to the phenotype of the diploid heterozygote. In this problem, the heterozygote is of normal phenotype; therefore, the *petite* gene is recessive.

6. Examine the text and notice that the inheritance patterns for the two, *segregational* and *neutral*, are quite different. The segregational mode is dependent on nuclear genes, while that of the neutral type is dependent on cytoplasmic influences, namely, mitochondria. If the two are crossed as stated in the problem, then one would expect, in the diploid zygote, the *segregational* allele to be "covered" by normal alleles from the neutral strain. On the other hand, as the nuclear genes are again "exposed" in the haploid state of the ascospores, one would expect a 1:1 ratio of normals to petites. The petite phenoytpe is caused by the nuclear, *segregational* gene.

7. In providing the answers to this question, remember that a *Paramecium* may be sensitive and carry the *K* gene. These are organisms that did not obtain kappa particles. There is a question as to whether cytoplasmic exchange has occurred. However, seeing the results in cross (b), one can assume that cytoplasmic exchange has occurred. In addition, one can assume that only the exconjugants are being described in the offspring. Under those conditions, the parental genotypes could be the following:

(a) *Kk* × *kk*

(b) any case where there is no *kk* such as:

$$KK \quad \times \quad KK$$

or

$$KK \quad \times \quad kk$$

(c) $\quad KK \quad \times \quad Kk$

8. (a) There are many similarities among mitochondrial, chloroplast, and prokaryotic molecular systems. It is likely that mitochondria and chloroplasts evolved from bacteria in a symbiotic relationship; therefore, it is not surprising that certain antibiotics that influence bacteria will also influence all mitochondria and chloroplasts.

(b) The mt^+ strain is the donor of the *cp*DNA since the inheritance of resistance or sensitivity is dependent on the status of the mt^+ gene.

9. The case with *Limnaea* involves a maternal effect in which the *genotype* of the mother influences the *phenotype* of the *immediate* offspring in a non-Mendelian manner. Notice that in the above statement, it is the maternal genotype that determines the phenoytpe of the offspring, regardless of its own genotype.

Since both of the parents are *Dd*, the parent contributing the eggs must be *Dd*. Therefore, all of the offspring must have the phenotype of the mother's genotype, which is dextral.

10. In a maternal effect, the *genotype* of the mother influences the *phenotype* of her immediate offspring in a non-Mendelian manner. The fact that all of the offspring (F_1) showed a dextral coiling pattern indicates that one of the parents (maternal parent) contains the *D* allele. Taking these offspring and seeing that their progeny (call these F_2) occur in a 1:1 ratio indicate that half of the offspring (F_1) are *dd*. In order to have these results, one of the original parents must have been *Dd*, while the other must have been *dd*.

Parents:	*Dd*	×	*dd*
Offspring (F_1):	1/2 *Dd*,		1/2 *dd*

(all dextral because of the maternal genotype)

Progeny (F_2):

All those from *Dd* parents will be dextral, while all those from *dd* parents will be sinistral.

11. It appears as if some factor normally provided by the *gs*[+] allele is necessary for normal development and/or functioning of the female offspring's gonads. Without this product, the daughters are sterile, thus the term *grandchildless.* Because the female provides so much vital material and information to the egg, including the cytoplasm necessary for germ-line determination, it is not surprising that such maternal effect genes exist.

12. Since there is no evidence for segregation patterns typical of chromosomal genes and Mendelian traits, some form of extranuclear inheritance seems possible. If the *lethargic* gene is dominant, then a maternal effect may be involved. In that case, some of the F_2 progeny would be hyperactive because maternal effects are only temporary, affecting only the immediate progeny. If the lethargic condition is caused by some infective agent, then perhaps injection experiments could be used. If caused by a mitochondrial defect, then the condition would persist in all offspring of lethargic mothers, through more than one generation.

13. In many cases, molecular components of mitochondria are recruited from the cytoplasm, having been synthesized from nuclear genes.

14. Since an initial mutation does not involve all copies of mtDNA within a mitochondrion, the original state is heteroplasmic and the mutated mtDNA is rare. If the new mutation confers no selective advantage to the host cell, the frequency of the mutation is likely to diminish. However, if the mutation confers a selective advantage to the cell, it is likely to gain in frequency. Depending on a number of factors, including chance as well as the extent of the selective advantage, an mtDNA mutation may become prominent and eventually establish homoplasmy.

15. The endosymbiotic theory states that mitochondria and chloroplasts arose independently around 2 billion years ago from free-living protobacteria. These bacteria brought the capacity for aerobic respiration and photosynthesis to primitive eukaryotic cells. Because such organelles have prokaryotic origins, a deeper understanding of extranuclear DNA is possible. As we understand more of the molecular biology of prokaryotes, we automatically gain insight into the behavior of extranuclear DNA.

16. Mitochondrial defects often involve processes of oxidative phosphorylation and/or other essential mitochondrial functions that are dependent not only on the mitochondrial genome, but also on the nuclear genome. When a nuclear genome is transferred, it may contain mutant genes that negatively influence mitochondrial function that were compensated for in the original donor cells, but not in the recipient. In addition, enucleated eggs invariably contain both normal and defective mitochondria. When a nuclear genome is transferred to an enucleated egg, mitochondrial defects may arise from an uncompensated defective nuclear genome, the heteroplasmic condition of the egg, or a combination of the two. A disease occurs when the mitochondrial mutational load exceeds a tissue-specific threshold that is generally low in highly metabolic tissues such as brain, heart, and muscle.

17. The results are consistent with an infectious agent that passes primarily through the maternal parent. Most (perhaps 84 percent) of the females of group A have the infective agent and produce offspring that are sensitive at the 10 percent threshold. Either some of the female parents in group A did not contain the sensitivity-producing agent, or they evolved genes resistant to that agent. Females in group B either carry fewer sensitivity-producing agents, or they have evolved a higher number or more effective genes that confer resistance to the agent. Without a specification of the sex of the offspring, it is not possible to rule out the presence of an X-linked dominant resistant mutation in strain B. Regardless, these data are similar to expectations of sigma infectivity in *Drosophila*.

18. (a) In general, organelle heredity is detected when the maternal parent has more influence over the phenotype of the offspring. In addition, assuming other factors, such as X-linked inheritance, can be eliminated, different results from reciprocal crosses support inheritance by extranuclear elements.

(b) While *segregational petites* exhibited Mendelian inheritance, both *neutral* and *suppressive petite* followed non-Mendelian patterns that were consistent with the involvement of an extranuclear agent.

(c) Electron micrographs show that DNA of mitochondria and chloroplasts looks like that seen in bacteria. In addition, the molecular components, notably ribosomal RNAs, are more like those in prokaryotes than eukaryotes.

(d) When eggs from a *Dd* (but sinistral because of its parent) snail are self-fertilized, all the offspring, even those that are *dd*, coil dextrally. Thus, the phenotype of the offspring is determined not by the mother's phenotype or its own phenotype, but by her mother's genotype. The genotype of the sperm is not influential in determining the direction of shell coiling in offspring.

19. Developmental phenomena that occur early are more likely to be under maternal influence than those occurring late. Anterior/posterior and dorsal/ventral orientations are among the earliest to be established, and in organisms where their study is experimentally and/or genetically approachable, they often show considerable maternal influence. Maternal effect genes yield products that are not carried over for more than one generation as is the case with organelle and infectious heredity. Crosses that illustrate the transient nature of a maternal effect could include the following. However, depending on particular biochemical/developmental parameters, not all crosses may give these types of patterns.

Female *Aa* × male *aa* ⟶ all offspring of the "A" phenotype. Take a female "A" phenotype from the above cross and conduct the following mating: *aa* × male *Aa*.

All offspring may be of the "a" phenotype because all of the offspring will reflect the *genotype* of the mother, not her *phenotype*. This cross illustrates that maternal effects last only one generation. In actual practice, the results of this cross may give a typical 1:1 ratio, depending on the biochemical/developmental characteristics of the system. However, the fact that the maternal effect only persists for one generation is clearly illustrated regardless of which set of results occurs.

20. (a) The presence of *bcd⁻/bcd⁻* males can be explained by the maternal effect: mothers were *bcd⁺/bcd⁻*.

(b) The cross

female *bcd⁺/bcd⁻* × male *bcd⁻/bcd⁻*

will produce an F_1 with normal embryogenesis because of the maternal effect. In the F_2, any cross having *bcd⁺/bcd⁻* mothers will have phenotypically normal embryos. Offspring from any cross involving homozygous *bcd⁻/bcd⁻* mothers will have problems with embryogenesis.

21. Because of sampling error due to relatively small numbers of offspring, this pedigree could represent a typical Mendelian dominant or recessive gene;

however, because the thrust of this chapter is on extranuclear inheritance, the condition is probably a case of extranuclear inheritance. The phenotype of the offspring will therefore follow the characteristics of the mother.

22. (a) A locus, *Segregation Distortion* (*SD*), is present on the wild-type chromosome. Some aspect of *SD* causes a shift in the segregation ratio by allowing sperm to carry the *SD* chromosome at the expense of the homolog.

(b) One could use this *SD* chromosome in a variety of crosses and determine that the abnormal segregation is based on a particular chromosomal element. One could even map the *SD* locus on the second chromosome (as has been done).

(c) Segregation Distortion describes a condition in which typical Mendelian segregation is distorted from the 50:50 ratio.

23. In all likelihood, a bacterium is causing the sex ratio distortion as suggested by the phrase "affected strains can be cured by antibiotics" and the identification of a PCR-amplifiable 16S rDNA. Bacteria would be expected to contain such DNA and be sensitive to antibiotics. The fact that mitochondria also contain a relatively small rDNA does, to some extent, complicate the conclusion. However, given that strains can be cured by antibiotics, one would again revert to a bacterial infection being involved.

24. Deficiencies that remove histone genes contribute to increased survival of progeny of *abo/abo* mothers. Since deficiencies in histone genes reduce the severity of the maternal effect it is likely that an overabundance of histones is involved. The observation that the addition of heterochromatin also reduces the severity of the maternal effect may be due to a sequestering of the histone overload by the heterochromatin. One might therefore speculate that the *abo* gene is a regulator of histone production. The normal allele specifies a negative regulator of histone

genes, while the mutant *abo* gene fails to exert such negative control.

25. (a) Note: to provide a meaningful pedigree, several individuals are added to the pedigree that are not listed in the table. Refer to Chapter 3 for information regarding symbols used.

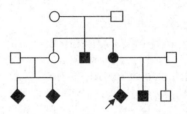

(b,c) If one looks solely at the above pedigree, one could argue that the pattern follows a typical Mendelian recessive. If that were the case, all individuals not showing the phenotype would be heterozygous. However, given that a mitochondrial DNA mutation was identified among affected family members, the pedigree is also consistent with organelle inheritance. Heteroplasmy explains variation in expression and transmission. While this may seem like an erroneous conclusion at first, consider the range of mutant mitochondria presented in the table. The maternal grandmother has 56 percent mutant mtDNA and could pass a mixed population of mitochondria to her offspring, two of which are symptomatic with percentages of mutant mtDNA above 90 percent. The two maternal cousins (of unknown sex) inherited, by chance, pools of mitochondria with relatively high frequencies (90 percent and 91 percent) of mutant mtDNA and are therefore symptomatic. It appears as if the threshold for phenotypic expression is 85 percent and above.

(d) Transmission of a trait by organelle heredity occurs primarily through the mother whereas single-gene mutations (albinism) can be transmitted through either parent. In addition, because of heteroplasmy, phenotypic expression may vary, and transmission patterns may complicate interpretations from pedigrees.

Chapter 10: DNA Structure and Analysis

Concept Areas	Corresponding Problems
Central Dogma	1, 2, 8, 9, 19, 35
Transformation	3, 4
Differential Labeling of Macromolecules	5, 6, 7
Genetic Variation	24, 33
Model Building	15, 16, 28, 31, 36
Nucleic Acid Structure	10, 11, 12, 13, 14, 17, 18, 20, 23, 27, 28, 29, 30, 32, 36, 37
Genomic Complexity	24, 41
Analytical Methods	20, 21, 22, 24, 25, 26, 27, 30, 34, 38, 39, 40, 41

Vocabulary: Organization and Listing of Terms and Concepts

Historical

1900–1944

    genetic material

        Miescher (nuclein)

        proteins

        nucleic acids

            tetranucleotide hypothesis

            base ratios, Erwin Chargaff

            transforming principle

            Avery et al. (1944)

            deoxycholate

        T2 bacteriophage (phage)

        Hershey and Chase (1952)

           ^{32}P, ^{35}S

Watson and Crick (1953)

Franklin

Wilkins

Structures and Substances

Messenger RNA (mRNA)

Transfer RNA (tRNA)

Ribosomal RNA (rRNA)

Ribonuclease

Deoxyribonuclease

Lysozyme

    Diplococcus serotype

Protoplasts (spheroplasts)

    ϕX174

Ultraviolet light action spectrum

Insulin

Interferon

Human β-globin gene

RNA core

Coat protein

Qβ RNA replicase

Retrovirus

Reverse transcriptase

Nucleic acids

    nucleotides

        nitrogenous base

purines

    adenine

    guanine

    pyrimidines

    cytosine

    thymine

    uracil

  pentose sugar

    ribose

    deoxyribose

  phosphoric acid

nucleoside

  monophosphate

  diphosphate

  triphosphate

    adenosine triphosphate

    guanosine triphosphate

phosphodiester bond (5'-3')

inorganic phosphate

  hydrolysis

oligonucleotide

polynucleotide

base composition

  $A = T, G = C$

  $(A + G) = (C + T)$

  $(A + T)/(C + G) = variable$

X-ray diffraction

antiparallel

0.34 nm (stacked bases) (3.4 Å)

3.4 nm (complete turn)

10 bases per turn

  10.4 bases per turn

  2.0nm diameter (20 Å)

hydrogen bonds

(A to T, G to C)

complementarity

major and minor grooves

hydrophobic bases

hydrophilic backbone

A-DNA

B-DNA

C-DNA

D-DNA

E-DNA

Z-DNA

P-DNA

RNA

  ribosomal RNA (rRNA)

    ribosomes

  messenger RNA (mRNA)

    primary transcripts

  transfer RNA (tRNA)

  small nuclear RNA

  telomerase RNA

  antisense RNA

  biotin

  avidin (strepavidin)

    fluorescent label

Processes/Methods

Replication (F10.1)

  mitosis

  meiosis

Storage of information (F10.1)

Expression (F10.1)

  transcription

  translation

    central dogma

Variation (mutation) (F10.1)

Transformation

  Diplococcus pneumoniae

    Streptococcus pneumoniae

    virulent

    avirulent

    serotypes (II, III)

    smooth, rough

    heat-killed IIIS

    rough, extremely rough (ER)

      ribonuclease

      proteolytic enzymes

      deoxyribonuclease

  transfection

  recombinant DNA research

    insulin

    interferon

    human β-globin gene

  transgenic mice

    growth hormone

  RNA as genetic material

    TMV (tobacco mosaic virus)

    Holmes ribgrass (HR)

      RNA core, coat protein

    Qβ phage

      Qβ RNA replicase

    retroviruses

    reverse transcription

Bonding

  sugar to purine

  sugar to pyrimidine

  nucleotide to nucleotide

Single crystal X-ray analysis

  Svedberg coefficient (S)

absorption of ultraviolet light (UV)

  254–260 nm

    sedimentation behavior

    gradient centrifugation

  sedimentation velocity

  sedimentation equilibrium

Denaturation (melting)

  heat, chemical treatment

Spectrophotometry

Melting profile

Melting temperature (T_m)

Hyperchromic effect

Renaturation (hybridization)

  DNA/DNA

  DNA/RNA

  in situ hybridization

  autoradiography

    FISH

    kinetics

    C_0t

    $C_0t_{1/2}$

    sequence complexity

  electrophoresis

    polyacrylamide

    agarose

Concepts

Central dogma

Characteristics of genetic material

Tetranucleotide hypothesis

Transformation

Differential labeling of macromolecules

Indirect evidence

  DNA content (n, $2n$)

mutagenesis	DNA double helix
action spectrum	storage of genetic information
absorption spectrum	information flow
260 nm, 280 nm	mutation
Direct evidence	Genomic complexity
recombinant DNA technology	reassociation kinetics
Genetic variation	Separation strategies
Model building	Labeling strategies

F10.1 Illustration of relationships between DNA, its functions, and related products.

Mutation

Replication

Information Storage

DNA   **DNA**

Reverse transcription (some viruses)   Transcription

RNA → **Protein**

Translation

Solutions to Problems and Discussion Questions

1. *Replication* is the process that leads to the production of identical copies of existing genetic information. Since daughter cells contain essentially exact copies (with some exceptions) of genetic information of the parent cell, and through the production and union of gametes, offspring contain copies (with variation) of parental genetic information, the genetic material must make copies of (replicate) itself. Replication is accomplished during the S phase of interphase.

The genetic material is capable of *expression* through the production of a phenotype. Through transcription and translation, proteins are produced that contribute to the phenotype of the organism. The genetic material must be stable enough to maintain information in "storage" from one cell to the next and from one organism to the next. Because the genetic material is not "used up" in the processes of transcription and translation, genetic information can be stored and used constantly. Above, it was stated that the genetic material must be stable enough to store genetic information; however, variation through *mutation* provides the raw material for evolution. The genetic material is capable of a variety of changes, at both the chromosomal and nucleotide levels. (See F10.1.)

2. Prior to 1940, most of the interest in genetics centered on the transmission of similarity and variation from parents to offspring (transmission genetics). While some experiments examined the possible nature of the hereditary material, abundant knowledge of the structural and enzymatic properties of proteins generated a bias that worked to favor proteins as the hereditary substance. In addition, proteins were composed of as many as 20 different subunits (amino acids), thereby providing ample structural and functional variation for the multiple tasks that must be accomplished by the genetic material.

The tetranucleotide hypothesis (structure) provided insufficient variability to account for the diverse roles of the genetic material.

3. Griffith performed experiments with different strains of *Diplococcus pneumoniae* in which a heat-killed pathogen, when injected into a mouse with a live nonpathogenic strain, eventually led to the mouse's death. A summary of this experiment is provided in the text. Examination of the dead mouse revealed living pathogenic bacteria. Griffith suggested that the heat-killed virulent (pathogenic) bacteria transformed the avirulent (nonpathogenic) strain into a virulent strain.

Avery and coworkers systematically searched for the transforming principle originating from the heat-killed pathogenic strain and determined it to be DNA. Taylor showed that transformed bacteria are capable of serving as donors of transforming DNA, indicating that the process of transformation involves a stable alteration in the genetic material (DNA).

4. Transformation is dependent on a macromolecule (DNA) that can be extracted and purified from bacteria. During such purification, however, other macromolecular species may contaminate the DNA. Specific degradative enzymes, proteases, RNase, and DNase were used to selectively eliminate components of the extract, and, if transformation is concomitantly eliminated, then the eliminated fraction is the transforming principle. DNase eliminates DNA and transformation; therefore, it must be the transforming principle.

5. Nucleic acids contain large amounts of phosphorus and no sulfur, whereas proteins contain sulfur and no phosphorus. Therefore, the radioisotopes ^{32}P and ^{35}S will selectively label nucleic acids and proteins, respectively.

The Hershey and Chase experiment was based on the premise that the substance injected into the bacterium is the substance responsible for producing the progeny phage and, therefore, must be the hereditary material. The experiment demonstrated that most of the ^{32}P-labeled material (DNA) was injected, while the phage ghosts (protein coats) remained outside the bacterium. Therefore, the nucleic acid must be the genetic material.

6. Actually, phosphorus is found in approximately equal amounts in DNA and RNA. Therefore, labeling with ^{32}P would "tag" both RNA and DNA. However, the T2 phage, in its mature state, contains very little, if any, RNA; therefore, DNA would be interpreted as being the genetic material in T2 phage.

7. In theory, the general design would be appropriate in that some substance, if labeled, would show up in the progeny of transformed bacteria. However, since the amount of transforming DNA is extremely small compared with the genomic DNA of the recipient bacterium and its progeny, it would be technically difficult to assay for the labeled nucleic acid. In addition, it would be necessary to know that the small stretch of DNA that caused the genetic transformation was actually labeled. This in itself would be relatively easy using present-day recombinant DNA techniques; however, in earlier times, such specific labeling would have been difficult.

8. The early evidence would be considered indirect in that at no time was there an experiment, like transformation in bacteria, in which genetic information in one organism was transferred to another using DNA. Rather, by comparing DNA content in various cell types (sperm and somatic cells) and observing that the *action* and *absorption* spectra of ultraviolet light were correlated,

DNA was considered to be the genetic material. This suggestion was supported by the fact that DNA was shown to be the genetic material in bacteria and some phages.

Direct evidence for DNA being the genetic material comes from a variety of observations, including gene transfer, which has been facilitated by recombinant DNA techniques.

9. Some viruses contain a genetic material composed of RNA. The tobacco mosaic virus is composed of an RNA core and a protein coat. "Crosses" can be made in which the protein coat and RNA of TMV are interchanged with another strain (Holmes ribgrass). The source of the RNA determines the type of lesion; thus, RNA is the genetic material in these viruses. Retroviruses contain RNA as the genetic material and use an enzyme known as *reverse transcriptase* to produce DNA that can be integrated into the host chromosome. See F10.1.

10. The structure of deoxyadenylic acid is given below and in the text. Linkages among the three components require the removal of water (H_2O).

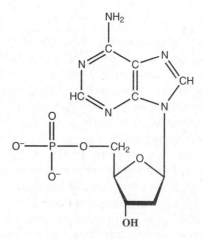

11. The numbering of the carbons on the sugar is especially important (see diagram below). Examine the text for the numbers on the carbons and nitrogens of the bases:

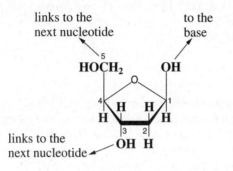

12. Examine the structures of the bases in the text. The other bases would be named as follows:

Guanine: 2-amino-6-oxypurine

Cytosine: 2-oxy-4-aminopyrimidine

Thymine: 2,4-dioxy-5-methylpyrimidine

Uracil: 2,4-dioxypyrimidine

13. Examine the text for the format for this drawing. Note that the complementary strand must be drawn in the antiparallel orientation.

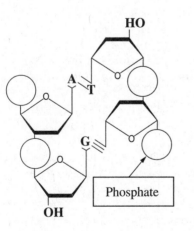

14. The following are characteristics of the Watson-Crick double-helix model for DNA:

The base composition is such that A = T, G = C and (A + G) = (C + T). Bases are stacked, 0.34 nm (3.4 Angstoms) apart, and in a plectonic, antiparallel manner. There is one complete turn for each 3.4 nm that constitutes 10 bases per turn. Hydrogen bonds hold the two polynucleotide chains together, each being formed by phosphodiester linkages between the five-carbon sugars and the phosphates. There are two hydrogen bonds forming the A to T pair and three forming the G to C pair. The double helix exists as a twisted structure, approximately 20 Angstroms in diameter, with a topography of major and minor grooves. The hydrophobic bases are located in the center of the molecule, while the hydrophilic phosphodiester backbone is on the outside.

15. In addition to creative "genius" and perseverance, model building skills, and the conviction that the structure would turn out to be "simple" and have a natural beauty in its simplicity, Watson and Crick employed the X-ray diffraction information of Franklin and Wilkins and the base ratio information of Chargaff.

16. Because in double-stranded DNA, A = T and G = C (within limits of experimental error), the data presented would have indicated a lack of pairing of these bases in favor of a single-stranded structure or some other nonhydrogen-bonded structure.

Alternatively, from the data it would appear that A = C and T = G, which would negate the chance for typical hydrogen bonding since opposite charge relationships do not exist. Therefore, it is quite unlikely that a tight helical structure would form at all. Watson and Crick might have concluded that hydrogen bonding is not a significant factor in maintaining a double-stranded structure.

17. A covalent bond is a relatively strong bond that involves the sharing of electrons between two or more atoms. Hydrogen bonds, much weaker than covalent bonds, are formed as a result of:

> . . . electrostatic attraction between a covalently bonded hydrogen atom and an atom with an unshared electron pair. The hydrogen atom assumes a partial positive charge, while the unshared electron pair—characteristic of covalently bonded oxygen and nitrogen atoms—assumes a partial negative charge. These opposite charges are responsible for the weak chemical attraction . . . (From page 260 in the textbook)

Complementarity, responsible for the chemical attraction between adenine and thymine (uracil) and guanine and cytosine, is responsible for DNA and RNA assuming their double-stranded character. Complementarity is based on hydrogen bonding.

18. Three main differences between RNA and DNA are the following:

(1) Uracil in RNA replaces thymine in DNA.

(2) Ribose in RNA replaces deoxyribose in DNA.

(3) RNA often occurs as both single- and partially double-stranded forms, whereas DNA most often occurs in a double-stranded form.

19. While there are many types of RNA, the three main types described in this section are presented below:

ribosomal RNA: rRNA combines with proteins to form ribosomes that function to align mRNA and charged tRNA molecules during translation.

transfer RNA: tRNAs are involved in protein synthesis in that they represent a "link" between the codes in DNA (as reflected in mRNA) and the ordering of amino acids in proteins. Transfer RNAs are specific in that each species is attached to only one type of amino acid.

messenger RNA: The genetic code in DNA is transferred to the site of protein synthesis by a relatively short-lived molecule called messenger RNA. In eukaryotes, mRNA carries genetic information from the nucleus to the cytoplasm. It is the sequence of bases in mRNA that specifies the order of amino acids in proteins.

20. The nitrogenous bases of nucleic acids (nucleosides, nucleotides, and single- and double-stranded polynucleotides), absorb UV light maximally at wavelengths 254 to 260 nm. Using this phenomenon, one can often determine the presence and concentration of nucleic acids in a mixture. Since proteins absorb UV light maximally at 280 nm, this is a relatively simple way of dealing with mixtures of biologically important molecules.

UV absorption is greater in single-stranded molecules (hyperchromic shift) as compared with double-stranded structures; therefore, by applying denaturing conditions, one can easily determine whether a nucleic acid is in the single- or double-stranded form. In addition, A-T rich DNA denatures more readily than G-C rich DNA; therefore, one can estimate base content by denaturation kinetics.

21. *Sedimentation velocity* centrifugation refers to an ultracentrifugation technique that monitors the velocity with which macromolecules move through a centrifugal field. Molecules move through the gradient on the basis of their mass and shape. If centrifuged long enough, such molecules will end up at the bottom of the tube.

Sedimentation equilibrium centrifugation is a technique that provides separation in a gradient on the basis of buoyant density. Macromolecules migrate through the gradient until they reach and subsequently remain at the point of equal density.

22. Guanine and cytosine are held together by three hydrogen bonds, whereas adenine and thymine are held together by two. Because G-C base pairs are more compact, they are denser than A-T pairs. The percentage of G-C pairs in DNA is thus proportional to the buoyant density of the molecule as illustrated in the text.

23. Various treatments, heat, and certain chemical environments cause separation of the hydrogen bonds, which hold together the complementary strands of DNA. Under these conditions, double-stranded DNA is changed to single-stranded DNA.

24. Carefully examine the text. First, understand the concept of molecular hybridization; then see that as the degree of strand uniqueness increases, the time required for reassociation increases. Repetitive sequences renature relatively quickly because the likelihood of complementary strands interacting increases.

For curve A in the problem, there is evidence for a rapidly renaturing species (repetitive) and a slowly renaturing species (unique). The fraction that reassociates faster than the *E. coli* DNA is highly repetitive and the last fraction (with the highest $C_0t_{1/2}$ value) contains primarily unique sequences. Fraction B contains mostly unique, relatively complex DNA.

25. *A hyperchromic effect* is the increased absorption of UV light as double-stranded.

DNA (or RNA for that matter) is converted to single-stranded DNA. As illustrated in the text, the change in absorption is quite significant, with a structure of higher G-C content *melting* at a higher temperature than an A-T rich nucleic acid. If one monitors the UV absorption with a spectrophotometer during the melting process, the hyperchromic shift can be observed. The T_m is the point on the profile (temperature) at which half (50 percent) of the sample is denatured.

26. Because G-C base pairs are formed with three hydrogen bonds, while A-T base pairs by two such bonds, it takes more energy (higher temperature) to separate G-C pairs.

27. The reassociation of separate complementary strands of a nucleic acid, either DNA or RNA, is based on hydrogen bonds forming between A-T (or U) and G-C.

28. In one sentence of their paper in *Nature*, Watson and Crick state:

> It has not escaped our notice that the specific pairing we have postulated immediately suggests a possible copying mechanism for the genetic material.

The model itself indicates that unwinding of the helix and separation of the double-stranded structure into two single strands immediately exposes the specific hydrogen bonds through which new bases are brought into place.

29. **(1)** As shown, the extra phosphate is not normally expected.

(2) In the adenine ring, a nitrogen is at position 8 rather than position 9.

(3) The bond from the C-1′ to the sugar should form with the N at position 9 (N-9) of the adenine.

(4) The dinucleotide is a "deoxy" form; therefore, each C-2′ should not have a hydroxyl group. Notice the hydroxyl group at C-2′ on the sugar of the adenylic acid.

(5) At the C-5 position on the thymine residue, there should be a methyl group.

(6) There are too many bonds between the N3-C2 of thymine.

(7) There are too few bonds (should be a double bond) between the C5 and C6 of thymine.

30. As shown in the text, a direct proportionality between $C_0t_{1/2}$ and the number of base pairs exists under certain conditions. The ratios for MS-2 would be as follows:

$0.5/10^5 = 0.001/X$

or $X/0.001 = 10^5/0.5$

$X = (0.001)(10^5)/0.5$

$X = 200$ base pairs

The ratios for *E. coli* would be as follows:

$0.5/10^5 = 10.0/X$ or

$X/10.0 = 10^5/0.5$

$X = (10.0)(10^5)/0.5$

$X = 2 \times 10^6$ base pairs

31. left side (a) = right, right side (b) = left

32. Since cytosine pairs with guanine and uracil pairs with adenine, the result would be a base substitution of G:C to A:T after two rounds of replication.

33. Under this condition, the hydrolyzed 5-methyl cytosine becomes thymine.

34. Fluorescence *in situ* hybridization employs fluorescently labeled DNA that hybridizes to metaphase chromosomes and interphase nuclei. A FISH survey is considered interpretable if hybridization is consistent in 70 percent or more cells examined. Results are available in one to two days after the sample is tested. Because of the relatively high likelihood of aneuploidy for chromosomes 13, 18, 21, X, and Y, they are routine candidates for analysis.

35. (a) Major lines of evidence that DNA is the genetic material originally came from experiments using bacteria and bacteriophages. Transformation studies showed that DNA is the genetic material in bacteria, and differential labeling (proteins and nucleic acids) of bacteriophage T2 showed that DNA is the genetic material in some viruses.

(b) Both direct and indirect studies have shown that DNA is the genetic material in eukaryotes. Other than in mitochondria and chloroplasts, DNA is localized in the nucleus where its quantity varies with ploidy (*n*, 2*n*) as one would predict for the genetic material. In addition, the action spectrum of UV light overlaps the absorption spectrum of DNA. Direct evidence comes from recombinant DNA studies where transgenic organisms can be generated with transferred DNA.

(c,d) Given base composition studies showing proportional amounts of A and T, and G and C, and X-ray diffraction studies, Watson and Crick showed that hydrogen bonding between the bases provided attraction and stability for a DNA double helix. DNA melting supports this arrangement.

(e) Rapidly renaturing sequences were discovered by Britten and Kohne. They suggested and later showed that such sequences were repetitive.

36. (i) The X-ray diffraction studies would indicate a helical structure, for it is on the basis of such data that a helical pattern is suggested. The fact that it is irregular may indicate different diameters (base pairings), additional strands in the helix, kinking, or bending.

(ii) The hyperchromic shift would indicate considerable hydrogen bonding, possibly caused by base pairing.

(iii) Such data may suggest irregular base pairing in which purines bind purines (all the bases presented are purines), thus giving the atypical dimensions.

(iv) Because of the presence of ribose, the molecule may show more flexibility, kinking, and/or folding. While several situations are possible for this model, the phosphates are still likely to be far apart (on the outside) because of their strong like charges. Hydrogen bonding probably exists on the inside of the molecule, and there is probably considerable flexibility, kinking, and/or bending.

37. Without knowing the exact bonding characteristics of hypoxanthine or xanthine, it may be difficult to predict the likelihood of each pairing type. Both are likely of the same class (purine or pyrimidine) because the names of the molecules indicate a similarity. In addition, the diameter of the structure is constant, which, under the model to follow, would be expected. In fact, hypoxanthine and xanthine are both purines.

Because there are equal amounts of A, T and H, one could suggest that they are hydrogen bonded to each other; the same may be said for C, G, and X. Given the molar equivalence of erythrose and phosphate, an alternating sugar-phosphate-sugar backbone, as in "earth-type" DNA, would be acceptable. A model of a triple helix would also be acceptable, since the diameter is constant. Given the chemical similarities to "earth-type" DNA, the unique creature's DNA probably follows the same structural plan.

38. (1) Heat application will yield a hyperchromic shift if the DNA is double-stranded. One could also get a rough estimation of the GC content from the kinetics of denaturation and the degree of sequence complexity from comparative renaturation studies.

(2) Determination of base content by hydrolysis and chromatography could be used for comparative purposes and could also provide evidence as to the strandedness of the DNA.

(3) Antibodies for Z-DNA could be used to determine the degree of left-handed structures, if present.

(4) Sequencing the DNA from both viruses would indicate sequence homology. In addition, through various electronic searches readily available on the Internet (Web site: blast@ncbi.nlm.nih.gov, for example) one could determine whether similar sequences exist in other viruses or in other organisms.

39. The way the question is stated suggests that DNA that is separated electrophoretically is of the same shape (long rod). DNA can exist in a variety of shapes as seen in supercoiled plasmids, relaxed (nicked) plasmids, and linear molecules. Size comparisons with DNA must be such that linear molecules are compared with linear molecules and supercoiled with supercoiled, and so on. In comparing DNA migration with RNA, even though RNA molecules have the same charge to mass ratios, they also exist in a variety of shapes. Complementary intrastrand base pairing can make more compact structures compared with the more relaxed, open conformation. For electrophoretic size comparisons, RNA molecules must be denatured to eliminate secondary structural variables.

40. The mobility of DNA through a gel is dependent on a number of factors, including the concentration of the gel, strength of the current, ionic strength of the buffer, and conformation of the DNA as stated in the problem. In general, superhelical/supercoiled DNA (form I) migrates the fastest, followed by linear DNA (form III). The slowest to migrate is usually the loose circle (form II).

41. In general, as the %GC pairs increase, the T_m increases. This is to be expected because three hydrogen bonds hold GC pairs together, whereas two bonds hold AT pairs. Therefore, it takes more energy to break GC pairs than AT pairs.

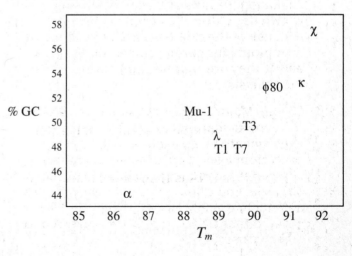

Chapter 11: DNA Replication and Recombination

Concept Areas	Corresponding Problems
Replication	1, 2, 3, 4, 5, 6, 7, 12, 13, 14, 18, 21, 22, 23, 24, 28, 29, 30, 31, 32, 33, 34, 35, 37
Nearest Neighbor Analysis	8, 9, 10, 11, 12, 23, 30, 36, 40
Enzymology	6, 15, 16, 17, 19, 20, 27, 28, 32, 36, 38
Conditional Mutations	25, 38
Gene Conversion	26

Vocabulary: Organization and Listing of Terms and Concepts

Structures and Substances

DNA polymerase I

Spleen phosphodiesterase (F11.1)

5′-nucleotides (F11.2)

3′-nucleotides (F11.2)

Phage φX174

  + strand, − strand

  replicative form (RF)

  5-bromouracil (BU)

DNA ligase (polynucleotide joining enzyme)

DNA polymerase II

DNA polymerase III

  primer

  exonuclease

  holoenzyme

  subunits

  dimer, γ complex

  replisome

DNA polymerase IV, V

Helicases, *dna*A, *dna*B, *dna*C

Single-stranded DNA binding proteins

DNA gyrase (topoisomerase)

RNA primer

  primase

  free 3′ hydroxyl group

DNA ligase

  ligase deficient mutant

  ori C, *ter*

  9mer, 13mer

  β-subunit clamp

Eukaryotic DNA polymerases

  six forms

  multiple replicons

Antonomously replicating sequence (ARS)

Origin replication complex (ORC)

Pre-replication complex

Nucleosome

Telomerase

  Tetrahymena

  TTGGGG

  hairpin loop

  catalytic ribonucleoprotein

Endonuclease

Heteroduplex DNA molecules

  Holliday structures

  chi form

  recombinant duplexes

  *rec*A, *rec*B, *rec*C, *rec*D

Processes/Methods

Replication of DNA
    semiconservative
    conservative
    dispersive
Meselson and Stahl (1958)
    E. coli
        equilibrium sedimentation
        $^{15}NH_4Cl$, $^{14}NH_4Cl$
    Taylor, Woods, and Hughes (1957)
        Vicia faba
        ^{3}H-thymidine
        autoradiography
        colchicine
        sister chromatid exchanges
    bidirectional *(vs. unidirectional)*
        origin of replication, *ori*
        termination, *ter*
        replicon
        replication fork
        continuous, discontinuous
            leading strand
            lagging strand
                Okazaki fragments
Synthesis of DNA *in vitro*
    Kornberg (1957)
    reaction mixture
    chain elongation
        fidelity
    base comparisons (template/product)
    nearest neighbor frequency test (F11.1)
    (see Problem 40 for explanation)

spleen phosphodiesterase
biologically active DNA
transfection of *E. coli*
faithful copying
Processivity
Polymerase switching
Exonuclease proofreading
Conditional mutation
    temperature sensitive
Genetic recombination
    homologous recombination
    single-stranded nick
    endonuclease and ligation
Gene conversion
    Neurospora
    nonreciprocal

Concepts

Replication
    semiconservative
    antiparallel
    continuous, discontinuous
    conservative (F11.4)
    dispersive (F11.4)
Biological activity
Nearest neighbor analysis
Repair
Proofreading
Eukaryotic DNA replication
Telomere replication
Conditional mutants (F11.3)
Genetic recombination
Gene conversion

F11.1 Illustration of the mode of action of spleen phosphodiesterase.

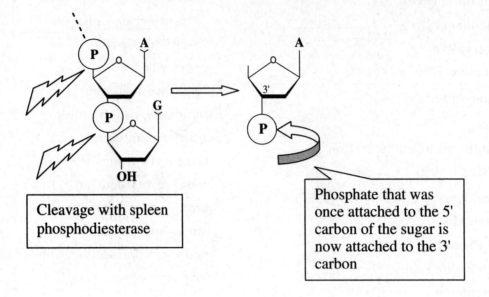

Cleavage with spleen phosphodiesterase

Phosphate that was once attached to the 5' carbon of the sugar is now attached to the 3' carbon

F11.2 Shorthand structures for 3' and 5' nucleotides.

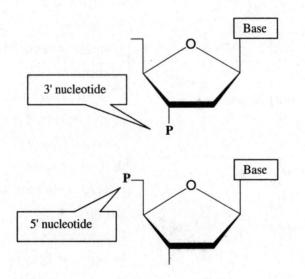

Base

3' nucleotide

Base

5' nucleotide

F11.3 Illustration of the influence of a conditional mutation on protein structure and function.

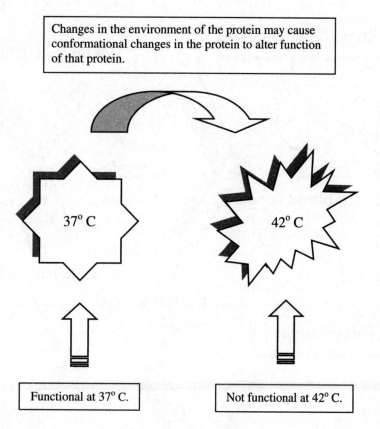

Changes in the environment of the protein may cause conformational changes in the protein to alter function of that protein.

37° C

42° C

Functional at 37° C.

Not functional at 42° C.

F11.4 Figure relating to question #4 in the problems section depicts labeling pattern under conservative and dispersive replication patterns.

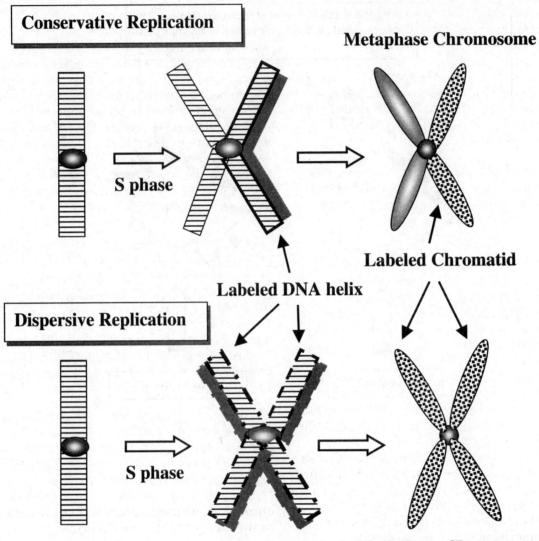

Conservative Replication

Metaphase Chromosome

S phase

Labeled Chromatid

Labeled DNA helix

Dispersive Replication

S phase

Metaphase Chromosome

Solutions to Problems and Discussion Questions

1. The differences among the three models of DNA replication relate to the manner in which the new strands of DNA are oriented as daughter DNA molecules are produced.

Conservative: In the conservative scheme, the original double helix remains as a complete unit and the new DNA double helix is produced as a single unit. The old DNA is completely conserved.

Semiconservative: Each daughter strand is composed of one old DNA strand and one new DNA strand. Separation of hydrogen bonds is required.

Dispersive: In the dispersive scheme, the original DNA strand is broken into pieces, and the new DNA in the daughter strand is interspersed among the old pieces. Separation of the individual covalent, phosphodiester bonds is required for this mode of replication.

2. The Meselson and Stahl experiment has the following components. By labeling the pool of nitrogenous bases of the DNA of *E. coli* with a heavy isotope ^{15}N, it would be possible to "follow" the "old" DNA. This was accomplished by growing the cells for many generations in medium containing ^{15}N. Cells were transferred to ^{14}N medium so that "new" DNA could be detected. A comparison of the density of DNA samples at various times in the experiment (initial ^{15}N culture and subsequent cultures grown in the ^{14}N medium) showed that after one round of replication in the ^{14}N medium, the DNA was half as dense (intermediate) as the DNA from bacteria grown only in the ^{15}N medium. In a sample taken after two rounds of replication in the ^{14}N medium, half of the DNA was of the intermediate density, and the other half was as dense as DNA containing only ^{14}N DNA.

3. Under a conservative scheme, the first round of replication in ^{14}N medium produces one dense double helix and one "light" double helix in contrast with the intermediate density of the DNA in the semiconservative mode. Therefore, after one round of replication in the ^{14}N medium, the conservative scheme can be ruled out.

After one round of replication in ^{14}N under a dispersive model, the DNA is of intermediate density, just as it is in the semiconservative model. However, in the next round of replication in ^{14}N medium, the density of the DNA is between the intermediate and "light" densities.

4. Refer to the text for an illustration of the labeling of *Vicia* chromosomes under a Taylor, Woods, and Hughes experimental design. Notice that only those cells that pass through the S phase in the presence of the ^{3}H-thymidine are labeled and that each double helix (per chromatid) is "half-labeled."

See Figure F11.4 in this book for a graphic description of these conservative and dispersive replication patterns.

(a) Under a conservative scheme, all of the newly labeled DNA will go to one sister chromatid, while the other sister chromatid will remain unlabeled. In contrast to a semiconservative scheme, the first replicative round would produce one sister chromatid, which has labels on both strands of the double helix (see F11.4).

(b) Under a dispersive scheme all of the newly labeled DNA will be interspersed with unlabeled DNA. Because these preparations (metaphase chromosomes) are highly coiled and condensed structures derived from the "spread out" form at interphase (which includes the S phase), it is impossible to detect the areas where label is not found. Rather, both sister chromatids would appear as evenly labeled structures (See F11.4.)

5. Because the semiconservative scheme predicts that *half* of the DNA in each daughter double helix is labeled, it would be difficult to envision a scheme where three strands are replicated in such a semiconservative manner. It would seem that either the conservative or dispersive scheme would fit more appropriately. To examine the nature of replication, one could devise an experiment similar to that of Meselson and Stahl or Taylor, Woods, and Hughes.

6. The *in vitro* replication requires a DNA template, a divalent cation (Mg^{++}), and all four of the deoxyribonucleoside triphosphates: dATP, dCTP, dTTP, and dGTP. The lower case "d" refers to the deoxyribose sugar.

7. Prior to the development of highly efficient methods of enzyme isolation, large cultures containing large numbers of bacterial cells were needed to yield even small quantities of enzymes.

8. Two general analytical approaches showed that the products of DNA polymerase I were probably copies of the template DNA. Because *base composition* can be similar without reflecting sequence similarity, the least stringent test was the comparison of base composition. By comparing *nearest neighbor frequencies*, Kornberg determined that there is a very high likelihood that the product is of the same base sequence as the template.

9. Because base composition can be similar without reflecting sequence similarity, the least stringent test was the comparison of base composition. By comparing nearest neighbor frequencies, Kornberg determined that there is a very high likelihood that the product is of the same base sequence as the template. However, since nearest neighbor analysis relates "neighbor frequency" and not base sequence, there is a chance that sequence differences are not detected.

10. The *in vitro* rate of DNA synthesis using DNA polymerase I is slow, being more effective at replicating single-stranded than double-stranded DNA. In addition, it is capable of degrading as well as synthesizing DNA. Such degradation suggests that it functioned as a repair enzyme. In addition, DeLucia and Cairns discovered a strain of *E. coli* (*pol*A1) that still replicates its DNA, but is deficient in DNA polymerase I activity.

11. See F11.1 and Problem 40 below to get started. The overall plan of the *nearest neighbor experiment* is to determine the frequency of neighbors of a given base, say adenine, in both the template DNA and the product DNA. Should the frequency of neighbors be similar, then the sequence of bases is likely to be the same. This argument is strengthened if the frequencies of neighbors of the other bases (G, C, and T) are also similar in the template and primer.

The procedure is to introduce labeled phosphate by use of labeled (innermost phosphate) 5'-nucleotides as shown in the text. In the example, cytidine has a ^{32}P attached to the C-5' atom. Spleen phosphodiesterase cleaves the polymer at the C-5' position (between the C-5' and the phosphate), thereby transferring the labeled phosphate to the C-3' atom of its 5' neighbor.

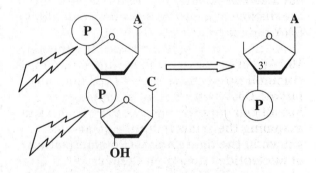

Chromatographic separation of the resulting 3´-nucleotides, followed by determination of the radioactivity of each, provides an estimate of the frequency of which each base is a neighbor of cytosine. By repeating this procedure using other bases and other templates, one can be somewhat confident that the template is similar in base sequence to the *in vitro* product.

12. As stated in the text, *biologically active* DNA implies that the DNA is capable of supporting typical metabolic activities of the cell or organism and is also capable of faithful reproduction.

13. ϕX174 is a well-studied single-stranded virus (phage) that can be easily isolated. It has a relatively small DNA genome (5500 nucleotides), which, if mutated, usually alters its reproductive cycle.

14. As shown in the text, DNA polymerase I and DNA ligase are used to synthesize and label an RF duplex. DNase is used to nick one of the two strands. The heavy (^{32}P/BU-containing) DNA is isolated by denaturation and centrifugation, and DNA polymerase and DNA ligase are used to make a synthetic complementary strand. When isolated, this synthetic strand is capable of transfecting *E. coli* protoplasts, from which new ϕX174 phages are produced.

15. The *polAI* mutation was instrumental in demonstrating that DNA polymerase I activity was not necessary for the *in vivo* replication of the *E. coli* chromosome. Such an observation opened the door for the discovery of other enzymes involved in DNA replication.

16. All three enzymes share several common properties. First, none can *initiate* DNA synthesis on a template, but all can *elongate* an existing DNA strand assuming there is a template strand as shown in the figure below. Polymerization of nucleotides occurs in the 5′ to 3′ direction where each 5′ phosphate is added to the 3′ end of the growing polynucleotide.

All three enzymes are large, complex proteins with a molecular weight in excess of 100,000 daltons, and each has 3′ to 5′ exonuclease activity. Refer to the text.

DNA polymerase I:
   exonuclease activity
   present in large amounts
   relatively stable
   removal of RNA primer

DNA polymerase II:
   possibly involved in repair function

DNA polymerase III:
   exonuclease activity
   essential for replication
   complex molecule

17. Refer to the text for a listing of the components of DNA polymerase III. The active form of the enzyme is called the holoenzyme. The region responsible for actual polymerization is called the "core" portion.

18. Given a stretch of double-stranded DNA, one could initiate synthesis at a given point and either replicate strands in one direction only (unidirectional) or in both directions (bidirectional) as shown below. Notice that in the text the synthesis of complementary strands occurs in a *continuous 5′>3′* mode on the leading strand in the direction of the replication fork, and in a *discontinuous 5′>3′* mode on the lagging strand opposite the direction of the replication fork. Such discontinuous replication forms Okazaki fragments.

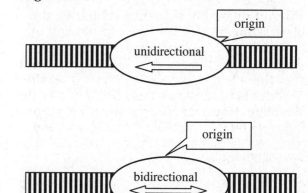

5′ ⊦——————————————3′

synthesis can initiate here

5′

19. *Helicase, dna*A and *single-stranded* DNA *binding* proteins initially unwind, open, and stabilize DNA at the initiation point. DNA *gyrase*, a DNA topoisomerase, relieves supercoiling generated by helix unwinding. This process involves breaking both strands of the DNA helix.

20. *Okazaki fragments* are relatively short (1000 to 2000 bases in prokaryotes) DNA fragments that are synthesized in a discontinuous fashion on the lagging strand during DNA replication. Such fragments appear to be necessary because template DNA is not available for 5'>3' synthesis until some degree of continuous DNA synthesis occurs on the leading strand in the direction of the replication fork. The isolation of such fragments provides support for the scheme of replication shown in the text. DNA *ligase* is required to form phosphodiester linkages in gaps, which are generated when DNA polymerase I removes RNA primer and meets newly synthesized DNA ahead of it. Notice in the text that the discontinuous DNA strands are ligated together into a single continuous strand. *Primer* RNA is formed by RNA primase to serve as an initiation point for the production of DNA strands on a DNA template. None of the DNA polymerases are capable of initiating synthesis without a free 3' hydroxyl group. The primer RNA provides that group and thus can be used by DNA polymerase III.

21. The synthesis of DNA is thought to follow the pattern described in the text. The model involves opening and stabilizing the DNA helix, priming DNA synthesis with RNA primer, and moving replication forks in both directions, which includes elongation of RNA primers in continuous and discontinuous 5'>3' modes and their removal by the exonucleolytic activity of DNA polymerase I. Okazaki fragments generated in the replicative process are joined together with DNA ligase. DNA gyrase relieves supercoils generated by DNA unwinding.

22. Eukaryotic DNA is replicated in a manner that is very similar to that of *E. coli*. Synthesis is bidirectional, continuous on one strand and discontinuous on the other, and the requirements of synthesis (four deoxyribonucleoside triphosphates, divalent cation, template, and primer) are the same. Okazaki fragments of eukaryotes are about one-tenth the size of those in bacteria.

Because a much greater amount of DNA is replicated and DNA replication is slower, there are multiple initiation sites for replication in eukaryotes (and increased DNA polymerase per cell) in contrast to the single replication origin in prokaryotes. Replication occurs at different sites during different intervals of the S phase. The proposed functions of four DNA polymerases are described in the text.

23. Even though the base composition between two species may be *similar*, sequences can vary considerably.

24. (a) In *E. coli*, 100 kb are added to each growing chain per minute. Therefore, the chain should be about 4,000,000 bp.

(b) Given $(4 \times 10^6 \text{ bp}) \times 0.34\text{nm/bp} =$

$$1.36 \times 10^6\text{nm or 1.3mm}$$

25. (a) no repair from DNA polymerase I and/or DNA polymerase III

(b) no DNA ligase activity

(c) no primase activity

(d) only DNA polymerase I activity

(e) no DNA gyrase activity

26. *Gene conversion* is likely to be a consequence of genetic recombination in which nonreciprocal recombination yields products in which it appears that one allele is "converted" to another. Gene conversion is now considered a result of heteroduplex formation, which is accompanied by mismatched bases. When these mismatches are corrected, the "conversion" occurs.

27. (a) Because DNA polymerase III is essential for DNA chain elongation, it is necessary for replication of the *E. coli* chromosome. Thus, strains that are mutant for this enzyme must contain conditional mutations.

(b) The 3′ – 5′ exonuclease activity is involved in proofreading. Thus, proofreading would be hampered in such mutant strains, and a higher than expected mutation rate would occur.

28. Telomerase activity is present in germ-line tissue to maintain telomere length from one generation to the next. In other words, telomeres cannot shorten indefinitely without eventually eroding genetic information.

29. (a) Two classic experiments, one using *E. coli* and the other using *Vicia faba*, using density and radioisotope labeling, respectively, demonstrated that replication is semiconservative in prokaryotes and eukaryotes. In both cases, daughter DNA molecules are each composed of one parental strand and one newly synthesized DNA strand.

(b) A mutant in DNA polymerase I (*polA1*) was nevertheless capable of synthesizing biologically active DNA, leading to the conclusion that at least one other enzyme is responsible for replicating DNA *in vivo*.

(c) *In vitro* studies by Kornberg and coworkers indicated that DNA strand elongation occurs by addition of nucleotides at the 3′ end. During chain elongation, two of the outer phosphates of the precursor dNTP are cleaved, and the remaining phosphate attaches to the 3′-OH group of the deoxyribose. *In vivo* or *in vitro*, DNA polymerases, including polymerase III, are only capable of 5′ to 3′ synthesis.

(d) Two lines of evidence indicated that DNA synthesis is discontinuous. First, in newly formed DNA, relatively short nucleotide fragments are hydrogen bonded to the template strands. Second, these short nucleotide fragments accumulate in ligase-deficient mutants of *E. coli*.

(e) Because eukaryotic chromosomes are linear rather than circular, free ends exist. It was predicted that such free ends would create the problem of shortening because of the 5′-3′ nature of DNA synthesis and the inability of DNA polymerases to initiate synthesis without a free 3′-OH. The finding of the telomerase enzyme and a number of terminal repeats at the ends of chromosomes supports the prediction of chromosome shortening and its solution.

30. Since synthesis is bidirectional, one can multiply the rate of synthesis by two to come up with a figure of 18,000 bases replicated per five minutes (30 bases/second $\times$ 300 seconds). Dividing 1.6×10^8 by 1.8×10^4 gives 0.88×10^4, or about 8800 replication sites.

31. If replication is conservative, the first autoradiographs (see metaphase I in the text) would have label distributed on only one side (chromatid) of the metaphase chromosome, as shown below.

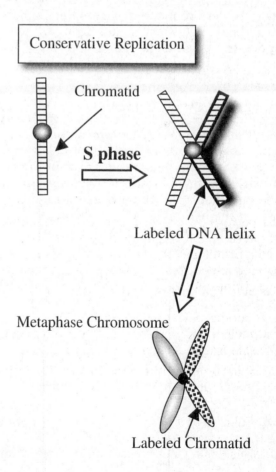

Conservative Replication

Chromatid

S phase

Labeled DNA helix

Metaphase Chromosome

Labeled Chromatid

32. (a) DNA polymerase would catalyze a bond between the 5′ end of the last nucleotide added and the 3′ end of the incoming nucleotide. In this reaction, the energy would be provided by the cleavage of the gamma- and beta phosphates of the last nucleotide added to the chain rather than of the incoming nucleotide.

(b) If DNA polymerase removed a base, it would not be able to add any more bases to the chain because the penultimate base would have a monophosphate rather than a triphosphate and there would be no source of energy for the polymerization reaction.

33. If the DNA contained parallel strands in the double helix and the polymerase would be able to accommodate such parallel strands, there would be continuous synthesis and no Okazaki fragments. The telomere problem would only be at one end. Several other possibilities exist. If the DNA strands were replicated as complete single strands, the synthesis could begin at the opposite free ends. In addition, if the DNA existed only as a single strand, the same results would occur.

34. (a) 5′ACCUAAGU **(b)** U

35. Conservative replication can be eliminated. This is because under a conservative mode of replication, both of the original DNA strands remain together in one chromatid and the two new strands form a single double helix in the other chromatid. Such is not the case in this figure.

36. (a) DNA, since one of the nitrogenous bases is T; also, notice the lack of an OH group at the 2′ carbon.

(b) 3′

(c) Since spleen diesterase cuts between the 5′ carbon and the phosphate, the original 5′ phosphate is transferred to

the 3′ carbon of the 5′ neighbor. Therefore, deoxyadenosine would obtain the phosphate at its 3′ position.

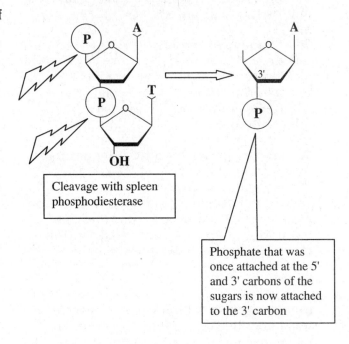

Cleavage with spleen phosphodiesterase

Phosphate that was once attached at the 5′ and 3′ carbons of the sugars is now attached to the 3′ carbon

37. First, given that label (^{3}H) is distributed on both ends of the structure, replication must be bidirectional. Second, since both upper and lower portions contain label, no restrictions to synthesis are apparent. The distribution of low-density grains in the center would indicate that replication begins in the middle and proceeds to the outward areas in both directions.

38. Notice in *strain A* that DNA synthesis is reduced at 42°C indicating that *strain A* is temperature sensitive. In addition, *strain A* is sensitive to novobiocin. Therefore, *strain A* is *gyr^{ts}*. Strain B is resistant to novobiocin but temperature sensitive, and is therefore *gyr$^{ts, r}$*. Strain C is sensitive to novobiocin but not temperature sensitive, and is therefore *wild type*. Strain D is resistant to novobiocin and not temperature sensitive and is therefore *gyr^r*.

39. The following table depicts similarities and differences in DNA replicative processes between *Pyrococcus abyssi*, bacteria, and eukaryotes.

Criterion	Eukaryotic	Bacteria
Circular chromosome	not similar	similar
Single origin	not similar	similar
RNA primer	similar	similar
RNA primer length	similar	not similar
Replicative proteins	similar	not similar
Replication rate	not similar	similar
Okazaki fragments	similar	similar
Okazaki fragment length	similar	not similar

40.

Initial Labeled Base	Labeled Base after Spleen Phosphodiesterase Digestion	
	ANTIPARALLEL	PARALLEL
G	A,T	C,T
C	G,A,G	G,A
T	C,T,G	C,T,A,G
A	T,C,A,T	T,C,A,G

One can determine which model occurs in nature by comparing the pattern in which the labeled phosphate is shifted following spleen phosphodiesterase digestion. Focus your attention on the antiparallel model and notice that the frequency of which "C" (for example) is the 5′ neighbor of "G" is not necessarily the same as the frequency of which "G" is the 5′ neighbor of "C." However, in the parallel model (b), the frequency of which "C" is the 5′ neighbor of "G" is the same as the frequency of which "G" is the 5′ neighbor of "C." By examining such "digestion frequencies," it can be determined that DNA exists in the opposite polarity.

Chapter 12: DNA Organization in Chromosomes

Concept Areas	Corresponding Problems
Viral and Bacterial Chromosomes	1, 2, 14, 15
Specialized Chromosomes	3, 4, 5, 7
Organization of DNA in Chromatin	6, 9, 10, 11, 12, 13, 16, 23, 24, 25, 26, 27, 28, 29, 30, 31, 32, 33, 34
Organization of the Eukaryotic Genome	6, 8, 21, 26, 27, 28, 29, 30, 31, 32, 33, 34

Vocabulary: Organization and Listing of Terms and Concepts

Structures and Substances

Viral chromosomes

  DNA, RNA

    double-stranded

    single-stranded

    often circular

  protein coat

  ϕX174

  polyoma

  lambda (λ)

Bacterial chromosomes

  DNA

  double-stranded

  nucleoid

  E. coli

  circular

DNA-binding proteins

  HU, H

  topoisomer

  topoisomerase

Eukaryotic chromosomes

  specialized chromosomes

    polytene chromosomes

chromomeres

  puff

lampbrush chromosomes

chromatin

mitotic chromosomes

  condensed chromatin

  folded fiber

Chromatin

  nucleoprotein

  histones

    amino acid composition

    tetramers, two types

      nucleosome core particle

  nonhistones

  micrococcal nuclease

    nucleosomes

    linker DNA

      histone H1

    solenoid

  chromatin remodeling

  5-methyl cytosine

  CpG island

Heterochromatin, euchromatin

  Barr body

136

telomere

  telomeric DNA sequences

  telomere-associated sequences

satellite and repetitive DNA

  middle (moderate) repetitive DNA

VNTRs

microsatellites

  SINES

  LINES

  retrotransposons

pseudogene

Centromeric DNA sequences

CEN

alphoid

Processes/Methods

Supercoiling

  supercoil

  linking number

    energetically relaxed

    energetically strained

Folded-fiber (eukaryotic chromosome)

  coiling-twisting-condensing

Chromatin remodeling

  acetylation

  methylation

  phosphorylation

Heterochromatin

  few genes

  late replicating

position effect

In situ hybridization

Chromosome banding

  C-banding

  G-banding

Repetitive DNA

  noncoding sequences

    satellite DNA

    highly repetitive DNA

  centromeric DNA (CEN)

    alphoid family

  telomeric DNA sequences

    telomeric-associated sequences

    telomerase

  moderately repetitive DNA

  short interspersed elements (SINEs)

    Alu family

  long interspersed elements (LINEs)

  variable number tandem repeats (VNTR)

  DNA fingerprinting

  repetitive transposed sequences

  moderately repetitive multicopy genes

Concepts

Variety of DNA conformations

Nucleosomes and chromatin structure

Heterochromatin/euchromatin

Centromeric structure

Repetitive DNA

Solutions to Problems and Discussion Questions

1. Bacteriophage λ has a linear, double-stranded DNA while in the phage coat, and upon infection, the DNA closes to form a circular chromosome. It contains about 50 kb. T2 phage also has a linear, double-stranded DNA chromosome; it is less than 200 kb. *E. coli* has a circular, double-stranded DNA chromosome of about 4.2×10^3 kb. Both intact phages are about 1/150 the size of *E.coli*. Since phages are obligate parasites of bacteria, they are dependent on their hosts for the manufacture of materials for their replication. Bacteria contain all genetic information for metabolism, replication, and *de novo* synthesis of numerous life-supporting materials. Phages, on the other hand, contain relatively few genes, namely, those needed to adsorb, inject, and produce progeny using primarily bacterial materials.

2. By having a circular chromosome, no free ends present the problem of linear chromosomes, namely, complete replication of terminal sequences.

3. Polytene chromosomes are formed from numerous DNA replications, pairing of homologs, and absence of strand separation or cytoplasmic division. Each chromosome contains about 1000 to 5000 DNA strands in parallel register. They appear in specific tissues, such as salivary glands, of many dipterans like *Drosophila*. They appear as comparatively long, wide fibers with sharp light and dark sections (bands) along their length. Such bands (chromomeres) are useful, among other things, in chromosome identification.

4. Since eukaryotic chromosomes are "multirepliconic" in that there are multiple replication forks along their lengths, one would expect to see multiple clusters of radioactivity if labeled for a short period of time.

5. Most puffs represent active genes as evidenced by staining and uptake of labeled RNA precursors as assayed by autoradiography.

6. Long interspersed elements (LINEs) are repetitive transposable DNA sequences in humans. The most prominent family, designated **L1**, is about 6.4 kb each and is represented about 100,000 times. LINEs are often referred to as retrotransposons because their mechanism of transposition resembles that used by retroviruses.

7. Lampbrush chromosomes are typically present in vertebrate oocytes and are so named because of their similar appearance to brushes used to clean kerosene lamp chimneys in the nineteenth century. They are also found in spermatocytes of some insects. They are found as diplotene stage structures and are active uncoiled versions of condensed meiotic chromosomes. Lampbrush chromosomes are typically viewed using light and electron microscopy.

8. While greater DNA content per cell is associated with eukaryotes, one cannot universally equate genomic size with an increase in organismic complexity. There are numerous examples where DNA content per cell varies considerably among closely related species. Because of the diverse cell types of multicellular eukaryotes, a variety of gene products is required, which may be related to the increase in DNA content per cell. In addition, the advantage of diploidy automatically increases DNA content per cell. However, seeing the question in another way, it is likely that a much higher *percentage* of the genome of a prokaryote is actually involved in phenotype production than in eukaryotes.

Eukaryotes have evolved the capacity to obtain and maintain what appear to be large amounts of "extra," perhaps "junk," DNA. This concept will be examined in subsequent chapters of the text. Prokaryotes, on the other hand, with their relatively short life cycles, are extremely efficient in their accumulation and use of their genome.

Given the larger amount of DNA per cell and the requirement that the DNA be partitioned in an orderly fashion to daughter cells during cell division, certain mechanisms and structures (mitosis, nucleosomes, centromeres, etc.) have evolved for packaging and distributing the DNA. In addition, the genome is divided into separate entities (chromosomes) to perhaps facilitate the partitioning process in mitosis and meiosis.

9. Digestion of chromatin with endonucleases, such as micrococcal nuclease, gives DNA fragments of approximately 200 base pairs or multiples of such segments.

X-ray diffraction data indicate a regular spacing of DNA in chromatin. Regularly spaced bead-like structures (nucleosomes) were identified by electron microscopy.

10. Nucleosomes are octomeric structures of two molecules of each histone (H2A, H2B, H3, and H4) except H1. Between the nucleosomes and complexed with linker DNA is histone H1. A 146-base-pair sequence of DNA wraps around the nucleosome.

11. As chromosome condensation occurs, a 300-Å fiber is formed. It appears to be composed of 5 or 6 nucleosomes coiled together. Such a structure is called a solenoid. These fibers form a series of loops that further condense into the chromatin fiber, which are then coiled into chromosome arms making up each chromatid.

12. *Heterochromatin* is chromosomal material that stains deeply and remains condensed when other parts of chromosomes, euchromatin, are otherwise pale and decondensed. Heterochromatic regions replicate late in S phase and are relatively inactive in a genetic sense because few genes are present, or if they are present, they are repressed. Telomeres and the areas adjacent to centromeres are composed of heterochromatin.

13. (a) Since there are 200 base pairs per nucleosome (as defined in this problem) and 10^9 base pairs, there would be 5×10^6 nucleosomes.

(b) Since there are 5×10^6 nucleosomes and 9 histones (including H1) per nucleosome, there must be $9(5 \times 10^6)$ histone molecules: 4.5×10^7.

(c) Since 10^9 base pairs are present and each base pair is 3.4 Å, the overall length of the DNA is 3.4×10^9 Å. Dividing this value by the packing ratio (50) gives 6.8×10^7 Å.

14. The first step of this solution is to convert all of the given values to cubic Å remembering that 1 μm = 10,000 Å. Using the formula πr^2 for the area of a circle and $4/3\ \pi r^3$ for the volume of a sphere, the following calculations apply:

Volume of DNA: 3.14×10 Å $\times 10$ Å $\times$
$$(50 \times 10^4 \text{ Å}) = 1.57 \times 10^8 \text{ Å}^3$$

Volume of capsid: $4/3\ (3.14 \times 400$ Å $\times$
$$400 \text{ Å} \times 400 \text{ Å}) = 2.67 \times 10^8 \text{ Å}^3$$

Because the capsid head has a greater volume than the volume of DNA, the DNA will fit into the capsid.

15. One base pair occupies 0.34 nm; therefore, the equation would be as follows:

52μm/(0.34 nm/bp) × 1000 nm/μm =

152,941 base pairs

16. Volume of the nucleus $= 4/3\pi r^3$

$$= 4/3 \times 3.14 \times (5 \times 10^3 nm)^3$$

$$= 5.23 \times 10^{11} nm^3$$

Volume of the chromosome $= \pi r^2 \times$ length

$$= 3.14 \times 5.5nm \times 5.5nm \times (2 \times 10^9 nm)$$

$$= 1.9 \times 10^{11} nm^3$$

Therefore, the percentage of the volume of the nucleus occupied by the chromatin is

$$= 1.9 \times 10^{11} nm^3/5.23 \times 10^{11} nm^3 \times 100$$

$$= \text{about } 36.3\%$$

17. When the w^+ locus is rearranged such that it is now positioned next to heterochromatin, activity becomes intermittent, leading to a variegated eye in a w^+/w heterozygote or w^+/Y male. Heterochromatin is characterized as gene-poor and relatively inaccessible to DNA-binding factors needed for transcription. Specific regions of heterochromatin recruit histone deacetylases that modify histones and essentially silence such regions. As with X chromosome inactivation in mammals, heterochromatic regions can spread until they reach specific sequences that signal a block to additional silencing. Such spreading can be continuous or discontinuous. When the w^+ gene is juxtaposed to heterochromatin, apparently the normal regulatory signals are altered and sporadic silencing that leads to variegation is the result. Once the w^+ gene is silenced, the w^+ gene in descendant cells is also silenced, leading to patches of white tissue.

18. (a) Since pseudogenes do not produce an observable phenotype, their identification by classical mutation analysis is not possible. In the absence of a product, the identification of pseudogenes depends mainly on extensive mining of DNA sequence databases to identify sections of DNA that resemble functional genes. In addition, the search for ORF and/or exon sequences is inhibited because of mutations that make up pseudogenes.

(b) Because gene spacing, chromatin folding, and various silencer/enhancer domains of chromosomes interact in normal genomic function, pseudogenes may play important roles by sponsoring or inhibiting such interactions. Recent evidence indicates that what can appear to be an inactive pseudogene in one setting (tissue or organism) may well have function in another. Some pseudogenes are transcribed and may serve in gene regulation.

19. Except for identical twins, each individual possesses a virtually unique set of numerous VNTRs. Such variety provides a dependable, consistent, and unique DNA fingerprint for forensic applications.

20. (a) Using radioactively labeled RNA precursors followed by autoradiography, researchers discovered a high rate of RNA incorporation indicating intense transcription.

(b) Higher level chromosome structures have been revealed through both chemical and observational analyses. In both prokaryotes and eukaryotes, chromosomal DNA is complexed with proteins that foster folding. Electron microscopic, X-ray, and neutron-scattering observations indicate the complex organization of DNA and proteins as chromatin transitions to individual chromosomes.

(c) Early evidence came from endonuclease digestion that yielded DNA fragments of about 200 base pairs in length. Electron microscopic, X-ray, and neutron-scattering observations revealed the structure of nucleosomes and their relationship to DNA.

(d) Base sequences and organizational motifs of satellite DNA are common to many regions within and flanking centromeric DNA. In humans, most satellite DNA is of the alphoid family found mainly in centromeric regions that total up to 3 million base pairs.

In addition, *in situ* hybridization of satellite DNA clusters in heterochromatic regions flanking centromeres. Rapid renaturation of DNA also indicates the presence of repetitive sequences.

21. Data by Sun et al. support the general observation that heterochromatic genes are less active than euchromatic genes and, more specifically, the possibility that heterochromatin may contain genes that are repressed. Heterochromatin is located in eukaryotic chromosomes as differentially staining compared with euchromatin. It is relatively inactive genetically either because of a lack of genes or the presence of repressed genes. Heterochromatin replicates later in S phase than euchromatic segments. Centromeric and telomeric regions of chromosomes are typically heterochromatic.

22. Chromosomes are not randomly distributed within nuclei. Homologous chromosomes tend to distribute themselves opposite each other and in an antiparallel manner, meaning that their positions are in reverse order on opposite sides of the nucleus. Assuming that such patterns are maintained throughout the entire cell cycle, it is possible that chromosomal positions may influence gene function and/or chromosomal behavior during mitosis and/or meiosis. If gene function is influenced not only by gene position in a chromosome, but also by gene position in a nucleus, then an alternative explanation for position effect exists.

23. The intimate relationships among histones, nucleosomes, and DNA in chromatin account for structural remodeling of chromosomes as the cell cycle proceeds from interphase to metaphase. That nucleosomes are associated with chromatin during periods of gene activity begs the question as to the possible roles they play in influencing not only chromosome structure but also gene function. The finding that natural chemical modification of nucleosomal components, as indicated in the question, increases gene activity

suggests that changes in the binding of nucleosomes to DNA (in this case due to methylation) enables genes to be more accessible to factors that promote gene function. In addition, the finding that heterochromatin, containing fewer genes and more repressed genes, is undermethylated, further supports the suggestion that histone modification is functionally related to changes in gene activity.

24. DNA replicates in a *semiconservative* fashion, with each daughter DNA double helix containing one new and one original single strand. Nucleosomes follow a *dispersive* pattern, with each daughter chromatid containing a mixture of new and original nucleosomes. One could test the distribution of nucleosomes by conducting an autoradiographic experiment similar to Taylor-Woods-Hughes, but instead of labeling the DNA with ^{3}H-thymidine, one would label some or all the histones H2A, H2B, H3, and H4 in nucleosomes.

25. Assuming a random distribution, dividing 3×10^9 base pairs by 10^6 gives approximately 3000 base pairs or 3 kbp between *Alu* sequences.

26. Bacteriophage lambda is composed of a double-stranded, linear DNA molecule of about 48,000 base pairs. It is capable of forming a closed, double-stranded circular molecule because of a 12-base pair, single-stranded, complementary "overhanging" sequence at the 5′ end of each single strand.

27. The distribution of microsatellites varies in a taxon-related manner. Microsatellites are more common within genes of yeast and fungi and quite infrequent in genes of mammals. There appears to be a general decrease in within-gene microsatellites in more recently evolved organisms.

28. The general frequency and pattern of various trinucleotide repeat motifs are similar in all taxonomic groups. Within-gene trinucleotide repeats are the most frequent repeat motif in all taxonomic groups followed by hexanucleotide repeats. One explanation might be that various microsatellite types (mono, di, tri, etc.) are generated at different rates in different genomic regions (within and between genes). A second possibility is that selection acts differentially depending on the type and location of a repeat. The correlation between the high frequency of tri- and hexanucleotide repeats within genes and a triplet code specifying particular amino acids within genes may not be coincidental.

29. (a) The microsatellite motif is imperfect and can be represented as $(GTCPy)_n$.

(b) The sequence of the nonmicrosatellite region is TCGATATAGC(PuPy)AT. It is not perfectly conserved in that there is one base difference among strains of *D. nigrodunni* and among strains of *D. dunni*.

30. If microsatellites, in general, are flanked by a conserved sequence, those conserved sequences may be involved in the generation and/or maintenance of the microsatellite. Alternatively, the microsatellite may generate the nonmicrosatellite region. Any hypothesis presented is in need of additional investigation before definitive statements can be made.

31. The basic issue here is to determine whether all the loci that are not from the mother can come from the father. That is, does the father's genotype provide the child's loci that are not provided by the mother? For example, at the *D9S302* locus, the mother contributed the child's 31 locus, and the alleged father could have contributed the child's 32 locus. Since other men also have the 32 locus, one cannot say that the alleged father is the father; rather, one could say that the alleged father cannot be excluded as the source of the sperm that produced the child. Notice that in every case, the child includes at least one locus from the father and one from the mother, which is expected if the alleged father is indeed the real father. Without information as to the frequency of each marker in the general population, it is difficult to draw definitive conclusions.

32. Generally, the higher the AT content of a DNA strand, the lower the temperature of melting or denaturation. Since one can monitor the degree of strand separation with absorption of ultraviolet light (optical density), one can get an estimate of the AT/GC content in a given stretch of uniform-length DNA. For relatively short strands of DNA, the temperature of melting is also related to strand length. Other factors being equal, the shorter the strand is, the lower the T_m.

33. By subjecting the satellite fraction to denaturation/renaturation studies, one could determine the degree of repetitiveness by reassociation kinetics. The DNA could be sequenced; in addition, one could use *in situ* hybridization to determine the origin of the satellite DNA. In this case, one would have to generate labeled probes and anneal these probes to chromosomes. Since polytene chromosomes of *Drosophila* are ideally suited for such studies, this would be a relatively straightforward analysis.

34. Since both genes mentioned in the problem are located near the end of chromosome 16, it is possible that erosion of the end of the chromosome is related to each disease. Examination of the gene by *in situ* hybridization and molecular cloning indicates that thalassemia involves a terminal deletion in the distal portion of 16p. To learn more about such conditions, visit the following site *http://www.ncbi.nlm.nih.gov/* and follow the OMIM link.

Chapter 13: Recombinant DNA Technology and Gene Cloning

Concept Areas	Corresponding Problems
Overview	1, 5, 9, 10, 30
Making DNA Clones	1, 3, 8, 9, 12, 26, 33
Restriction Endonucleases	4, 6, 7, 9, 10, 11, 20, 31
Constructing DNA Libraries	2, 8, 13, 15, 16, 17, 18, 21, 25
Identifying Specific Cloned Sequences	12, 13, 18, 19, 20, 24, 31
Methods of Analysis of Cloned Sequences	12, 14, 19, 20, 31, 34, 35
DNA Sequencing	19, 28, 29
Polymerase Chain Reaction	26, 27, 32, 34, 35, 36
Applications	36

Vocabulary: Organization and Listing of Terms and Concepts

Structures and Substances

Recombinant DNA, clone

Restriction endonucleases

  palindrome

  "sticky" ends

  Eco R1, Smal

Vector

  cloning vehicle, plasmids

    pUC18

      multiple cloning polylinker site

      *lac*Z, X-gal

    bacteriophage, λ

  cosmids

    shuttle vector

Bacterial artificial chromosome (BAC)

Yeast artificial chromosome (YAC)

  selectable marker

Agrobacterium tumifaciens

  Ti plasmid

  callus

Expression vector

  T7

  lac operator

  IPTG

Cloned DNA fragments

Probe

Oligonucleotide

  primers

  Taq polymerase

    gene specific, random

Restriction map

Dideoxynucleotide

Processes/Methods

Recombinant DNA technology

  gene splicing

  genetic engineering

    restriction endonucleases

    vector

      plasmids

      selection (antibiotic resistance)

bacteriophage

  transfection

  DNA sequencing

cosmids

  cos sequences (lambda)

 hosts

  E. coli K12 transformation

polymerase chain reaction (PCR)

library construction

  genomic libraries

   $N = \ln(1 - P)/\ln(1 - f)$

  chromosome-specific libraries

pulse field gel electrophoresis

  cDNA libraries

   reverse transcriptase

   DNA polymerase I

  selection of recombinant clones

   probes

  colony and plaque

hybridization

  nitrocellulose or nylon filter

Analytical methods

 expression vector

 open reading frame (ORF)

 restricting mapping

  restriction fragment length
  polymorphism (RFLP)

 gel electrophoresis

 nucleic acid blotting

  Southern blot

  northern blot

  western blot

DNA sequencing

  applications

  gene mapping

PCR analysis

  denaturation

  annealing of primers

  extension of primers

   heat stable polymerase

   Taq polymerase

yeast

  plasmid

  yeast artificial chromosome (YAC)

plants

  Agrobacterium tumifaciens

  tumor-inducing plasmid (Ti)

T-DNA

  callus

  transgenic

  mammals

Concepts

Cloning

  selection strategies

  expression vector

Polymerase chain reaction

Probes

Restriction mapping

Gene mapping

Gene engineering

  research

  clinical applications

Transgenic organism

Solutions to Problems and Discussion Questions

1. Recombinant DNA technology, also called genetic engineering or gene splicing, involves the creation of associations of DNA that are not typically found in nature. Particular enzymes, called *restriction endonucleases*, cut DNA at specific sites and often yield "sticky" ends for additional interaction with DNA molecules cut with the same class of enzyme.

Isolated from bacteria, restriction enzymes fall into several classes, each having peculiarities as to structure and interaction with DNA. A vector may be a plasmid, bacteriophage, or cosmid that receives, through ligation, a piece or pieces of foreign DNA. The recombinant vector can transform (or transfect) a host cell (bacterium, yeast cell, etc.) and be amplified in number.

2. *Reverse transcriptase* is often used to promote the formation of cDNA (complementary DNA) from an mRNA molecule. Eukaryotic mRNAs typically have a 3′ polyA tail as indicated in the following diagram. The poly-dT segment provides a double-stranded section, which serves to prime the production of the complementary strand.

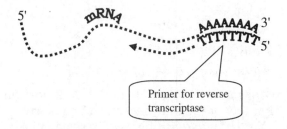

Primer for reverse transcriptase

3. Even though the human gene coding for insulin contains a number of introns, a cDNA generated from insulin mRNA is free of introns. Plasmids containing insulin genes (from cDNA) are free of introns, so no processing issue surfaces.

4. The question of protein/DNA recognition and interaction is a difficult one to answer. Much research has been done to attempt to understand the nature of the specificity of such interactions. It is believed that the protein interacts with the major groove of the DNA helix. This information comes from the structure of the proteins that have been sufficiently studied to suggest that the DNA major groove and "fingers" or extensions of the protein form the basis of interaction.

5. There are several reasons, some stemming from the original use of bacteria as the "workhorse" of molecular biologists, as well as the ease with which bacteria and yeast can be manipulated. In addition, intense interest has arisen in understanding the biology of mammalian cells for obvious reasons, and such cells have been manipulated in culture for many years. Perhaps one of the most important reasons is the fact that higher plants lack a suitable variety of vectors that are common to the other cell types mentioned above.

6. This segment contains the palindromic sequence of GGATCC, which is recognized by the restriction enzyme *Bam* HI. The double-stranded sequence is the following:

CCTAGG

GGATCC

7. The simple answer to this question is to assume that one is asking about the advantage to the scientist of having restriction enzyme sites recognize palindromic sites. In this case, the answer would be that single-stranded overhanging ends are often generated, which allow DNA from different sources cut with the same restriction enzyme to generate complementary overhangs, which can anneal to form recombinant molecules.

If one considers the question from a bacterial standpoint, the answer is much more involved. In fact, bacterial chromosomes actually have fewer palindromic sites than expected based on chance. This adaptation stems from the fact that restriction sites cleave at palindromic sequences, and one way to keep them from cleaving the host DNA is to evolve away from such sequences. So why do restriction enzymes often cleave at palindromic sites in the first place? First, the classical Type II restriction enzymes are dimers of identical units that recognize identical sequences. To protect such sequences in the bacterial chromosome from attack, a modification enzyme, a methyltransferase, must fully methylate certain bases on both strands of the DNA at the site of a particular restriction endonuclease attack.

Methyltransferases are typically monomers consistent with the process of methylating newly replicated DNA strands. In order for both strands to be protected by methylation, the sequence must be read the same in both directions on the double helix. So, returning to the original question, the advantage to the bacterium of having palindromic sites for restriction enzymes is more related to the protection of such sites from cleavage.

8. Plasmids were the first to be used as cloning vectors, and they are still routinely used to clone relatively small fragments of DNA. Because of their small size, they are relatively easy to separate from the host bacterial chromosome, and they have relatively few restriction sites. They can be engineered fairly easily (i.e., polylinkers and reporter genes added). For cloning larger pieces of DNA such as entire eukaryotic genes, cosmids are often used. For instance, when modifications are made in the bacterial virus lambda (λ), relatively large inserts of about 20 kb can be cloned. This is an important advantage when one needs to clone a large gene or generate a genomic library from a eukaryote.

In addition, some cosmids will only accept inserts of a limited size, which means that small, less meaningful perhaps, fragments will not be cloned unnecessarily. Both plasmids and cosmids suffer from the limitation that they can only use bacteria as hosts.

Yeast artificial chromosomes (YACs) contain telomeres, an origin of replication, and a centromere and are extensively used to clone DNA in yeast. With selectable markers (TRP1 and URA3) and a cluster of restriction sites, DNA inserts ranging from 100 kb to 1000 kb can be cloned and inserted into yeast. Since yeast, being a eukaryote, undergoes many of the typical RNA and protein processing steps of other, more complex eukaryotes, the advantages are numerous when working with eukaryotic genes.

9. Assuming a random distribution of all four bases, the four-base sequence would occur (on average) every 256 base pairs (4^4) and the six-base sequence would occur every 4096 base pairs (4^6). This is akin to calculating the probability of any particular sequence of bases occurring in row (of 4 or 6).

10. This problem can be solved by the following expressions:

*Not*I	4^8
*Hin*fI	$4 \times 4 \times 1 \times 4 \times 4$
*Xho*II	$2 \times 4 \times 4 \times 4 \times 4 \times 2$

The reason for using a "1" in the *Hin*fI portion is that any of the four bases can be inserted for the "N," whereas only two bases can be used for "Pu" and "Py" in the *Xho*II portion.

11. One might use an eight-base restriction enzyme to produce relatively few large fragments. If one wanted to construct a eukaryotic genomic library, such large fragments would have to be cloned into special vectors, such as yeast artificial chromosomes.

12. (a) Because the *Drosophila* DNA has been cloned into the *Pst*I site in the ampicillin resistance gene of the plasmid, the gene will be mutated, and any bacterium with the recombinant plasmid will be ampicillin sensitive. The tetracycline resistance gene remains active, however. Bacteria that have been transformed with the recombinant plasmid will be resistant to tetracycline; therefore, tetracycline should be added to the medium.

(b) Colonies that grow on a tetracycline medium should be tested for growth on an ampicillin medium either by replica plating or by some similar controlled transfer method. Those bacteria that do not grow on the ampicillin medium probably contain the *Drosophila* DNA insert.

(c) Resistance to both antibiotics by a transformed bacterium could be explained in several ways. First, if cleavage with the *Pst*I was incomplete, then no change in biological properties of the uncut plasmids would be expected. Also, it is possible that the cut ends of the plasmid were ligated together in the original form with no insert.

13. The question states that the average insert size is 5 kb (5000 bp) and that the genome is 1.5×10^5bp. Apply the formula:

$$= \ln(1 - 0.99)/\ln[1 - (5000/1.5 \times 10^5)]$$
$$= \ln(0.01)/\ln(0.9999667)$$
$$= -4.605/-0.0033886782$$
$$= 1.38 \times 10^3$$

14. Given that there is only one site for the action of *Hind*III, the following will occur: Cuts will be made such that a four-base single-stranded set of sticky ends will be produced. For the antibiotic resistance to be present, the ligation will reform the plasmid into its original form. However, two of the plasmids can join to form a dimer as indicated in the following diagram.

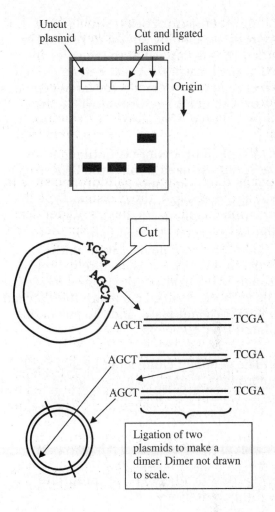

15. Using the human nucleotide sequence, one can produce a probe to screen the library of the African okapi. Second, one can use the amino acid sequence and the genetic code to generate a complementary DNA probe for screening the library. The probe is used, through hybridization, to identify the DNA that is complementary to the probe and allow one to identify the library clone containing the DNA of interest. Cells with the desired clone are then picked from the original plate, and the plasmid is isolated from the cells.

16. Because of complementary base pairing, the 3' end of the DNA strand often loops back onto itself, thereby providing a primer for DNA polymerase I.

17. All other factors being equal (appropriate cloning sites and selectable markers), it is important to consider the size of the foreign DNA that can be cloned into the vector. Generally, for large genomes it is best to use a vector that will accept relatively large fragments.

18. A typical procedure is outlined in the text. A filter is used to bind the DNA from the colonies containing recombinant plasmids. A labeled probe is constructed for the protein sequence of EF1a. Since it is highly conserved, it should show considerable complementation to the human EF-1a cDNA. It is used to detect, through hybridization, the DNA of interest. Cells with the desired clone are then picked from the original plate, and the plasmid is isolated from the cells.

19. The genomic clone most likely contains numerous introns, which are spliced out during RNA processing. Such sections of DNA (introns) are not represented in cDNAs.

20. The problem can be best solved by drawing out the strands and then placing the restriction sites in the appropriate positions as follows:

enzyme I ___350_|____950_____

enzyme II 200|____1100_____

   To determine the orientation of the restriction sites to each other, examine the results of the double-digested DNA and note that there is a 150 bp fragment, meaning that enzyme II cuts within the 350 bp fragment of enzyme I. Therefore, the final map is as follows:

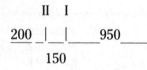

         II I
200 _|__|____950_____
        150

21. Several factors may contribute to the lack of representation of the 5′ end of the mRNA. One has to deal with the possibility that the reverse transcriptase may not completely synthesize the DNA from the RNA template. The other reason may be that the 3′ end of the copied DNA tends to fold back on itself, thus providing a primer for the DNA polymerase. Additional preparation of the cDNA requires some digestion at the folded region. Since this folded region corresponds to the 5′ end of the mRNA, some of the message is often lost.

22. Option (b) fits the expectation because the thick band in the offspring probably represents the bands at approximately the same position in both parents. The likelihood of such a match is expected to be low in the general population.

23. (a) Starting with zero at the top, the various patterns tell us that there is an E site at 1000 bp because a new E site was brought in by the *Drosophila* fragment. By comparing the lanes of the double digests, one can see that there is an A site at 500 bp and a B site at 2500 bp. For the 2000 bp band of the E + B double digest, there are actually two fragments.

(b) Notice that the probe hybridizes consistently to the 2000 bp fragment between the A and B restriction sites, so the *rosy* gene is somewhere in that region.

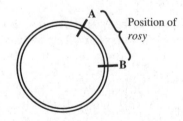

24. Assuming that one has knowledge of the amino acid sequence of the protein product or the nucleotide sequence of the target nucleic acid, a degenerate set of DNA strands can be made that can be prepared for cloning into an appropriate vector or amplified by PCR. A variety of labeling techniques can then be used, through hybridization, to identify complementary base sequences contained in the genomic library. One must know at least a portion of the amino acid sequence of the protein product or its nucleic acid sequence in order for the procedure to be applied. Some problems can occur through degeneracy in the genetic code (not allowing construction of an appropriate probe), the possible existence of pseudogenes in the library (hybridizations with inappropriate related fragments in the library), and variability of DNA sequences in the library due to introns (causing poor or background hybridization). To overcome some of these problems, one can construct a variety of relatively small probes of different types that take into account the degeneracy in the code. By varying the conditions of hybridization (salt and temperature) one can reduce undesired hybridizations.

25. Taking the number of bases recognized by *Bam*HI as 6, there would be approximately 4096 base pairs between sites. Given that lambda DNA contains approximately 48,500 base pairs, there would be about 11.8 sites (48,500/4096).

26. (a) Heating to 90–95°C denatures the double-stranded DNA so that it dissociates into single strands. It usually takes about five minutes, depending on the length and GC content of the DNA.

(b) Lowering the temperature to 50–70°C allows the primers to bind to the denatured DNA.

(c) Bringing the temperature to 70–75°C allows the heat-stable DNA polymerase an opportunity to extend the primers by adding nucleotides to the 3′ ends of each growing strand. Each PCR is designed with specific temperatures (not ranges) based on the characteristics of the DNAs (template and primers).

27. *Taq* polymerase is from a bacterium called *Thermus aquaticus*, which typically lives in hot springs. It is heat stable like some other enzymes used in PCR that are isolated from thermal vents in the ocean floor.

28. ddNTPs are analogs of the "normal" deoxyribonucleotide triphosphates (dNTPs), but they lack a 3′-hydroxyl group. As DNA synthesis occurs, the DNA polymerase occasionally inserts a ddNTP into a growing DNA strand. Since there is no 3′-hydroxyl group, chain elongation cannot take place and resulting fragments are formed, which can be separated by electrophoresis. Where the ddNTP was incorporated, the length of each strand, and therefore the position of the particular ddNTP, is established and used to eventually provide the base sequence of the DNA.

29. It is likely that the DNA that served as the template in the sequencing reaction was not pure so that at the same position (length) more than one type of ddNTP could be incorporated. This could be due to natural polymorphisms, often called single-nucleotide polymorphisms (or SNPs) or impure samples.

30. (a) Restriction endonucleases cut DNA reproducibly at given recognition sequences. The frequency that a given sequence appears in the DNA is dependent on the frequency of each base and the complexity (length) of the sequence. If all bases are equally frequent, the longer the sequence, the less frequent a cut will occur.

(b) Identity of the restriction sites is determined by the restriction enzyme used. There are two methods for determining the location of restriction sites. First, if the sequence is known, one could sequence the DNA of interest and search for the recognition sites. Second, one could electrophorese the DNA fragments produced by restriction and then align the sites in order based on the sizes of the restriction fragments. Both double and partial digestions are required.

(c) Northern and western blots are often used to detect the production of RNA and protein, respectively, from particular sources. Such products usually indicate the expression of different sets of genes in different tissues and cells. RNA profiles can also be detected by PCR and microarray analysis.

(d) Bacterial artificial chromosomes (BACs) contain F factor genes for replication and copy number, at least one selectable marker, and a polylinker that is flanked by promoter sequences that can be used to generate RNA molecules for expression and characterization of the cloned segment. A yeast artificial chromosome (YAC) has telomeres, an origin of replication, a centromere, selectable markers, and restriction recognition sequences for insertion of foreign DNA. Artificial chromosomes are constructed by recombining various segments using recombinant DNA technology.

(e) To be amplified by PCR, DNA is first denatured by relatively high temperature. Specificity of amplification depends on the association (annealing) of specific primers to or flanking a target DNA. Once the primers are annealed, they are extended using a heat-stable DNA polymerase. Repeated 25–35 times yields millions to billions of copies of the target DNA.

31. (a) The overall size of the fragment is 12 kb. From the A + N digest, sites A and N must be 1 kb apart. N must be 2 kb from an E site. Pattern #5 is the likely choice. Notice that digest A + N breaks up the 6 kb E fragment.

(b) By drawing lines though sections that hybridize to the probe, one can see that the only place of consistent overlap to the probe is the 1 kb fragment between A and N.

32. $T_m(°C) = 81.5 + 0.41(\%GC) - (675/N) = 81.5 + 0.41(33.3) - (675/21) =$ about 63°C. Subtracting 5°C gives us a good starting point of about 58°C for PCR with this primer. Notice that as the % of GC and length increase, the $T_m(°C)$ increases. GC pairs contain three hydrogen bonds rather than two as between AT pairs.

33. Notice that the middle "integration, excision, and recombination" region is related to the lysogenic process in λ. If one wanted to clone a gene, integration and related activities associated with lysogeny would be undesirable. Progeny phage generation and lysis would be desirable outcomes of a cloning experiment.

34. Applying the following formula with the concentrations of Na^+ and formamide in the table gives the following T_m.

$$T_m = 81.5 + 16.6(\log M[Na^+]) + 0.41(\%G + C) - 0.72(\%F)$$

(a)

MNa^+	% Formamide(F)	T_m
0.825	20	84.16
0.825	40	69.76
0.165	20	72.56
0.165	40	58.16

(b) Sodium, a monovalent cation, interacts with the negative phosphates that make up the nucleic acid backbone. The repulsive forces between negative phosphates are reduced, and the double helix becomes more stable, therefore requiring a higher temperature for melting. Formamide competes for hydrogen bond locations of the bases and lessens the attractions that hold each double helix together. As the competition for hydrogen bonding increases with increased formamide, the lower the melting temperature.

35. By examining the equations in Questions 32 and 34 it is clear that a variety of factors influence T_m and therefore annealing of primers with DNA. Primers with different percentages of GC and/or length will have different annealing temperatures. To factor these variables into a single T_m given a number of other factors (divalent and monovalent cation concentrations, primer and target concentrations) has, to date, been a complex problem that is often unresolvable.

36. (a) Short tandem repeats of the Y chromosome (Y-STRs) vary considerably among individuals and populations. By amplifying Y-STRs by PCR and separating the amplified products by electrophoresis, one can genotypically type an individual as one does with a standard fingerprint. Because tissue samples are often left at the scene of a violent crime, DNA fingerprints are sometimes more available than standard fingerprints. Linking an individual with the time and place of a significant event has multiple forensic applications. Eliminating an individual as a suspect also has important forensic applications.

(b) The nonrecombining region of the Y is maintained strictly in the male population. Of special relevance in forensic applications would be the elimination of half the population (females) from a suspect group.

(c) Because different ethnic groups show different levels of Y-STR polymorphism, different final probabilities occur as products of individual probabilities. Since these probabilities are used to match individuals in forensics, ethnic variations must be taken under consideration.

(d) While DNA samples have many potential uses, generally a "match" is determined by multiplying the occurrence probabilities of each haplotype to arrive at the overall probability (product) of a genotype occurring in a population. If an individual's genotype matches that found in DNA at a crime scene, depending on the frequencies of the haplotypes, one might be able to say that the individual was at the crime scene. However, contamination, inappropriate genotyping, and laboratory expertise may give both false-positive or negative results. Identical twins will have identical DNA fingerprints and may complicate forensic applications.

Chapter 14: The Genetic Code and Transcription

Concept Areas	Corresponding Problems
Genetic Code	1, 5, 9, 10, 12, 13, 14, 15, 16, 17, 26
Deciphering the Code	3, 4, 6, 7, 8, 11, 26, 28
Characteristics of the Code	2, 5, 6, 14, 16, 27, 29, 30
Information Flow	18, 19, 20, 21, 22, 23, 31
RNA Structure and Function	14, 16, 32, 33, 34
RNA Processing	24, 25, 35

Vocabulary: Organization and Listing of Terms and Concepts

Structures and Substances

Codon

  triplet

Messenger RNA

  *r*II, β cistron

Proflavin

Phage T4

Strain B of *E. coli*

Strain K12 of *E. coli*

Tobacco mosaic virus (TMV)

  adaptor molecule

Polynucleotide phosphorylase

  random assembly of nucleotides

Homopolymer codes

  RNA homopolymers

  RNA heteropolymers

   anticodon

N-formylmethionine (fmet)

Ribosome

RNA polymerase

  holoenzyme

  (α, β, β′, σ)

  consensus sequences

Pribnow box (-10) TATA

-35 region

  termination factor (rho)

Messenger RNA (mRNA)

  polycistronic mRNA

  monocistronic mRNA

RNA polymerase (eukaryotic) – I, II, III

  RNP II

  heterogeneous nuclear RNA (hnRNA)

  heterogeneous nuclear

  ribonucleoprotein (hnRNP)

  nucleoside triphosphates (NTPs)

  nucleoside monophosphates (NMPs)

  nucleotides

  promoters (promoter sequences)

Consensus sequences

  adenine and thymine richness

  cis-acting elements

  Goldberg-Hogness (-30, TATA box)

  CCAAT sequence

  enhancers

  trans-acting factors

  transcription factors

TATA-factor (TFIIA, B)

TATA-binding protein (TBP)

pre-mRNAs

split genes (intervening sequences)

  introns

  exons

  heteroduplexes

β-globin gene

ovalbumin gene

dystrophin

poly-A

cap (7mG)

  5′ to 5′

isoforms

Double-stranded RNA adenosine deaminase

ADAR (adenosine deaminase acting on RNA)

Processes/Methods

Transcription, translation

Frameshifts

Cell-free protein-synthesizing system

  ribosomes, tRNAs, amino acids, etc.

  artificial mRNAs

Triplet binding assay

Split genes

Overlapping genes

  multiple initiation

Transcription

  RNA polymerase II

    cleft, clamp

    active center

abortive transcription

  lid, pore

(mRNA, evidence for)

template binding

  template strand, partner strand

denaturation (unwinding)

DNA footprinting

initiation

chain elongation (5′ to 3′)

chain termination

gene amplification

RNA processing

  split genes

  posttranscriptional changes

    poly-A (3′), cap (5′)

  mechanisms

    rRNA self-excision (ribozyme)

    spliceosome

      snRNAs, snurps (snRNP)

    branch point

    alternative splicing

      isoform

RNA editing

  substitution

  insertion/deletion

  guide RNA (gRNA)

Concepts

Genetic code

  triplet codon

    frameshift mutations (r_{II})

    (+++)(− − −)

      nonsense triplets

Chapter 14 The Genetic Code and Transcription

codon assignments

   artificial mRNAs

   triplet binding assay

   repeating copolymers

  ordered codons

  confirmation of codon assignments

   MS2 sequencing

  colinearity

unambiguous

degenerate, wobble

  support for degenerate code

punctuation

  start, AUG, GUG (rare)

  stop, UAA, UAG, UGA

nonoverlapping

  support for nonoverlapping

code

universal, exceptions

ordered

Hypotheses

  adaptor molecule

  messenger RNA

  wobble hypothesis

   pattern of degeneracy

Information flow (F14.1)

  transcription

   primary transcript

   an intermediate molecule

   RNA polymerases (I, II, III)

  translation (F14.2)

gene amplification

RNA splicing

  beta-globin gene

  ovalbumin gene

  pro-α-2(I) collagen

  mechanisms

Alternative splicing, RNA editing

Comparisons (eukaryotic, **prokaryotic**)

F14.1 Illustration of the processes, transcription, and translation, involved in protein synthesis. Such relationships are often called the Central Dogma.

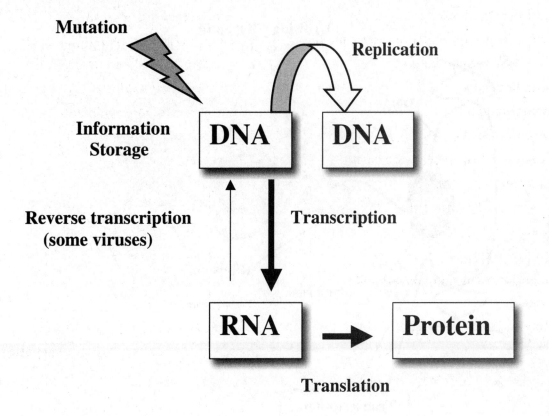

F14.2 Illustration of transcription in prokaryotes coupled with translation. Transcription involves production of RNA from a DNA template.

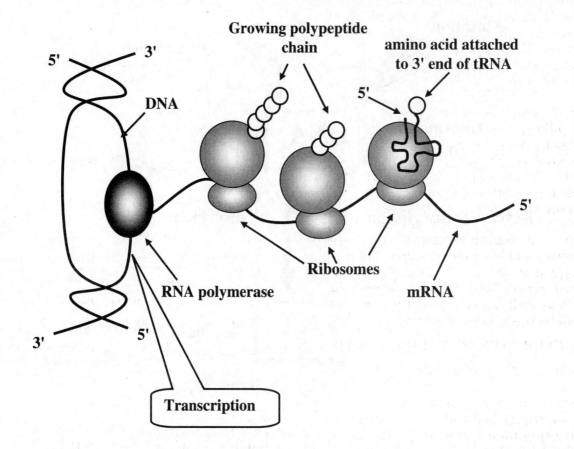

Solutions to Problems and Discussion Questions

1. In eukaryotes, protein synthesis occurs primarily in the cytoplasm, far from the location of DNA and the encoded information. In addition, while some of the basic amino acids would be able to associate directly with DNA, the acidic amino acids would be unable to do so. Thus, some sort of "adaptor" system was needed for DNA to direct amino acid assembly.

2. The reason (+++) or (− − −) restored the reading frame is that the code is triplet. By having the (+++) or (− − −), the translation system is "out of phase" until the third "+" or "−" is encountered. If the code contained six nucleotides (a sextuplet code), then the translation system is "out of phase" until the sixth "+" or "−" is encountered. In this case, the "out-of-phase" region would probably be longer and would likely cause more amino acid alterations. Given a sextuplet code, restoration of the reading frames would only occur with the addition or loss of six nucleotides. Lay out a sequence such as

CATDOGPIGOWLCATDOGPIGOWLCAT. . .

and test this explanation.

3. (a) The way to determine the fraction of each triplet that will occur with a random incorporation system is to find the likelihood that each base will occur in each position of the codon (first, second, third), and then multiply the individual probabilities (fractions) for a final probability (fraction).

$$GGG = 3/4 \times 3/4 \times 3/4 = 27/64$$
$$GGC = 3/4 \times 3/4 \times 1/4 = 9/64$$
$$GCG = 3/4 \times 1/4 \times 3/4 = 9/64$$
$$CGG = 1/4 \times 3/4 \times 3/4 = 9/64$$
$$CCG = 1/4 \times 1/4 \times 3/4 = 3/64$$

$$CGC = 1/4 \times 3/4 \times 1/4 = 3/64$$
$$GCC = 3/4 \times 1/4 \times 1/4 = 3/64$$
$$CCC = 1/4 \times 1/4 \times 1/4 = 1/64$$

(b) Glycine:

GGG and one G_2C (adds up to 36/64)

Alanine:

one G_2C and one C_2G (adds up to 12/64)

Arginine:

one G_2C and one C_2G (adds up to 12/64)

Proline:

one C_2G and CCC (adds up to 4/64)

(c) With the wobble hypothesis, variation can occur in the third position of each codon.

Glycine:	GGG, GGC
Alanine:	CGG, GCC, CGC, GCG
Arginine:	GCG, GCC, CGC, CGG
Proline:	CCC.CCG

4. Assume that you have introduced a copolymer (ACACACAC. . .) to a cell-free protein-synthesizing system. There are two possibilities for establishing the reading frames: ACA, if one starts at the first base, and CAC, if one starts at the second base. These would code for two different amino acids (ACA = threonine; CAC = histidine) and would produce repeating polypeptides that would alternate *thr-his-thr-his*. . . or *his-thr-his-thr*. . . .

Because of a triplet code, a trinucleotide sequence will, once initiated, remain in the same reading frame and produce the same code all along the sequence regardless of the initiation site.

Given the sequence CUACUACUACUA, notice the different reading frames producing three different sequences, each containing the same amino acid.

Codons:	CUA	CUA	CUA	CUA...
Amino Acids:	leu	leu	leu	leu...
	UAC	UAC	UAC	UAC...
	tyr	tyr	tyr	tyr...
	ACU	ACU	ACU	ACU...
	thr	thr	thr	thr...

If a tetranucleotide is used, such as ACGUACGUACGU...

Codons:	ACG	UAC	GUA	CGU	ACG
Amino Acids:	thr	tyr	val	arg	thr
	CGU	ACG	UAC	GUA	CGU
	arg	thr	tyr	val	arg
	GUA	CGU	ACG	UAC	GUA
	val	arg	thr	tyr	val
	UAC	GUA	CGU	ACG	UAC
	tyr	val	arg	thr	tyr

Notice that the sequences are the same except that the starting amino acid changes.

5. The UUACUUACUUAC tetranucleotide sequence will produce the following triplets depending on the initiation point: UUA = leu; UAC = tyr; ACU = thr; CUU = leu. Notice that because of the degenerate code, two codons correspond to the amino acid leucine.

The UAUCUAUCUAUC tetranucleotide sequence will produce the following triplets depending on the initiation point: UAU = tyr; AUC = ile; UCU = ser; CUA = leu. Notice that, in this case, degeneracy is not revealed and all the codons produce unique amino acids.

6. From the repeating polymer ACACA..., one can say that threonine is either CAC or ACA. From the polymer CAACAA... with ACACA..., ACA is the only codon in common. Therefore, threonine would have the codon ACA.

7. As in the previous problem, the procedure is to find those sequences that are the same for the first two bases but that vary in the third base. Given that AGG = arg, then information from the AG copolymer indicates that AGA also codes for arg and GAG must therefore code for glu.

Coupling this information with that of the AAG copolymer, GAA must also code for glu and AAG must code for lys.

8. The basis of the technique is that if a trinucleotide contains bases (a codon) that are complementary to the anticodon of a charged tRNA, a relatively large complex is formed that contains the ribosome, the tRNA, and the trinucleotide. This complex is trapped in the filter, whereas the components by themselves are not trapped. If the amino acid on a charged, trapped tRNA is radioactive, then the filter becomes radioactive.

9. List the substitutions; then from the code table, apply the codons to the original amino acids. Select codons that provide single-base changes.

Original		*Substitutions*
threonine	$\longrightarrow$	*alanine*
<u>A</u>C(U, C, A, or G)		<u>G</u>C(U, C, A, or G)
glycine	$\longrightarrow$	*serine*
<u>G</u>G(U or C)		<u>A</u>G(U or C)
isoleucine	$\longrightarrow$	*valine*
<u>A</u>U(U, C or A)		<u>G</u>U(U, C or A)

10. Apply the most conservative pathway of change.

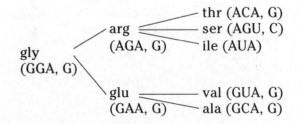

158

11. The enzyme generally functions in the degradation of RNA; however, in an *in vitro* environment, with high concentrations of the ribonucleoside diphosphates, the direction of the reaction can be forced toward polymerization. *In vivo*, the concentration of ribonucleoside diphosphates is low, and the degradative process is favored.

12. Because Poly U is complementary to Poly A, double-stranded structures will be formed. In order for an RNA to serve as a messenger RNA, it must be single-stranded, thereby exposing the bases for interaction with ribosomal subunits and tRNAs.

13. Applying the coding dictionary, the following sequences are "decoded":

Sequence 1: met-pro-asp-tyr-ser-(term)

Sequence 2: met-pro-asp-(term)

The 12th base (a uracil) is deleted from Sequence #1, thereby causing a frameshift mutation, which introduced a terminating triplet UAA.

14. (a)

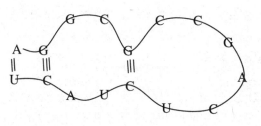

(b) TCCGCGGCTGAGATGA (use complementary bases, substituting T for U)

(c) GCU

(d) Assuming that the AGG. . . is the 5′ end of the mRNA, then the sequence would be

arg-arg-arg-leu-tyr

15. Given the sequence GGA, by changing each of the bases to the remaining three bases, then checking the code table, one can determine whether amino acid substitutions will occur.

G G A gly	G G U gly
U G A **term**	G G C gly
C G A **arg**	G G A gly
A G A **arg**	G G G gly
G U A **val**	U G U **cys**
G C A **ala**	C G U **arg**
G A A **glu**	A G U **ser**
G G U gly	G U U **val**
G G C gly	G C U **ala**
G G A gly	G A U **asp**

16. (a) Starting from the 5′ end and locating the AUG triplets, one finds two initiation sites leading to the following two sequences:

met-his-thr-tyr-glu-thr-leu-gly

met-arg-pro-leu-asp (or glu)

(b) In the shorter of the two reading sequences (the one using the internal AUG triplet), a UGA triplet was introduced at the second codon. While not in the reading frames of the longer polypeptide (using the first AUG codon), the UGA triplet eliminates the product starting at the second initiation codon.

17. By examining the coding dictionary, one will notice that the number of codons for each particular amino acid (synonyms) is directly related to the frequency of amino acid incorporation stated in the problem.

18. The central dogma of molecular genetics and, to some extent, all of biology states that DNA produces, through transcription, RNA, which is "decoded" (during translation) to produce proteins. See F14.2 for a graphic description.

19. Several observations indicated that a "messenger" molecule exists. First, DNA, the genetic material, is located in the nucleus of a eukaryotic cell, whereas protein synthesis occurs in the cytoplasm. DNA, therefore, does not directly participate in protein synthesis. Second, RNA, which is chemically similar to DNA, is synthesized in the nucleus of eukaryotic cells. Much of the RNA migrates to the cytoplasm, the site of protein synthesis. Third, there is generally a direct correlation between the amounts of RNA and protein in a cell. More direct support was derived from experiments showing that an RNA other than that found in ribosomes was involved in protein synthesis and, shortly after phage infection, an RNA species is produced that is complementary to phage DNA.

20. RNA polymerase from *E. coli* is a complex, large (almost 500,000 daltons) molecule composed of subunits ($\alpha,\beta,\beta',\sigma$) in the proportion $\alpha2,\beta,\beta'$, σ for the holoenzyme. The β subunit provides catalytic function, while the sigma (σ) subunit is involved in recognition of specific promoters. The core enzyme is the protein without the sigma.

21. Ribonucleoside triphosphates and a DNA template in the presence of RNA polymerase and a divalent cation (Mg^{++}) produce a ribonucleoside monophosphate polymer, DNA, and pyrophosphate (diphosphate). Equimolar amounts of precursor ribonucleoside triphosphates, and product ribonucleoside monophosphates and pyrophosphates (disphosphates) are formed. In *E. coli,* transcription and translation can occur simultaneously. Ribosomes add to the 5′ end nascent mRNA and progress to the 3′ end during translation. While transcription/translation can be "visualized" in the *E. coli* (F14.2), the predominant components "visualized" are the strings of ribosomes (polysomes).

22. While some folding (from complementary base pairing) may occur with mRNA molecules, they generally exist as single-stranded structures, which are quite labile. Eukaryotic mRNAs are generally processed such that the 5′ end is "capped" and the 3′ end has a considerable string of adenine bases. It is thought that these features protect the mRNAs from degradation. Such stability of eukaryotic mRNAs probably evolved with the differentiation of nuclear and cytoplasmic functions. Because prokaryotic cells exist in a more unstable environment (nutritionally and physically, for example) than many cells of multicellular organisms, rapid genetic response to environmental change is likely to be adaptive. To accomplish such rapid responses, a labile gene product (mRNA) is advantageous. A pancreatic cell, which is developmentally stable and exists in a relatively stable environment, could produce more insulin on stable mRNAs for a given transcriptional rate.

23. Apply complementary bases, substituting U for T:

(a)

Sequence 1: 3′-GAAAAAACGGUA-5′

Sequence 2: 3′-UGUAGUUAUUGA-5′

Sequence 3: 3′-AUGUUCCCAAGA-5′

(b)

Sequence 1: *met-ala-lys-lys*

Sequence 2: *ser-tyr-(ter)*

Sequence 3: *arg-thr-leu-val*

(c) Apply complementary bases:

3′-GAAAAAACGGTA-5′

24. The immediate product of transcription of an RNA destined to become an mRNA often involves modification of the 5′ end to which a 7-methylguanosine cap is added.

In addition, a stretch of as many as 250 adenylic acid residues is often added to the 3′ end after removal of an AAUAAA sequence. The vast majority of eukaryotic pre-mRNAs also contain intervening sequences that are removed, often in a variety of combinations, during the maturation process. In some organisms, RNA editing occurs in one of two ways: substitution editing where nucleotides are altered and insertion/deletion editing that changes the total number of bases.

Processing location	Example
5′-end	-addition of 7-mG
3′-end	-poly-A addition
internal	-removal of internal sequences
	-RNA editing
	-substitution
	-insertion/deletion

25. RNA editing falls into two general categories. Substitution editing occurs when individual nucleotide bases are altered. It is very common in mitochondrial and chloroplast RNAs as well as some nuclear-derived eukaryotic RNAs. Apolipoprotein B occurs in a long and short form, even though a single gene encodes both forms. The initial transcript is edited, which generates a stop codon that terminates the polypeptide at about half its length. The other category is insertion/deletion editing. The parasite that causes African sleeping sickness uses insertion/deletion editing of its mitochondrial RNAs in forming the initiation codon that then places the remaining sequence in proper reading frame.

26. (a) The triplet nature of the code was suggested because, given 20 amino acids, minimal use of the four DNA bases would require three bases per amino acid, thus providing 64 possible code words. The nonoverlapping nature of the code was suggested because of the limitations that an overlapping code would place on peptide sequences. In addition, with an overlapping code, single-nucleotide substitutions would often alter two adjacent amino acids, which was not observed in the mutant proteins examined at the time. The triplet, nonoverlapping nature of the code, along with other characteristics, were demonstrated primarily by studies on frameshift mutations in the *rII* locus of phage T4.

(b) An initial understanding about the composition (unordered) of codons came from homopolymer and heteropolymer RNA introduced into an *in vitro* system. Assays of the relative amino acid composition of resulting polypeptides indicated the composition of the bases in codons, but not their actual sequence.

(c) The specific sequences of the triplet codes were determined by the triplet binding assay and repeating copolymers of known sequence. When added to a cell-free system, a direct analysis of codon assignments was possible.

(d) Since the complete sequence of the RNA phage MS2 was known, scientists matched that sequence with protein products of MS2 that supported the code as derived from previous studies.

(e) Work with *E. coli* infected with phage showed that the synthesis of proteins was under the direction of newly synthesized RNA. Others were able to show that newly synthesized RNA formed during a phage infection of bacteria would hybridize only with phage DNA, thus demonstrating the dependence of RNA on the template nature of DNA.

(f) The most direct evidence for the presence of noncoding sequences in RNA and therefore the presence of split genes comes from hybridization experiments. When mature mRNAs are hybridized to DNA containing the genes specifying that mRNA, heteroduplexes form indicating that sequences in the DNA are not always represented in mRNA products. In addition, studies that compare the sequences of DNAs to their corresponding RNAs and proteins show that DNA often contains sequences that are not represented in RNA and protein products.

27. (a) Notice that the first two bases in the triplet code are common to more codons than the last base. If fewer amino acids were used in earlier times, perhaps the first two bases were primarily involved.

(b) Interestingly, all the amino acids mentioned as primitive use guanine as the first base in each codon. We might therefore suppose that the GNN configuration was the starting point of the present-day code. Within the GNN format, the second base is used to distinguish among the amino acids mentioned as primitive.

(c) Interestingly, the amino acids considered to be the most primitive are GNN coded, while the later-arriving amino acids are U(U,A,G)(U,C) coded. It would seem that some phenomenon could explain the differences in codon structure between primitive and late-arriving amino acids. The addition of new amino acids to the codon field was likely a slow and mutation-prone process. Did the addition of late-arriving amino acids displace earlier codon assignments, or were some of the late-arriving amino acids able to make use of codons that originally did not code for an amino acid? If this is the case, fewer and more restricted codon assignments would be available for late-arriving amino acids. Notice that each of the late-arriving amino acids have the same starting nucleotide as the present-day stop codons. Is it possible that what were once stop codons were used for late-arriving amino acids because this would be less disruptive to protein synthesis than displacing assignments at the time of their introduction? Much is left to be discovered regarding the structure of the genetic code.

28. First, compute the frequency (percentages would be easiest to compare) for each of the random codons.

For 4/5 C: 1/5 A:

$CCC = 4/5 \times 4/5 \times 4/5 = 64/125$ (51.2%)

$C_2A = 3(4/5 \times 4/5 \times 1/5) = 48/125$ (38.4%)

$CA_2 = 3(4/5 \times 1/5 \times 1/5) = 12/125$ (9.6%)

$AAA = 1/5 \times 1/5 \times 1/5 = 1/125$ (0.8%)

For 4/5 A: 1/5 C:

$AAA = 4/5 \times 4/5 \times 4/5 = 64/125$ (51.2%)

$A_2C = 3(4/5 \times 4/5 \times 1/5) = 48/125$ (38.4%)

$AC_2 = 3(4/5 \times 1/5 \times 1/5) = 12/125$ (9.6%)

$CCC = 1/5 \times 1/5 \times 1/5 = 1/125$ (0.8%)

Proline:	C_3 and one of the C_2A triplets
Histidine:	one of the C_2A triplets
Threonine:	one C_2A triplet and one A_2C triplet
Glutamine:	one of the A_2C triplets
Asparagine:	one of the A_2C triplets
Lysine:	A_3

29. (a) #1: *nonsense mutation*

#2: *missense mutation*

#3: *frameshift mutation*

(b) #1: mutation in third position to A or G

#2: change U to C in third triplet

#3: removal of a G in the UGG triplet (trp)

(c) termination

(d) All of the amino acids can be assigned specific triplets, including the third base of each triplet. Compare the sequences for the wild type and mutant #2. After removal of a G in the UUG triplet of tryptophan, the frameshift mutation shifts the first base of the following triplet to the third (often ambiguous) base of the previous triplet. The only tricky solution is with serine, which has six triplet possibilities, but it can still be resolved.

AUG UGG UAU CGU GGU AGU CCA ACA

(e) The mutation may be in a promoter or an enhancer, although many posttranscriptional alterations are possible. Depending on the gene and the organism, the mutation may be in an intron/exon splice site, and so on.

30. (a,b) Use the code table to determine the number of triplets that code each amino acid; then construct a graph and plot such as this one below:

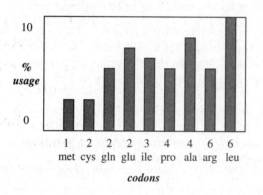

(c) There appears to be a weak correlation between the relative frequency of amino acid usage and the number of triplets for each.

(d) To continue to investigate this issue, one might examine additional amino acids in a similar manner. In addition, different phylogenetic groups use code synonyms differently. It may be possible to find situations in which the relationships are more extreme. One might also examine more proteins to determine whether such a weak correlation is stronger with different proteins.

31. Consider the following diagram representing the possibility described in the problem. If the promoter is not transcribed, as is the case of typical protein-coding genes, retrotransposition will produce a "daughter" *Alu* void of a promoter. Such an *Alu* would be a "dead-end" because it would not be capable of giving rise to its own *Alu* sequences. Perhaps an *Alu* sequence inserted 3′ to a promoter would produce daughters, but this would likely be rare.

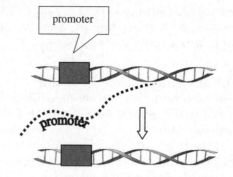

32.

(a)

gucccaaccaugcccaccgaucuuccgccugcuucuga
agAUGCGGGCCCAG

(b)

5′ gtc cca acc **atg** ccc acc gat ctt ccg cct gct
tct gaa gAT GCG GGC CCA G

(c)

5′ gtcccaaccatgcccaccgatcttccgcctgcttctgaag
ATG CGG GCC CAG

The two initiator codons are not in phase.

(d)

5′ gtc cca acc **atg** ccc acc gat ctt ccg cct gct
tct gaa gAT GCG GGC CCA G

            **met pro thr asp leu pro pro ala
ser glu asp ala gly pro**

5′ gtcccaaccatgcccaccgatcttccgcctgcttctgaag
ATG CGG GCC CAG

met arg ala gln

The amino acid sequences in the region of overlap are not the same.

(e) One might argue for the conservation of DNA by having the same region code for a multiple of products, and that might be the case in viruses and prokaryotes where genomic efficiency is more of an issue. However, eukaryotes appear to be much less likely to evolve strategies that conserve DNA sequences per se. However, if functionally and/or structurally related products can be conveniently regulated by such an arrangement, then perhaps an evolutionary advantage exists. The most obvious disadvantage is that if a mutation occurs in the common region, then two gene products are altered instead of one.

33. The advantage would be that if sequence homologies can be identified for a variety of HIV isolates, then perhaps a single or a few vaccines could be developed for the multitude of subtypes that infect various parts of the world. In other words, the wider the match of a vaccine to circulating infectives is, the more likely the efficacy. On the other hand, the more finely aligned a vaccine is to the target, the more likely it is that new or previously undiscovered variants will escape vaccination attempts.

34.

(a)

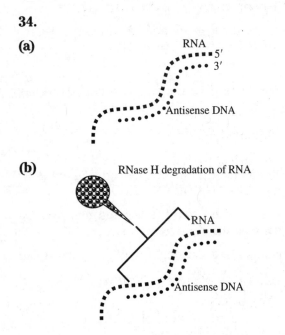

(b)

(c) Since the antisense strand is relatively short, under physiological conditions, nonspecific binding of the antisense strand to other RNAs in the cell may cause the degradation of nontargeted RNAs.

(d) Since the exact behavior of antisense DNA in a cell is not completely known, the answer to this question is elusive. However, given the complexity of intracellular events, it is likely that reduction of expression of a repressor gene group may induce other genes by eliminating such repressors.

(e) One of the major drawbacks to antisense therapy is the lack of specificity described here and the relatively unknown behavior of DNA oligodeoxynucleotides in living cells.

35. (a, b) Alternative splicing occurs when pre-mRNAs are spliced in more than one way to yield various combinations of exons in the final mRNA product. Upon translation of a group of alternatively spliced mRNAs, a series of related proteins, called isoforms, are produced. It is likely that alternative splicing evolved to provide a variety of functionally related proteins in a particular tissue from one original source. In other words, varieties of similar proteins can be produced by alternative splicing rather than by independent evolution.

Chapter 15: Translation and Proteins

Vocabulary: Organization and Listing of Terms and Concepts

Structures and Substances

Polypeptide, protein

Signal sequence

Chaperone

Ribosome

  monosome

rRNA

  5S, 16S, 23S RNA (single transcript)

    proteins

  5.8S, 18S, 28S RNA (single transcript)

    5S

    proteins

    tandem repeats and spacer DNA

    clustered on chromosomes: 13, 14, 15, 21, 22

    ribosomal proteins

Ribosome complex

  peptidyl (P site)

  aminoacyl (A site)

  exit (E site)

tunnel

peptidyl transferase

Transfer RNAs – tRNA

  75–90 nucleotides

  unusual bases

  cloverleaf model

  cognate amino acid

    anticodon, codon

    pCpCpA (3′)

    pG (5′)

  aminoacyl tRNA synthetases

    charging

    activated form

      (aminoacyladenylic acid)

    isoaccepting tRNAs

Initiation factors

  initiation complex

  Shine-Delgarno sequence

Formylmethionine (N-formylmethionine)

  tRNA^{fmet}

Elongation factors

GTP-dependent release factors

   termination (nonsense)

   stop codons UAA, UAG, UGA

Polyribosomes (polysomes)

  mRNA

Heterogeneous RNA (hnRNA)

  poly-A

  cap (7mG)

    5′ to 5′

  Kozak sequences

  5′-ACCAUGG

Inborn Errors of Metabolism

  alkaptonuria

    homogentisic acid

    (alkapton 2,5-dihydrophenylacetic acid)

  phenylketonuria

    phenylalanine hydroxylase

  Neurospora

  arginine

  citrulline

  ornithine

  sickle-cell anemia (trait)

    HbA, HbS, HbA$_2$

    heme group

    globin portion

Hemoglobin structure

  HbA, HbA$_2$, HbF

    α, β, δ, γ, ζ, ε

Amino acid

  carboxyl group

  amino group

  R (radical) group

  central carbon

  hydrophobic

  polar (hydrophilic)

    negative, positive

Peptide bond

Primary structure

Secondary structure

  α-helix

  β-pleated sheet

Tertiary structure

Quaternary structure

  collagen

  keratin

  actin, myosin

  immunoglobin

  transport proteins

    hemoglobin, myoglobin

  enzyme (active site)

  hormone, receptor

    anabolic, catabolic

      energy of activation

    protein domain

    LDL receptor protein

    epidermal growth factor

Processes/Methods

Transcription, translation

RNA processing

  posttranscriptional modification

Translation

  codon, anticodon

  tRNA charging

  aminoacyl tRNA synthetases

  chain initiation

chain elongation

translocation

chain termination, UAG, UAA, UGA

Simultaneous transcription and translation

(Prokaryotes, F15.1)

wobble hypothesis

Starch gel electrophoresis

Colinear relationships

Exon shuffling

Post-translational modification

protein targeting

modification, trimming

Concepts

Information flow

Transcription, translation (F15.1)

Comparisons (eukaryotic, prokaryotic)

One-gene: one-enzyme hypothesis

One-gene: one-protein

One-gene: one-polypeptide chain

Pathway analysis

Colinearity, protein structure

Post-translational modification

Structure/function relationships

Intron-early

Intron-late

F15.1 Polarity constraints associated with simultaneous transcription and translation in prokaryotes. The RNA polymerase is moving downward (arrow) in this sketch.

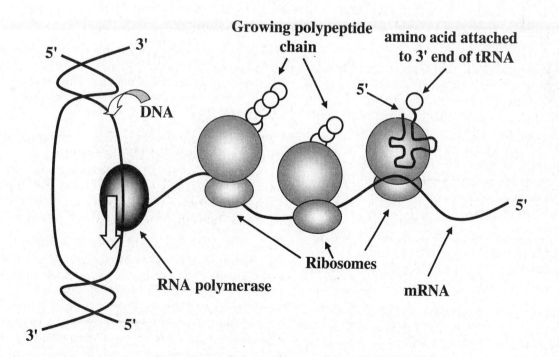

Solutions to Problems and Discussion Questions

1. A functional polyribosome will contain the following components: mRNA, charged tRNA, large and small ribosomal subunits, elongation and perhaps initiation factors, peptidyl transferase, GTP, Mg^{++}, nascent proteins, and possibly GTP-dependent release factors.

2. Transfer RNAs are "adaptor" molecules in that they provide a way for amino acids to interact with sequences of bases in nucleic acids. Amino acids are specifically and individually attached to the 3' end of tRNAs, which possess a three-base sequence (the anticodon) that can base-pair with three bases of mRNA (codons). Messenger RNA, on the other hand, contains a copy of the triplet codes, which are stored in DNA. The sequences of bases in mRNA interact, three at a time, with the anticodons of tRNAs.

Enzymes involved in transcription include the following: RNA polymerase (*E. coli*) and RNA polymerase I, II, III (eukaryotes). Those involved in translation include the following: aminoacyl tRNA synthetases, peptidyl transferase, and GTP-dependent release factors.

3. It was reasoned that there would not be sufficient affinity between amino acids and nucleic acids to account for protein synthesis. For example, acidic amino acids would not be attracted to nucleic acids. With an adaptor molecule, specific hydrogen bonding could occur between nucleic acids, and specific covalent bonding could occur between an amino acid and a nucleic acid tRNA.

4. The sequence of base triplets in mRNA constitutes the sequence of codons. A three-base portion of the tRNA constitutes the anticodon.

5. Since three nucleotides code for each amino acid, there would be 423 code letters (nucleotides), 426 including a termination codon. This assumes that other features, such as the polyA tail, the 5' cap, and noncoding leader sequences, are omitted.

6. Dividing 20 by 0.34 gives the number of nucleotides (about 59) occupied by a ribosome. Dividing 59 by 3 gives the approximate number of triplet codes, approximately 20.

7. The steps involved in tRNA charging are outlined in the text. An amino acid in the presence of ATP, Mg^{++}, and a specific aminoacyl synthetase produces an amino acid-AMP enzyme complex (+ PP$_i$). This complex interacts with a specific tRNA to produce the aminoacyl tRNA.

8. The four sites in tRNA that provide for specific recognition are the following: attachment of the specific amino acid, interaction with the aminoacyl tRNA synthetase, interaction with the ribosome, and interaction with the codon (anticodon).

9. Phenylalanine is an amino acid that, like other amino acids, is required for protein synthesis. While too much phenylalanine and its derivatives will cause PKU in phenylketonurics, too little will restrict protein synthesis.

10. Both phenylalanine and tyrosine can be obtained from the diet. Even though individuals with PKU cannot convert phenylalanine to tyrosine, it is obtained from the diet.

11. Tyrosine is a precursor to melanin, skin pigment. Individuals with PKU fail to convert phenylalanine to tyrosine, and even though tyrosine is obtained from the diet, at the population level, individuals with PKU have a tendency for less skin pigmentation.

12. When an expectant mother resumes consuming phenylalanine as part of her diet, she subjects her baby to higher than normal levels of phenylalanine throughout its development. Since increased phenylalanine is toxic, many (approximately 90 percent) newborns are severely and irreversibly retarded at birth. Expectant mothers (who are genetically phenylketonurics) should return to a low-phenylalanine intake during pregnancy.

13. **(a)** In this cross, two gene pairs are operating because the F_2 ratio is a modification of a 9:3:3:1 ratio, which is typical of a dihybrid cross. If one assumes that homozygosity for either or both of the two loci gives white, then let strain *A* be *aaBB* and strain *B* be *AAbb*. The F_1 is *AaBb* and pigmented (purple). The typical F_2 ratio would be as follows:

9/16	*A_B_*	purple
3/16	*aaB_*	white
3/16	*A_bb*	white
1/16	*aabb*	white

If a pathway exists that has the following structure, then the genetic and biochemical data are explained.

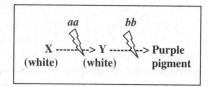

(b) For this condition, with the pink phenotype present, leave the symbols the same. However, change the Y compound such that when accumulated, a pink phenotype is produced:

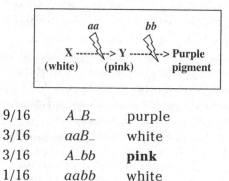

9/16	*A_B_*	purple
3/16	*aaB_*	white
3/16	*A_bb*	**pink**
1/16	*aabb*	white

14. The best way to approach these types of problems, especially when the data are organized in the form given, is to realize that the substance (supplement) that "repairs" a strain, as indicated by a (+), is *after* the metabolic block for that strain. In addition, and most important, the substance

that "repairs" the highest number of strains is either *the end product* or is *closest to the end product*.

Looking at the table, notice that the supplement tryptophan "repairs" all the strains. Therefore, it must be at the end of the pathway or at least after all the metabolic blocks (defined by each mutation). Indole "repairs" the next highest number of strains (3); therefore, it must be second from the end. Indole glycerol phosphate "repairs" two of the four strains, so it is third from the end. Anthranilic acid "repairs" the least number of strains, so it must be early (first) in the pathway.

Minimal medium is void of supplements, and mutant strains involving this pathway would not be expected to grow (or be "repaired"). The pathway, therefore, would be as follows:

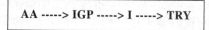

To assign the various mutations to the pathway, keep in mind that if a supplement "repairs" a given mutant, the supplement must be after the metabolic block. Applying this rationale to the above pathway, we see that the metabolic blocks are created at the following locations.

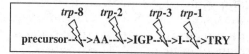

15. In general, the rationale for working with a branched chain pathway is similar to that stated in the previous problem. Since thiamine "repairs" each of the mutant strains, it must, as stated in the problem, be the final synthetic product.

Remembering the "one-gene: one-enzyme" statement, each metabolic block should only occur in one place, so even though pyrimidine and thiazole supplements each "repair" only one strain, they will not occupy the same step; rather, a branched pathway is suggested. Consider that pyrimidine and thiazole are products of distinct pathways and that both are needed to produce the end product, thiamine, as indicated in the following:

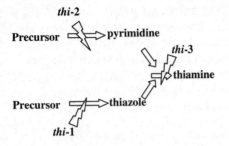

16. The fact that enzymes are a subclass of the general term *protein*, a *one-gene: one-protein* statement might seem to be more appropriate. However, some proteins are made up of subunits, each different type of subunit (polypeptide chain) being under the control of a different gene. Under this circumstance, the *one-gene: one-polypeptide* statement might be more reasonable.

It turns out that many functions of cells and organisms are controlled by stretches of DNA that either produce no protein product (operator and promoter regions, for example) or have more than one function as in the case of overlapping genes and differential mRNA splicing. A simple statement regarding the relationship of a stretch of DNA to its physical product is difficult to justify.

17. The electrophoretic mobility of a protein is based on a variety of factors, primarily the net charge of the protein and, to some extent, the conformation in the electrophoretic environment. Both are based on the type and sequence (primary structure) of the component amino acids of a protein.

The interactions (hydrogen bonds) of the components of the peptide bonds, hydrophobic, hydrophilic, and covalent interactions (as well as others) are all dependent on the original sequence of amino acids and take part in determining the final conformation of a protein. A change

in the electrophoretic mobility of a protein would therefore indicate that the amino acid sequence had been changed.

18. The following types of normal hemoglobin are presented in the text:

Hemoglobin	Polypeptide chains
HbA	$2\alpha2\beta$ (alpha, beta)
HbA$_2$	$2\alpha2\delta$ (alpha, delta)
HbF	$2\alpha2\gamma$ (alpha, gamma)
Gower 1	$2\zeta2\varepsilon$ (zeta, epsilon)

The *alpha* and *beta* chains contain 141 and 146 amino acids, respectively. The *zeta* chain is similar to the alpha chain, while the other chains are like the beta chain. Each chain represents a primary structure of amino acids connected by covalent peptide bonds. Secondary structures are determined by hydrogen bonding between components of the peptide bonds. Alpha helices and pleated sheets result. Tertiary structures are formed from interactions between the amino acid side chains, while the quaternary level results from the associations of chains shown above.

19. Sickle-cell anemia is coined a *molecular* disease because it is well understood at the molecular level; there is a base change in DNA, which leads to an amino acid change in the β chain of hemoglobin. It is a *genetic* disease in that it is inherited from one generation to the next. It is not contagious as might be the case of a disease caused by a microorganism. Diseases caused by microorganisms may not necessarily follow family blood lines, whereas genetic diseases do.

20. In the late 1940s, Pauling demonstrated a difference in the electrophoretic mobility of HbA and HbS (sickle-cell hemoglobin) and concluded that the difference had a chemical basis. Ingram determined that the chemical change occurs in the primary structure of the globin portion of the molecule using the fingerprinting technique. He found a change in the sixth amino acid in the β chain.

21. It is possible for an amino acid to change without changing the electrophoretic mobility of a protein under standard conditions. If the amino acid is substituted with an amino acid of like charge and similar structure, there is a chance that factors that influence electrophoretic mobility (primarily net charge) will not be altered. Other techniques such as chromatography of digested peptides may detect subtle amino acid differences.

22. One would expect individuals with HbC to suffer some altered hemoglobin function and perhaps be resistant to malaria as well. In fact, HbC homozygotes suffer mild hemolytic anemia (a benign hemoglobinopathy). The *HbC* gene is distributed particularly in malarial-infested areas, suggesting that some resistance to malaria is conferred. Recent studies indicate that HbC may be protective against severe forms of malaria, but not against more uncomplicated forms.

23. All of the substitutions involve one base change.

24. "Fine-mapping," meaning precise mapping of mutations *within* a gene, is possible in some phage systems because many recombinants can often be generated relatively easily. Having the precise intragenic location of mutations as well as the ability to isolate the products, especially mutant products, allows scientists to compare the locations of lesions within genes. Mutations occurring near the 5' end of a gene will produce proteins with defects near the N-terminus. In this problem, the lesions cause chain termination. Therefore, the nearer the mutations are to the 5' end of the mRNA, the shorter will be the polypeptide product

and thus demonstrate the colinear relationship of genes and proteins.

25. *Colinearity* refers to the sequential arrangement of subunits, amino acids, and nitrogenous bases in proteins and DNA, respectively. Sequencing of genes and products in MS2 phages and studies on mutations in the A subunit of the *tryptophan synthetase* gene indicate a colinear relationship.

26. Yanofsky's work on the *trp* A locus in bacteria involved the mapping of mutations and the finding that a relationship exists between the position of the mutation in a gene and the amino acid change in a protein. Work with the MS2 by Fiers showed, by sequencing of the coat protein (129 amino acids) and the gene (387 nucleotides), a linear relationship as predicted by the code word dictionary. Because Fiers showed a direct relationship between codons, amino acids, and punctuation (initiation and termination), one would consider it direct evidence for colinearity.

27. As stated in the text, the four levels of protein structure are the following:

Primary: the linear arrangement or sequence of amino acids. This sequence determines the higher level structures.

Secondary: α-helix and β-pleated sheet structures generated by hydrogen bonds between components of the peptide bond.

Tertiary: folding that occurs as a result of interactions between the amino acid side chains. These interactions include, but are not limited to, the following: covalent disulfide bonds between cysteine residues, interactions of hydrophilic side chains with water, and interactions of hydrophobic side chains with each other.

Quaternary: the association of two (dimer) or more polypeptide chains. Called *oligomeric*, such a protein is made up of more than one protein chain.

28. There are probably as many different types of proteins as there are different types of structures and functions in living systems. Your text lists the following:

Oxygen transport: hemoglobin, myoglobin

Structural: collagen, keratin, histones

Contractile: actin, myosin

Immune system: immunoglobins

Cross-membrane transport: a variety of proteins in and around membranes, such as receptor proteins

Regulatory: hormones, perhaps histones

Catalytic: enzymes

29. Enzymes function to regulate catabolic and anabolic activities of cells. They influence (lower) the *energy of activation,* thus allowing chemical reactions to occur under conditions that are compatible with living systems. Enzymes possess active sites and/or other domains that are sensitive to the environment. The active site is considered to be a crevice, or pit, which binds reactants, thus enhancing their interaction. The other domains mentioned above may influence the conformation and, therefore, function of the active site.

30. An exon often encodes a functional domain within a protein, rather than some random part of the protein. Exon shuffling hypothesizes that such an arrangement facilitates the mixing of domains. Evidence supporting exon shuffling comes from discoveries of DNA sequences related to functional domains of proteins that appear to have been recruited during evolution. In addition, the partial architectures of genes with respect to exons appear to be conserved but also modified as if altered by shuffling. The "intron-early" theory suggests that introns appeared early in evolution but were selected against. This model is supported by DNA sequence data whereby similar gene architecture is shared by distantly related species. The "intron-late" theory suggests that introns arose late in evolution with the origin of eukaryotes. The fact that introns are almost totally absent in prokaryotes and infrequent in yeast supports this view.

31. (a) The base sequences in tRNA suggested a cloverleaf secondary structure due to within-strand complementary base pairing. Such a model was later supported by X-ray crystallography and denaturation studies.

(b) When UAA, UGA, or UAG triplets occur at internal sites in genes, premature translation termination takes place and verifies the chain-terminating function of these triplets.

(c) Examination of nutritional mutations in *Neurospora* showed that upsets in metabolic pathways could result from mutant genes that segregated and assorted in typical fashion. In some cases, sufficient information was available to show that defective enzymes caused the metabolic upset. Thus, mutant genes must be responsible for the production of defective enzymes.

(d) Since enzymes are proteins, it is reasonable to conclude that genes make proteins. In addition, early work on hemoglobin showed that one gene was responsible for making one of the polypeptide chains in hemoglobin.

(e) A variety of experiments, ranging from sequencing of DNA and respective proteins to transformation and transfection experiments with known DNAs, directly confirm the genetic code.

(f) Mutations that alter the amino acid sequence of a protein often alter its structure and surface chemistry. Since phenotypes (functions) are altered by mutations, structural changes in proteins are usually accompanied by alterations in function. The classic example that demonstrates the structure/function relationship of proteins is the comparison between normal (HbA) and mutant (HbS) hemoglobin. An amino acid substitution alters the structure of HbS as well as its function.

32. One can conclude that the amino acid is not involved in recognition of the codon.

33. Even though three gene pairs are involved, notice that because of the pattern of mutations, each cross may be treated as monohybrid **(a)** or dihybrid **(b,c)**.

(a) F$_1$:   *AABbCC* = speckled

F$_2$: 3   *AAB_CC* = speckled

1   *AAbbCC* = yellow

(b) F$_1$:   *AABbCc* = speckled

F$_2$: 9   *AAB_C_* = speckled

3   *AAB_cc* = green

3   *AAbbC_* = yellow $\left.\begin{array}{c} \\ \end{array}\right\}4$

1   *AAbbcc* = yellow

(c) F$_1$:   *AaBBCc* = speckled

F$_2$: 9   *A_BBC_* = speckled

3   *A_BBcc* = green

3   *aaBBC_* = colorless $\left.\begin{array}{c} \\ \end{array}\right\}4$

1   *aaBBcc* = colorless

34. Because cross **(a, b)** is essentially a monohybrid cross, there would be no difference in the results if crossing over occurred (or did not occur) between the *A* and *B* loci.

35. With the codes for valine being GUU, GUC, GUA, and GUG, single-base changes from glutamic acid's GAA and GAG can cause the glu>>>val switch. The normal glutamic acid is a negatively charged amino acid, whereas valine carries no net charge and lysine is positively charged. Given these significant charge changes, one would predict some, if not considerable, influence on protein structure and function. Such changes could stem from internal changes in folding or interactions with other molecules in the RBC, especially other hemoglobin molecules.

36. (a) Outcomes from the last cross with its 9:4:3 ratio suggest two gene pairs.

(b) orange   =   *Y_R_*

yellow   =   *yyrr, yyR_*

red   =   *Y_rr*

(c) white —-> yellow — *y* -> red — *r* -> orange (pathway V)

37. A cross of the following nature would satisfy the data:

AABBCC   ×   *aabbcc*

Offspring in the F$_2$:

27	*A_B_C_*	= purple
9	*A_B_cc*	= pink
9	*A_bbC_*	= rose
9	*aaB_C_*	= orange
3	*A_bbcc*	= pink
3	*aaB_cc*	= pink
3	*aabbC_*	= rose
1	*aabbcc*	= pink

$$\text{pink} \xrightarrow{\;c\;} \text{rose} \xrightarrow{\;b\;} \text{orange} \xrightarrow{\;a\;} \text{purple}$$

The above hypothesis could be tested by conducting a backcross as given below:

AaBbCc   ×   *aabbcc*

The cross should give a

4(pink):2(rose):1(orange):1(purple) ratio

38.

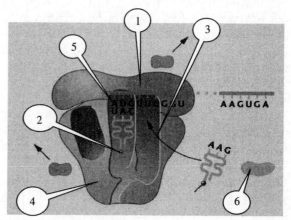

39.

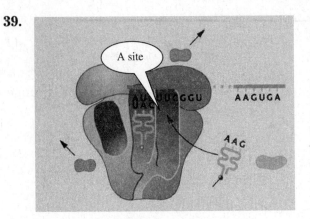

40. (a) Since protein synthesis is dependent on the passage of mRNA from DNA to ribosomes, any circumstance that compromises the flow will cause a reduction in protein synthesis. The more specific the binding of the antisense oligonucleotide to the target mRNA is, the more specific the influence on protein synthesis. The ideal situation would be where a particular species of antisense oligonucleotide impacted on one and only one protein population.

(b) Clearly, a length of around 15–16 nucleotides is most effective in causing RNA degradation.

(c) A number of factors, including length of the oligonucleotide, are probably involved *in vivo*. It is likely that stability of the oligonucleotide is dependent on its base composition and length. The oligonucleotide must be small enough to diffuse effectively throughout the cell in order to "locate" the targeted mRNA, and it must not assume a folded conformation, which blocks opportunities for base pairing.

Since the oligonucleotide is so much smaller than the target mRNA, it is also likely that the actual location of binding to the target is important in mRNA degradation. One of the main problems of antisense therapy is the introduction of the oligonucleotide into the interior of target cells.

41. (a) Considering the pedigree, it would appear that the gene is inherited as a dominant because to be recessive, all three individuals from outside the blood line would have to be heterozygous, an unlikely event. In addition, one would expect that a mutation in a tRNA synthetase would have considerable negative impact on glycine-bearing protein synthesis.

(b) On the other hand, because affected individuals in the pedigree are heterozygous, sufficient glycyl tRNA synthetase activity must be present to provide vital functions.

(c) Mutational and physiological perturbations, especially when occurring early in development, often cause neuropathologies. This is because of the highly sensitive nature of nerve cell development, and perhaps because axons are typically quite long, reduction of synthesis of glycine-bearing proteins inhibits required widespread distribution of such proteins within axons.

Chapter 16: Gene Mutation and DNA Repair

Concept Areas	Corresponding Problems
Overview	23
Mutations as Genetic Tools	1
Random and Adaptive Mutations	3, 4
Classes of Mutations	2, 6, 21
Detection of Mutations	15, 17, 30
Induced Mutations	19
Molecular Basis of Mutation	5, 7, 8, 9, 10, 11, 19, 21, 25, 27
Case Studies, Human Impact	13, 14, 16, 18, 19, 20, 22, 25, 26, 28, 29
Complementation	24
Repair of DNA	12, 27
UV Radiation and Skin Cancer	29

Vocabulary: Organization and Listing of Terms and Concepts

Structures and Substances

Somatic cells

Gamete-forming cells

  germ line

  gametes

  missense

5-Bromouracil

2-Amino purine

Acridine dyes

Acridine orange

Proflavin

Mustard gas

Ethylmethane sulfonate

6-Methylguanine

Apurinic site

ABO antigens

  H substance

  glycosyltransferase

Dystrophin

Pyrimidine dimers

FMR-1

uvr gene product

DNA polymerase I (*pol*A1)

AP endonuclease

DNA glycosylases

XPA, XPF, XPG

TFIIH

*rec*A

*lex*A

Photoreactivation enzyme

Adenine methylase

Heterokaryon

Processes/Methods

Variation by mutation

  adaptation hypothesis

    Luria-Delbruck fluctuation test

adaptive mutations

replication

repair errors

background radiation

cosmic sources

mineral sources

ultraviolet light

rates

induced

X rays

gametic, germ line

autosomal dominant

X-linked recessive

autosomal recessive

haploinsufficiency

loss-of-function

gain-of-function

null mutations

gene knockouts

neutral

somatic

Detection

bacteria and fungi

minimal medium

complete medium

prototrophs, auxotrophs

segregation (1:1)

humans

pedigree analysis

cell culture (*in vitro*)

molecular basis

direct sequencing of DNA

ABO antigens

H substance modification

muscular dystrophy

Duchenne muscular dystrophy

Becker muscular dystrophy

dystrophin

trinucleotide

reading frame hypothesis

fragile-X syndrome

repeats

myotonic dystrophy (DM)

chromosome 19

MDPK

(serine-threonine protein kinase)

Huntington disease

spinobulbar muscular dystrophy
(Kennedy disease)

Genetic anticipation

Ames test

Salmonella typhimurium

Molecular basis

base substitution or point mutations

transition

transversion

frameshift

tautomeric shifts (forms)

base analogs

5-bromouracil

2-amino purine

reverse mutation

alkylation

mustard gases

ethylmethane sulfonate

frameshift mutations

acridine dyes (acridines)

acridine orange

proflavin

apurinic sites

deamination

oxygen radicals

H_2O_2

OH^- (hydroxyl radical)

superoxide (O_2^-)

ultraviolet light

pyrimidine dimers

T-T

recA, lexA, uvr

SOS response

high-energy radiation

ionizing radiation

X rays

gamma radiation

cosmic radiation

free radicals

reactive ions

intensity of dose

roentgen

Repair

ultraviolet radiation (260 nm)

pyrimidine dimers

T-T, C-C, T-C

photoreactivation

photoreactivation enzyme (PRE)

excision repair

base excision repair (BER)

nucleotide excision repair (NER)

uvr gene product

DNA polymerase I

DNA ligase

AP endonuclease

DNA glycosylases

proofreading and mismatch repair

strand discrimination

DNA methylation

GATC sequence

mutH, L, S and *U*

postreplication repair

homologous recombinational repair

(also nonhomologous)

RAD52

double-stranded break repair (DSBR)

xeroderma pigmentosum (XP)

unscheduled DNA synthesis

photoreactivation enzyme

heterokaryon

somatic cell genetics

Concepts

Mutation

basis of organismic diversity (F16.1)

somatic, germ line (F16.2)

dominant autosomal

X-linked, autosomal recessive

morphological

nutritional or biochemical

behavioral

regulatory

lethal

conditional, temperature-sensitive

Sources

exogenous (environmental)

endogenous

spontaneous

Anticipation

Detection of mutations

Complementation

Molecular diversity of mutations

Mutation analysis of gene function

Repair

F16.1 Graphic representation of the relationship between mutation and Darwinian evolutionary theory. Mutation provides the original source of variation on which natural selection operates.

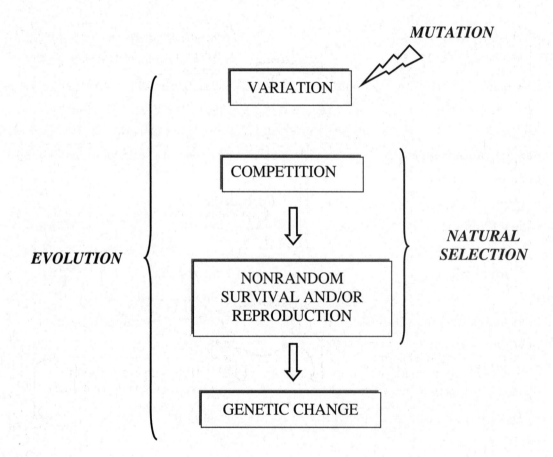

F16.2 Illustration of the difference between somatic and germ-line mutations. Somatic mutations are not passed to the next generation, whereas those in the germ line may be passed to offspring.

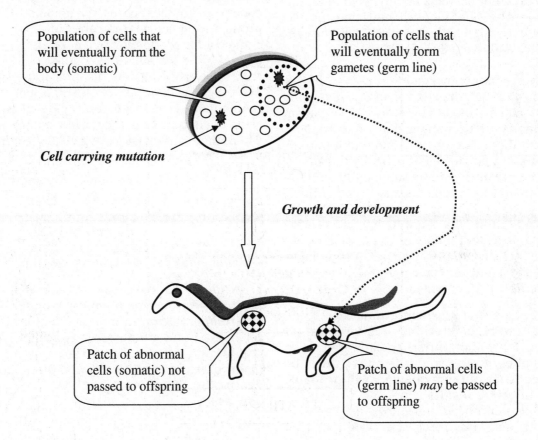

Solutions to Problems and Discussion Questions

1. Mutations are the "windows" through which geneticists look at the normal function of genes, cells, and organisms. When a mutation occurs, it allows the investigator to formulate questions as to the function of the normal allele of that mutation. For example, hemophilia is an inherited blood-clotting disease. Because there are three different inherited forms of the disease, two X-linked and one autosomal, all determined by nonallelic genes, one can say that at least three different proteins are involved in blood clotting. At a different level, mutations provide "markers" with which biologists can study the genetics and dynamics of populations.

2. When conducting genetic screens, one assumes that all the cells of an organism are genetically identical. Therefore, the organism responds to the screen-enabling detection of the mutation. Since a somatic mutation first appears in a single cell, it is highly unlikely that the organism will be sufficiently altered to respond to a screen because none of the other cells in that organism will have the same mutation. That's not to say that somatic mutations cannot influence the organism. Cancer cells generally originate from a single altered cell and can have a profound influence on the fate of an organism.

3. It is true that *most* mutations are thought to be deleterious to an organism. A gene is a product of perhaps a billion or so years of evolution, and it is only natural to suspect that random changes will probably yield negative results.

However, not *all* mutations may be deleterious. Those few, rare variations that are beneficial will provide a basis for possible differential propagation of the variation. Such changes in gene frequency represent the basis of the evolutionary process. See F16.1 in this book.

4. As stated in the previous question, a functional sequence of nucleotides, a gene, is likely to be the product of perhaps a billion or so years of evolution. Each gene

and its product function in an environment that has also evolved, or coevolved. A coordinated output of each gene product is required for life. Deviations from the norm, caused by mutation, are likely to be disruptive because of the complex and interactive environment in which each gene product must function. However, on occasion a beneficial variation occurs.

5. A diploid organism possesses at least two copies of each gene (except for "hemizygous" genes), and in most cases, the amount of product from one gene of each pair is sufficient for production of a normal phenotype. Recall that the condition of "recessive" is defined by the phenotype of the heterozygote. If output from one normal (nonmutant) gene in a heterozygote gives the same phenotype as in the normal homozygote, where there are two normal genes, the normal allele is considered "dominant."

	Phenotype, if mutant is:	
Genotypes	*recessive*	*dominant*
wild/wild	wild	wild
wild/mutant	wild	mutant
mutant/mutant	mutant	mutant

6. A *conditional* mutation is one that produces a wild-type phenotype under one environmental condition and a mutant phenotype under a different condition. A conditional *lethal* is a gene that under one environmental condition leads to premature death of the organism.

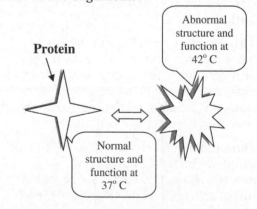

7. Watson and Crick recognized that various tautomeric forms, caused by single proton shifts, could exist for the nitrogenous bases of DNA. Such shifts could result in mutations by allowing hydrogen bonding of normally noncomplementary bases. As stated in the text, important tautomers involve keto-enol pairs for thymine and guanine, and amino-imino pairs for cytosine and adenine.

8. All three of the agents are mutagenic because they cause base substitutions. Deaminating agents oxidatively deaminate bases such that cytosine is converted to uracil and adenine is converted to hypoxanthine. Uracil pairs with adenine, and hypoxanthine pairs with cytosine.

Alkylating agents donate an alkyl group to the amino or keto groups of nucleotides, thus altering base-pairing affinities. 6-ethyl guanine acts like adenine, thus pairing with thymine. Base analogs such as 5-bromouracil and 2-amino purine are incorporated as thymine and adenine, respectively, yet they base pair with guanine and cytosine, respectively.

9. Frameshift mutations are likely to change more than one amino acid in a protein product because as the reading frame is shifted, new codons are generated. In addition, there is the possibility that a nonsense triplet could be introduced, thus causing premature chain termination. If a single pyrimidine or purine has been substituted, then only one amino acid is influenced.

10. X rays are of higher energy and shorter wavelength than UV light. They have greater penetrating ability and can create more disruption of DNA.

11. The delay or arrest of cell division provides an opportunity for normal DNA repair mechanisms to operate. Apoptosis is an organismic survival mechanism that eliminates a cell and its descendants, which may eventually harm the organism.

12. *Photoreactivation* can lead to repair of UV-induced damage. An enzyme, photoreactivation enzyme, will absorb a photon of light to cleave thymine dimers.

Excision repair involves the products of several genes, DNA polymerase I and DNA ligase, to clip out the UV-induced dimer, fill in, and join the phosphodiester backbone in the resulting gap. The excision repair process can be activated by damage that distorts the DNA helix.

Recombinational repair is a system that responds to DNA that has escaped other repair mechanisms at the time of replication. If a gap is created on one of the newly synthesized strands, a "rescue operation or SOS response" allows the gap to be filled. Many different gene products are involved in this repair process: *rec*A and *lex*A. In SOS repair, the proofreading by DNA polymerase III is suppressed, and this therefore is called an "error-prone system."

13. Because mammography involves the use of X rays and X rays are known to be mutagenic, it has been suggested that frequent mammograms may do harm. This subject is presently under considerable debate. At the 2002 World Health Organization conference in Barcelona, Spain, the conclusion was that "mammograms can prevent breast cancer deaths in one in 500 women ages 50 to 69."

14. Each involves a ballooning of trinucleotide repeats. See the text for a detailed description of the role of trinucleotide repeats in a variety of human diseases. Genetic anticipation is the occurrence of an earlier age of onset of a genetic disease in successive generations.

15. In the *Ames assay*, the compound to be tested is incubated with a mammalian liver extract to simulate an *in vivo* environment. This solution is then placed on culture plates with an indicator microorganism, *Salmonella typhimurium*, which is defective in its normal repair processes. The frequency of mutations in the tester strains is an indication of the mutagenicity of the compound.

16. *Xeroderma pigmentosum* is a form of human skin cancer caused by perhaps several rare autosomal genes, which interfere with the repair of damaged DNA. Studies with heterokaryons provided evidence for complementation, indicating that as many as seven different genes may be involved.

The photoreactivation repair enzyme appears to be involved. Since cancer is caused by mutations in several types of genes, interfering with DNA repair can enhance the occurrence of these types of mutations.

17. Given that the cells were treated, then allowed to complete one round of replication, the final computation of the mutation rate should be divided by two (two cells are plated for each cell treated). The general expression for the mutation rate is the number of mutant cells divided by the total number of cells. In this case, the equation would be as follows:

$$\frac{18 \times 10^1}{6 \times 10^7}$$

$$\text{or} \quad 3 \times 10^{-6}$$

Now dividing by two (as stated above) gives

$$1.5 \times 10^{-6}$$

18. It is possible that through the reduction of certain environmental agents that cause mutations, mutation rates might be reduced. On the other hand, certain industrial and medical activities actually concentrate mutagens (radioactive agents and hazardous chemicals). Unless human populations are protected from such agents, mutation rates might actually increase. If one asks about the accumulation of mutations (not rates) in human populations as a result of improved living conditions and medical care, then it is likely that as the environment becomes less harsh (through improvements), more mutations will be tolerated as selection pressure decreases. In addition, as individuals live longer and have children at a later age, some studies indicate that older males accumulate more gametic mutations.

19. Any agent that inhibits DNA replication, either directly or indirectly, through mutation and/or DNA crosslinking, will suppress the cell cycle and may be useful in cancer therapy. Since guanine alkylation often leads to mismatched bases, they can often be repaired by a variety of mismatched repair mechanisms. However, DNA crosslinking can be repaired by recombinational mechanisms; thus, for such agents to be successful in cancer therapy, suppressors of DNA repair systems are often used in conjunction with certain cancer drugs. See: Wang, Z., et al. 2001. *J Nat'l Cancer Inst.* 93(19):1434–436.

20. Both major forms of muscular dystrophy include muscular wasting of differing severity and age of onset. Both forms are caused by mutations in the *dystrophin* gene, which is very large, composed of 97 exons and 2.6 Mb. Given the size of this gene and the number of exons/introns, many opportunities exist for mutational upset. Interestingly, the severity of the phenotype is not always connected with the size of a deleted segment. What seems to be quite important in determining expression is whether a frameshift is introduced. See: http://compbio.berkeley.edu/people/ed/rust/Dystrophin.html.

21. Replication slippage is a process that generates small deletions and insertions during DNA replication. While it can occur anywhere in the genome, it is most prevalent in regions already containing repeated sequences. Thus, repeated sequences are hypermutable.

22. An unexpected mutant gene may enter a pedigree in several ways. If a gene is incompletely penetrant, it may be present in a population and only express itself under certain conditions. It is unlikely that the gene for hemophilia behaved in this manner. If a gene's expression is suppressed by another mutation in an individual, it is possible that offspring may inherit a given gene and not inherit its suppressor. Such offspring would have hemophilia. Since all genetic variations must arise at some point, it is possible that the mutation in the Queen Victoria family was new, arising in the father.

Lastly, is it possible that the mother was heterozygous and by chance, no other individuals in her family were unlucky enough to receive the mutant gene.

23. (a) When no known agents are involved and a mutation occurs and there is no indication of a mutation in the "family line," that mutation is considered to have arisen spontaneously.

(b) Numerous studies, beginning with those of Muller (1927) and Stadler (1928), showed that the occurrence of mutations could be associated with X rays. Since that time, various chemicals and radiation have been tested by a number of screening strategies. When the frequency of mutation in a test organism increases after exposure to a given agent, that agent is classified as a mutagen.

(c) In addition to postreplication, SOS, photoreactivation, and excision repair, various proofreading functions have been discovered in polymerases. Each has provided evidence that many mutations, once generated, may trigger repair.

24. Unscheduled DNA synthesis represents DNA repair. One can determine complementation groupings by placing each heterokaryon giving a "–" into one group and those giving a "+" into a separate group. For instance, *XP1* and *XP2* are placed in the same group because they do not complement each other. However, *XP1* and *XP5* do complement ("+"); therefore, they are in different groups. Completing such pairings allows one to determine the following grouping:

XP1	*XP4*	*XP5*
XP2		*XP6*
XP3		*XP7*

The groupings (complementation groups) indicate that at least three "genes" form products necessary for unscheduled DNA synthesis. All of the cell lines that are in the same complementation group are defective in the same product.

25. (a) (1). When a region of DNA contains repeated segments, it is possible that the alignment of these segments may be offset

as pictured below. Should there be a crossover between the elements within a segment, shortening and lengthening of the segments can occur. (*Note:* Both of the figures below were obtained from http://biol.lf1.cuni.cz/ucebnice/en/repetitive_dna.htm.)

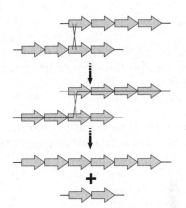

(2). When a loop forms because of within-strand base pairing of complementary repeats within a repetitive segment, it provides an opportunity for the polymerase to add repeats by continuing to replicate beyond the loop as shown below.

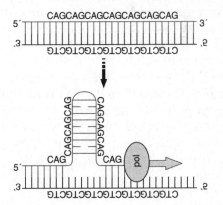

(b) A variety of regulatory signals occur both upstream and downstream from the coding regions of genes. Repeats often upset such regulatory signals. Although introns are normally removed from RNAs during maturation, repeats with introns may upset the splicing process or may actually influence regulatory sequences that are contained in introns.

(c) The coding region of a gene specifies a sequence of amino acids in a protein. Having a stretch of repetitive amino acids, even if short, may have a profound influence on protein function. Trinucleotide repeat expansion probably occurs to the same degree within and outside exons, but there is stronger selection against protein sequence changes. Changes in upstream and downstream sequences would also be significantly influenced by repeat expansion and be selected against.

26. The cystic fibrosis gene produces a complex membrane transport protein that contains several major domains: a highly conserved ATP binding domain, two hydrophobic domains, and a large cytoplasmic domain, which probably serves in a regulatory capacity. The protein is like many ATP-dependent transport systems, some of which have been well studied. When a mutation causes clinical symptoms, fluid secretion is decreased and dehydrated mucus accumulates in the lungs and air passages. Mutations that radically alter the structure of the protein (frameshift, splicing, nonsense, deletions, duplications, etc.) would probably have more influence on protein function than those that cause relatively minor amino acid substitutions, although this generalization does not always hold true. A protein with multiple functional domains would be expected to react to mutational insult in a variety of ways.

27. (a) For those organisms that generate energy by aerobic respiration, a process occurs that involves the reduction of molecular oxygen. Partially reduced species are produced as intermediates and by-products of such molecular action: O_2^-, H_2O_2, and OH^-. These species are potent electrophilic oxidants that escape mitochondria and attack numerous cellular components. Collectively, these are called reactive oxygen species (ROS).

(b)

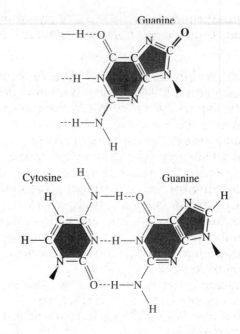

When casually examining the structures in the above diagrams, it is not immediately obvious that oxoG:A pairs should occur. However, hydrogen bonding can occur to any other base, including self pairs. Homopurine (A:A, G:G) and heteropurine (A:G) pairs represent anomalous base-pairing possibilities even with nonaltered bases. While G:C is undoubtedly the most stable, several mispairs are actually stronger than the A-T pair.

Base pairing is complicated by the fact that the purines possess two H-bonding faces: the Watson-Crick face, involving ring positions 1 and 6 for adenine and 1, 2, and 6 for guanine, and the Hoogsteen face involving ring positions 6 and 7. The typical pairing mode is indicated as *wc* where pairing occurs on the Watson-Crick face in the normal orientation, even for the mispair A:G. Alteration of pairing and favoring of the Hoogsteen face can occur with oxoGuanine. Indeed, triple helix configurations commonly involve the Hoogsteen face.

(c) If not repaired (see below), the first round of replication involves the pairing of oxoG to adenine (see above), while in the next round of replication, adenine pairs with

184

its normal thymine. Therefore, if one starts with a G:C pair, one ends up with an A:T pair.

(d) It turns out that G:G>T:A transversions are quite commonly found in human cancers and are especially prevalent in the tumor-suppressor gene *p53*. Thus, the cellular defense system has been extensively studied. One component is a triphosphatase that cleanses the nucleotide precursor pool by removing the two outermost phosphates from oxo-dGTP. Another involves a DNA glycosylase that initiates repair of misreplicated oxoG:A by hydrolyzing the glycosidic bond linking the adenine base to the sugar. Another is a DNA gycosylase/lyase system that recognizes oxoG opposite cytosine. Of the three systems, the DNA glycosylases are probably the most effective.

28. Nonsense mutation in coding regions: shortened product somewhat less than 375 amino acids depending on where the chain termination occurred. Insertion in Exon 1, causing frameshift: a variety of amino acid substitutions, and possible chain termination downstream. Insertion in Exon 7, causing frameshift: a variety of amino acid substitutions, and possible chain termination downstream involving less of the protein than the insertion in Exon 1. Missense mutation: an amino acid substitution. Deletion in Exon 2, causing frameshift: depending on the size of the deletion, a few too many amino acids may be missing. The frameshift would cause additional amino acid changes and possible termination. Deletion in Exon 2, in frame: amino acids missing from Exon 2 without additional changes in the protein. Large deletion covering Exons 2 and 3: significant loss of amino acids toward the N-terminal side of the protein.

29. Individuals with *xeroderma pigmentosum (XP)* are much more likely to contract skin cancer in youth than non-XP individuals. By age 20, approximately 80 percent of the XP population has skin cancer compared with approximately 4 percent in the non-XP group. XP individuals lack one or more genes involved in DNA repair.

30. (a, b, c) Although a positive Ames test does not prove carcinogenicity, it is highly likely to be the case. The control plate indicates that some mutations occur as normal background when the buffer-soaked filter was added. In Test #1, the relatively high concentration of compound Z is so mutagenic that all bacteria were killed. In Test #3, while the extract partially reduced the mutagenicity of compound Z, it is still mutagenic. Test #2 shows some clearing (killing) of bacteria around the disk because of considerable mutagenicity. As the more dilute solution of compound Z diffuses out to the periphery of the plate, some *his$^+$* bacteria survive.

(d) There is no clear space around the disk in Test #3 because the extract reduced the mutagenicity of compound Z to a considerable degree. The similarity of the control plate with Test #3 indicates that the extract is quite effective in reducing the mutagenicity of compound Z.

(e) The Ames test is useful as a preliminary screen for testing the mutagenicity of compounds. However, within an organism, compounds are metabolized differentially. In addition, different organisms metabolize compounds in different ways.

(f) Because the extract was apparently capable of altering the mutagenicity of compound Z, one might fractionate the extract into its components to determine the nature and concentration of the component(s) involved in reducing the mutagenicity of compound Z. Mixing each liver component individually and in combination with compound Z in the Ames assay system would be an approach.

Chapter 17: Regulation of Gene Expression in Prokaryotes

Concept Areas	Corresponding Problems
Overview	1, 2, 3, 17
Lactose Metabolism in E. coli: *Inducible*	4, 5, 6, 7, 8, 9, 10, 11, 27
Positive and Negative Control	2, 3, 18, 19, 20, 21, 22, 23, 26
Tryptophan Operon	12, 13, 25
Attenuation	24, 25
Arabinose Operon	16
Model Systems	14, 15, 21, 22, 23

Vocabulary: Organization and Listing of Terms and Concepts

Structures and Substances

Lactose

  structural genes

  lac operon

    cis-acting

    trans-acting

    lac Z

      β-galactosidase

    lac Y

      permease

    lac A

      transacetylase

  polycistronic mRNA

  gratuitous inducers

    isopropylthiogalactoside (IPTG)

  constitutive mutants

    lac I⁻

    lac O^c

      merozygote

      regulatory units

repressor gene

repressor molecule

repression loop

diffusible cellular product (F17.2)

operator region

no diffusible product

adjacent control (F17.2)

  lac I ^{s}

  lac I ^{q}

catabolite activating protein (CAP)

  promoter region

  glucose

  CAP binding site

cyclic adenosine monophosphate (cAMP)

  adenyl cyclase

arabinose

  *ara*B, A, D, I, O$_2$

  *ara*C regulatory protein

tryptophan

tryptophan synthetase

trp R⁻, *trp R⁺*

  co-repressor

structural genes

  trp E, D, C, B, A

trp P-*trp* O region

leader sequence

  attenuator

  tRNA^{trp}

  termination loop

  antitermination hairpin

  Bacillus subtilis

  TRAP (trpRNA-binding attenuating protein)

  AT (anti-TRAP)

Processes/Methods

Genetic regulation

  adaptive

    inducible

      inducer, lactose

  equilibrium dialysis

    catabolite repression

cooperative binding

repressible

  tryptophan

    attenuation, ribosome "stall"

  negative, positive control

    catabolite repression

    arabinose regulation

constitutive

allosteric

superrepression

Concepts

Genetic regulation

  efficiency

Cis-acting, *trans*-acting

Positive control (F17.1)

  catabolite repression

Negative control (F17.1)

  lactose operon

  tryptophan operon

    repression

    attenuation, "stalling"

F17.1 Illustration of general processes of *negative* and *positive* control. If *negative* control is operating, the regulatory protein inhibits transcription. With *positive* control, transcription is stimulated.

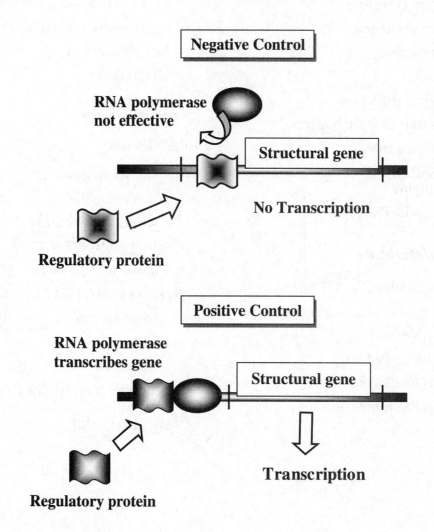

F17.2 Illustration of the nature of the product of the *I* gene. If can act "at a distance" because it is a protein that can diffuse through the cytoplasm and thus act in *trans*. There is no protein product of the operator gene; therefore, it can only act in *cis*.

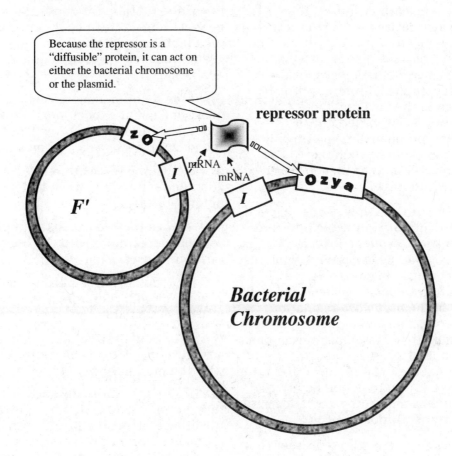

Solutions to Problems and Discussion Questions

1. The answer to this question is a key to enhancing a student's understanding of the Jacob-Monod model as related to lactose and tryptophan metabolism. The enzymes of the lactose operon are needed to break down and use lactose as an energy source. If lactose is the sole carbon source, the enzymes are synthesized to use that carbon source. With no lactose present, there is no "need" for the enzymes. The tryptophan operon contains structural genes for the *synthesis* of tryptophan. If there is little or no tryptophan in the medium, the tryptophan operon is "turned on" to manufacture tryptophan. If tryptophan is abundant in the medium, then there is no "need" for the operon to be manufacturing "tryptophan synthetases."

2. Refer to F17.1 to see that under *negative* control, the regulatory molecule interferes with transcription, while in *positive* control, the regulatory molecule stimulates transcription. Negative control is seen in the *lactose* and *tryptophan* systems, as well as a portion of the *arabinose* regulation. Catabolite repression and a portion of the *arabinose* regulatory systems are examples of positive control. Negative control requires a molecule to be removed from the DNA for transcription to occur. Positive control requires a molecule to be added to the DNA for transcription to occur.

3. In an *inducible system*, the repressor that normally interacts with the operator to inhibit transcription is inactivated by an *inducer*, thus permitting transcription. In a *repressible system*, a normally inactive repressor is *activated* by a *co-repressor*, thus enabling the activated repressor to bind to the operator to inhibit transcription. Because the interaction of the protein (repressor) has a negative influence on transcription, the systems described here are forms of *negative control* (see F16.).

4. (a) Due to the deletion of a base early in the *lac Z* gene, there will be "frameshift" of all the reading frames downstream from the deletion. It is likely that either premature chain termination of translation will occur (from the introduction of a nonsense triplet in a reading frame) or the normal chain termination will be ignored. Regardless, a mutant condition for the *Z* gene will be likely. If such a cell is placed on a lactose medium, it will be incapable of growth because β-galactosidase is not available.

(b) If the deletion occurs early in the *A* gene, one might expect impaired function of the *A* gene product, but it will not influence the use of lactose as a carbon source.

5. Refer to the text and to F17.1,2 to get a good understanding of the lactose system before starting.

$I^+ O^+ Z^+$ = **Inducible** because a repressor protein can interact with the operator to turn off transcription.

$I^- O^+ Z^+$ = **Constitutive** because the repressor gene is mutant; therefore no repressor protein is available.

$I^+ O^c Z^+$ = **Constitutive** because even though a repressor protein is made, it cannot bind with the mutant operator.

$I^- O^+ Z^+ / F' I^+$ = **Inducible** because even though there is one mutant repressor gene, the other I^+ gene, on the F factor, produces a normal repressor protein that is diffusible and capable of interacting with the operon to repress transcription. (See F17.2 in this book.)

$I^+ O^c Z^+ / F' O^+$ = **Constitutive** because there is a constitutive operator (O^c) next to a normal *Z* gene. Remembering that this operator functions in *cis* and is not influenced by the repressor protein, constitutive synthesis of β-galactosidase will occur.

$I^s O^+ Z^+$ = **Repressed** because the product of the I^s gene is *insensitive* to the inducer lactose and thus cannot be inactivated. The repressor will continually interact with the operator and shut off transcription regardless of the presence or absence of lactose.

$I^s\ O^+\ Z^+\ /F'\ I^+$ = **Repressed** because, as in the previous case, the product of the I^s gene is insensitive to the inducer lactose and thus cannot be inactivated. The repressor will continually interact with the operator and shut off transcription regardless of the presence or absence of lactose. The fact that there is a normal I^+ gene is of no consequence because once a repressor from I^s binds to an operator, the presence of normal repressor molecules will make no difference.

6. Before starting, refer to the text and to F17.2 to get a good understanding of the lactose system.

$I^+\ O^+\ Z^+$ = Because of the function of the active repressor from the I^+ gene, and no lactose to influence its function, there will be **No Enzyme Made.**

$I^+\ O^c\ Z^+$ = There will be a **Functional Enzyme Made** because the constitutive operator is in *cis* with a Z gene. The lactose in the medium will have no influence because of the constitutive operator. The repressor cannot bind to the mutant operator.

$I^-\ O^+\ Z^-$ = There will be a **Nonfunctional Enzyme Made** because with I^- the system is constitutive, but the Z gene is mutant. The absence of lactose in the medium will have no influence because of the nonfunctional repressor. The mutant repressor cannot bind to the operator.

$I^-\ O^+\ Z^-$ = There will be a **Nonfunctional Enzyme Made** because with I^- the system is constitutive, but the Z gene is mutant. The lactose in the medium will have no influence because of the nonfunctional repressor. The mutant repressor cannot bind to the operator.

$I^-\ O^+\ Z^+\ /F'\ I^+$ = There will be **No Enzyme Made** because in the absence of lactose, the repressor product of the I^+ gene will bind to the operator and inhibit transcription.

$I^+\ O^c\ Z^+\ /F'\ O^+$ = Because there is a constitutive operator in *cis* with a normal Z gene, there will be **Functional Enzyme Made**. The lactose in the medium will have no influence because of the mutant operator.

$I^+\ O^+\ Z^-\ /F'\ I^+\ O^+\ Z^+$ = Because there is lactose in the medium, the repressor protein will not bind to the operator and transcription will occur. The presence of a normal Z gene allows a **Functional and Nonfunctional Enzyme to Be Made**. The repressor protein is diffusible, working in *trans*.

$I^-\ O^+\ Z^-\ /F'\ I^+\ O^+\ Z^+$ = Because there is no lactose in the medium, the repressor protein (from I^+) will repress the operators and there will be **No Enzyme Made**.

$I^s\ O^+\ Z^+\ /\ F'\ O^+$ = With the product of I^s there is binding of the repressor to the operator and therefore **No Enzyme Made**. The lack of lactose in the medium is of no consequence because the mutant repressor is insensitive to lactose.

$I^+\ O^c\ Z^+\ /F'\ O^+\ Z^+$ = The arrangement of the constitutive operator (O^c) with the Z gene will cause a **Functional Enzyme to Be Made**.

7. The mutations described are consistent with the structure of the *lac* repressor. The N-terminal portion of the repressor is involved in DNA binding, while the C-terminal portion is more involved in association with lactose and its analogs.

8. A single *E. coli* cell contains very few molecules of the *lac* repressor. However, the *lac* I^q mutation causes a $10\times$ increase in repressor protein production, thus facilitating its isolation. With the use of dialysis against a radioactive gratuitous inducer (IPTG), Gilbert and Muller-Hill were able to identify the repressor protein in certain extracts of *lac* I^q cells.

The material that bound the labeled IPTG was purified and shown to be heat labile and have other characteristics of protein. Extracts of *lac* I^- cells did not bind the labeled IPTG.

9. First, mutations could be isolated, suggesting that these mutations functioned in *trans*. At that time, gene products were assumed to be proteins, and the *trans* aspect strengthened the thought that a protein was involved. The IPTG-binding protein was labeled with sulfur-containing amino acids and mixed with DNA from λ phage, which contained the *lac O⁺* section of DNA. By glycerol gradient centrifugation, it was shown that the labeled repressor protein binds only to DNA that contained the *lac O⁺* region, thus indicating a specific binding to DNA.

10. In order to understand this question, it is necessary that you understand the negative regulation of the *lactose* operon by the *lac* repressor as well as the positive control exerted by the CAP protein. Remember, if lactose is present, it inactivates the *lac* repressor. If glucose is present, it inhibits adenyl cyclase, thereby reducing, through a lowering of cAMP levels, the positive action of CAP on the *lac* operon.

(a) With no lactose and no glucose, the operon is off because the *lac* repressor is bound to the operator, and although CAP is bound to its binding site, it will not override the action of the repressor.

(b) With lactose added to the medium, the *lac* repressor is inactivated and the operon is transcribing the structural genes. With no glucose, the CAP is bound to its binding site, thus enhancing transcription.

(c) With no lactose present in the medium, the *lac* repressor is bound to the operator region, and since glucose inhibits adenyl cyclase, the CAP protein will not interact with its binding site. The operon is therefore "off."

(d) With lactose present, the *lac* repressor is inactivated; however, since glucose is also present, CAP will not interact with its binding site. Under this condition transcription is severely diminished, and the operon can be considered to be "off."

11. (a) Because activated CAP is a component of the cooperative binding of RNA polymerase to the *lac* promoter, absence of a functional *crp* would compromise the positive control exhibited by CAP.

(b) Without a CAP binding site there would be a reduction in the inducibility of the *lac* operon.

12. Attenuation functions to reduce the synthesis of tryptophan when it is in full supply. It does so by reducing transcription of the *tryptophan* operon. The same phenomenon is observed when tryptophan activates the repressor to shut off transcription of the *tryptophan* operon.

13. It is likely that attenuation evolved as yet another means to regulate gene output. It provides a fine level of control over gene expression, and it attests to the complex measures that organisms have taken to effectively regulate their genomes. Attenuation can be achieved in a rather straightforward manner with amino acids, since their availability determines the availability of corresponding charged tRNAs. It is the availability, or lack of, those charged tRNAs that regulates transcription. Overall, then, attenuation provides a direct route for amino acids to control gene expression.

14. Neelaredoxin appears to be a protein that defends anaerobic and perhaps aerobic organisms from oxidative stress brought on by the metabolism of oxygen. The generation of oxygen-free radicals (creates the oxidative stress) is dependent on several molecular species including O_2 and H_2O_2. Apparently, relatively high levels of neelaredoxin are produced at all times (*constitutively expressed*) even when potential inducers of gene expression are not added to the system. Additional neelaredoxin gene expression is not responsive (*induced*) as a result of O_2 and H_2O_2 treatment.

15. Since selection was for rapid fermentation of lactose, one would expect the operon to be in the "on" or constitutive state because lactose must be converted to glucose and galactose for lactic acid to be formed through fermentation. Several types of mutations could cause the constitutive state: a mutation in the operator such that it may not recognize the repressor protein; a mutation in the repressor gene such that an ineffective (or no) repressor protein is made. In both cases, the term *mutation* would include not only base alterations, but also larger scale changes such as deletions, duplications, or insertions.

16. When arabinose is present in the medium, the structural genes for the *arabinose* operon are transcribed. If the structural genes for the *lac* operon replaced the structural genes for the *ara* operon, then in the presence of arabinose, the *lac* structural genes would be transcribed and β-galactosidase would be produced at induced levels.

17. (a) Since 1900, scientists have known that when certain additives are supplied to growth media, organisms respond with the production of certain enzymes. Such enzymes were referred to as adaptive in contrast to constitutive enzymes that are produced regardless of particular medium additives.

(b) Beginning with studies by Monod in 1946, it was determined that when lactose is added to medium, *E. coli* respond with the production of enzymes involved in lactose metabolism. When lactose was removed, the concentration of such enzymes decreased.

(c) While a repressor molecule was originally suggested by Jacob and Monod from *cis*-acting O^c mutations, its isolation was achieved by others. Using a mutant of *E. coli* that produces relatively large amounts of the repressor, Gilbert and his colleagues were able to show that a repressor binds specifically to DNA containing the operator portion of the *lac* operon.

(d) Radioactive IPTG, a sulfur-containing analog of lactose, was shown to bind to the *lac* repressor. Extracts of I^- constitutive cells, having no *lac* repressor activity, did not bind IPTG.

(e) Contrary to the *lac* system where a material in the medium (lactose) causes the synthesis of *lac* structural proteins, addition of tryptophan to the medium represses the synthesis of proteins for the synthesis of tryptophan.

18. Since a substance supplied in the medium (the antibiotic) causes the synthesis of the efflux pump components, two situations seem appropriate. Under a *negative control* system, the antibiotic would interrupt the repressor to bring about induction (this would be an inducible system). Under *positive control,* the antibiotic would activate an activator (this again would be an inducible system).

19. First, notice that in the first row of data, the presence of *tm* in the medium causes the production of active enzyme from the wild-type arrangement of genes. From this, one would conclude that the system is *inducible*. To determine which gene is the structural gene, look for the *IE* function and see that it is related to *C*. Therefore, *C* codes for the **structural gene**. Because when *B* is mutant, no enzyme is produced, *B* must be the **promoter**.

Notice that when genes *A* and *D* are mutant, constitutive synthesis occurs; therefore, one must be the operator, and the other gene codes for the repressor protein. To distinguish these functions, one must remember that the repressor operates as a diffusible substance and can be on the host chromosome or the F factor (functioning in *trans*). However, the operator can only operate in *cis*. In addition, in *cis*, the constitutive operator is dominant to its wild-type allele, while the mutant repressor is recessive to its wild-type allele.

Notice that the mutant *A* gene is dominant to its wild-type allele, whereas the mutant *d* allele is recessive (behaving as wild type in the first row). Therefore, the *A* locus is the **operator** and the *D* locus is the **repressor** gene.

20. Because the deletion of the regulatory gene causes a loss of synthesis of the enzymes, the regulatory gene product can be viewed as one exerting *positive control*.

When <u>tis</u> is present, no enzymes are made; therefore, <u>tis</u> must inactivate the positive regulatory protein. When <u>tis</u> is absent, the regulatory protein is free to exert its positive influence on transcription. Mutations in the operator negate the positive action of the regulator. F17.3 is a model that illustrates these points.

F17.3 Model of regulatory system described in Problem 20. This is an example of *positive* control.

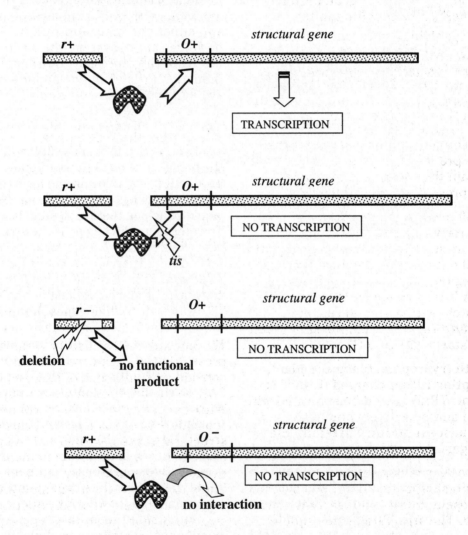

21. The first two sentences in the problem indicate an inducible system in which oil stimulates the production of a protein, which turns on (positive control) genes to metabolize oil. The different results in strains #2 and #4 suggest a *cis*-acting system. Because the operon by itself (when mutant as in strain #3) gives constitutive synthesis of the structural genes, a *cis*-acting system is also supported. The *cis*-acting element is most likely part of the operon.

22. (a) Call one constitutive mutation *lex*A$^-$ (mutation in the repressor gene product) and the other O^{uvrA-} (mutation in the operator).

(b) One can make partial diploid strains using F′. O^{uvrA-} will (given the other genes brought in by the F′ element) be dominant to O^{uvrA+} and *lex*A$^-$ will be recessive to *lex*A$^+$. O^{uvrA-} will act in *cis*.

23. If one could develop an assay for the other gene products under SOS control, with a *lex*A$^-$ strain the other gene products should be present at induced levels.

24. You will need to identify the complementary regions. This is one of the rare cases in this handbook where the entire answer will not be directly given. You will find four regions that "fit." To get started, find the CACUUCC sequence. It pairs, with one mismatch, with a second region. *Hint:* The third region is composed of seven bases and starts with an AG.

25. (a) With tryptophan being abundant, the assumption is that charged tRNA^{trp} is also present. TRAP should be saturated with tryptophan and be actively bound to the 5′ end of the nascent mRNA. Therefore, the structural genes should not be expressed.

(b) If tryptophan is scarce, even though tRNA^{trp} is present it should not be charged. TRAP is present, but it is not saturated with tryptophan. The structural genes should be expressed.

(c) The answer to this situation needs some qualification. If tryptophan is abundant, but tRNA^{trp} is scarce, the assumption is that charged tRNA^{trp} is being described. This could be due to a nonfunctional tryptophanyl-tRNA synthetase. In that case, the uncharged tRNA^{trp} can induce AT, which then binds to tryptophan-saturated TRAP. This prevents TRAP from binding to the leader RNA sequence, thus allowing expression of the tryptophan operon.

(d) With no TRAP, there can be no termination of transcription. Therefore under this condition, even with abundant tryptophan, there is expression of the operon.

26. (a) The simplest model for the action of R and D in *Chlamydia* would be to have the repressor element (R) become ineffective in binding the *cis*-acting element (D) when heat-shocked. This could happen in two ways. Either the supercoiled DNA alters its conformation and becomes ineffective at binding R, or the D-binding efficiency of the R protein is altered by heat. In either case, the genes for infectivity are transcribed in the presence of the heat shock.

(b) The most straightforward comparison between the heat-shock R and D system in *Chlamydia* and the heat-shock sigma factor in *E. coli* would be where the R-D system is inactivated in *Chlamydia* and a sigma factor is activated by heat in *E. coli*.

27. Since all the regulatory elements are present in the engineered plasmid, one must consider the influence of glucose, through CAP, on the production of structural genes. With glucose present, there will be limited (considered here as no) synthesis of the structural genes regardless of the presence of lactose. I^s will act as a dominant to I^+ because, being insensitive to lactose, once it binds to an operator it will shut it off. O^c will only act in *cis* and allow production of its structural genes regardless of the presence or absence of lactose unless there is glucose in the medium. With glucose in the medium, an operon with O^c will be shut off because of catabolite repression. Expected results are presented below.

Medium Condition

Genotype	Lactose	Glucose	β-galactosidase	Green Colonies
$I^+O^+Z^+/pI^+O^+GFP$	−	+	−	−
	+	+	−	−
	+	−	+	+
$I^+O^+Z^-/pI^+O^cGFP$	−	+	−	−
	+	−	−	+
$I^+O^+Z^+/pI^sO^cGFP$	−	+	−	−
	+	−	−	+
$I^+O^cZ^+/pI^sO^+GFP$	−	+	−	−
	+	−	+	−

196

Chapter 18: Regulation of Gene Expression in Eukaryotes

Vocabulary: Organization and Listing of Terms and Concepts

Structures and Substances

Chromosome territories

Transcription factories

  interchromosomal compartments

Chromatin

  remodeling components

Histones

  nucleosome

  DNase I

  histone acetyltransferase enzymes

    HAT

  histone deacetylases (HDAC)

  insulator element

  histone code

    SWI/SNF

  HpaII

  CpG-rich region

  GC doublet

  5′-azacytidine

  methyl group

Promoters

  CAAT box

consensus sequence

Transcription factors

  cis-acting

    metallothionein IIA

      hMTIIA

      TATA

  positive/negative factors

  functional domains

    DNA-binding domains

    trans-

  activating domains

    motif, GAL4, UAS$_G$

  TFIID, TFIIB, TFIIF, TFIIA

  TBP, TAFs (TATA), others

  zinc fingers

  helix-turn-helix (HTH)

    homeobox

    homeodomain

  leucine zippers (bZIP)

    coactivator

  enhanceosome

RNA polymerases

Enhancers

   positive

Silencers

   negative

cis-acting, *trans*-acting

   thyrotropin-β gene

   Oct-1 gene

Transcription complex

Yeast

   GAL genes

   DNase hypersensitive sites

     UAS$_G$

   Proteome

     Dscam gene

     para gene

Intron

Exon

Sex-determining genes in *Drosophila*

   Sxl, tra, dzx

RNAi

   siRNA

   RISC

   Dicer

   microRNAs (miRNAs)

   RITS

Tubulin

Iron response element (IRE)

p53

Processes/Methods

Chromosome painting

Chromosome remodeling

Epigenetic processes

Histone modification

Gene regulation

DNA methylation

   X chromosome inactivation

   transcription

     upstream (5′) organization

       promoters

         TATA box

         CAAT box or CCAAT

         GC box

       enhancers

       silencers

         variable position

         variable orientation

         cis-acting

         upstream and downstream

   basal, induced states

     positive, negative

   DNA binding

     cis, trans-activating

       galactose metabolism

       catabolite repression

       positive control

       DNase hypersensitivity

   gene alterations

     DNA methylation

     tissue specificity

   processing (posttranscriptional regulation)

     intron removal

     exon splicing

     alternative splicing

       CT/CGRP gene

     3′-polyadenylation (polyA tail)

   transport

mRNA stability

adenosine-uracil rich element (ARE)

translational control

autoregulation

tubulin regulation

RNase action and degradation

post-translational modification

alternative processing

transport

stability

half-life

nonsense-mediated decay

translation

post-translational modification

RNA silencing

Stimulation of transcription

positive control

catabolite repression

relationships to transcription factors

relationships to enhancers

relationships to silencers

Autoregulation

Sex determination in *Drosophila*

Concepts

Chromosome territories

Comparison to prokaryotes

Epigenetic modifications

Genetic regulation

methylation

transcription

posttranscriptional

processing

Solutions to Problems and Discussion Questions

1. There are several reasons for anticipating a variety of different regulatory mechanisms in eukaryotes as compared with prokaryotes. Eukaryotic cells contain greater amounts of DNA, and this DNA is associated with various proteins, including histones and nonhistone chromosomal proteins. *Chromatin* as such does not exist in prokaryotes. In addition, whereas there is usually only one chromosome in prokaryotes, eukaryotes have more than one chromosome all enclosed in a membrane (nuclear membrane). This nuclear membrane separates, both temporally and spatially, the processes of transcription and translation, thus providing an opportunity for post-transcriptional, pre-translational regulation.

While prokaryotes respond genetically to changes in their external environment, cells of multicellular eukaryotes interact with each other as well as the external environment. The structural and functional diversity of cells of a multicellular eukaryote, coupled with the finding that all cells of an organism contain a complete complement of genes, suggests that certain genes are active in some cells but not in others.

It is often difficult to study eukaryotic gene regulation because of the complexities mentioned above, especially tissue specificity and the various levels at which regulation can occur (as indicated in question #2 below). Obtaining a homogeneous group of cells from a multicellular organism often requires a significant alteration of the natural environment of the cell. Thus, results from studies on isolated cells must be interpreted with caution. In addition, because of the variety of intracellular components (nuclear and cytoplasmic), it is difficult to isolate, free of contamination, certain molecular species. Even if such isolation is accomplished, it is difficult to interpret the actual behavior of such molecules in an artificial environment.

2. *Chromatin remodeling*: Changes in DNA/chromosome structure can influence overall gene output. DNA methylation also influences transcription efficiency.

Transcription: Several factors are known to influence transcription: *promoters*, TATA, CAAT, and GC boxes, as well as other upstream regulatory sequences: *enhancers*, which are *cis*-acting sequences that act at various locations and orientations; *transcription factors*, with various structural motifs (zinc fingers, homeodomains, and leucine zippers) that bind DNA and influence transcription; and *receptor-hormone complexes* that influence transcription.

Processing and transport: These types of regulation involve the efficiency of hnRNA maturation as related to capping, polyA tail addition, intron removal, and mRNA stability.

Translation: After mRNAs are produced from the processing of hnRNA, they have the potential of being translated. The stability of the mRNAs appears to be an additional regulatory control point. Certain factors, such as protein subunits, may influence a variety of steps in the translational mechanism. For instance, a protein or protein subunit may activate an RNase, which will degrade certain mRNAs, or a particular regulatory element may cause a ribosome to stall, thus decreasing the speed of translation and increasing the exposure of an mRNA to the action of RNAses.

3. Determining the location of individual chromosomes in the interphase nucleus has been made possible by chromosome-painting techniques whereby fluorescent markers attach to specific chromosomes. Each chromosome occupies a discrete domain called a territory, between which are interchromosomal compartments. Transcription factories are nuclear sites where RNA polymerase II is most prevalent.

4. When DNA is transcriptionally active, it is in a less condensed state and, as such, is more open to DNase digestion.

5. Epigenetic modifications include a host of factors that influence gene function other than those directly related to the sequence of bases in a stretch of DNA. DNA methylation alters the efficiency at which transcription occurs and chromatin remodeling alters the association of nucleosomes to DNA. Both processes regulate gene activity. Other factors, including chromosome territories and transcription factories, influence gene activity by nuclear position. Eukaryotic cell structure is more complex than prokaryotic cell structure, thereby providing a variety of opportunities for epigenetic modifications, even in single-celled eukaryotes. Complexities associated with multicellularity require a sophisticated regulatory environment, and in some ways, cell structure that includes a membrane-bound nucleus enhances regulatory opportunities within that environment.

6. In general, chromatin is remodeled when there are significant changes in chromatin organization. Such remodeling involves changes in DNA methylation and interaction of DNA with histones in nucleosomes. Nucleosome remodeling complexes alter nucleosome structure and position by a number of processes, including histone modification.

7. *Promoters* are conserved DNA sequences that influence transcription from the "upstream" side (5′) of mRNA coding genes. They are usually fixed in position and within 100 base pairs of the initiation site for mRNA synthesis. Examples of such promoter sites are the following: TATA, CAAT, and GC boxes.
   Enhancers are *cis*-acting sequences of DNA that stimulate the transcription from most, if not all, promoters. They are somewhat different from promoters in that the position of the enhancer need not be fixed; it may be significantly upstream, downstream, or within the gene being regulated. The orientation may be inverted without significantly influencing its action. Enhancers can work on different genes; that is, they are not gene-specific.

8. Transcription factors are proteins that are *necessary* for the initiation of transcription. However, they are not *sufficient* for the initiation of transcription. To be activated, RNA polymerase II requires a number of transcription factors. Transcription factors contain at least two functional domains: one binds to the DNA sequences of promoters and/or enhancers, while the other interacts with RNA polymerase or other transcription factors. Some transcription factors bind to other transcription factors without themselves binding to DNA.

9. Basic differences that are known to occur when comparing genetic regulation in prokaryotes and eukaryotes include the following:

—differences in basic chromosome structure

—chromosome remodeling

—histone acetylation

—differences in gene structure

—cell structure (nucleus in eukaryotes)

—levels of potential regulation

  . . .transcriptional

  . . .mRNA processing

  . . .transport

  . . .selection for processing and translation

  . . .mRNA stability

—genomic aspects (amplification, etc.)

—biological context in terms of multicellular interactions versus single-cell survival

10. Generally, one determines the influence of various regulatory elements by removing necessary elements or adding extra elements. In addition, examining the outcome of mutations within such elements often provides insight as to function. Assay systems determine the relative levels of gene expression after such alterations.

11. Both the *lac* and *gal* systems are influenced by catabolite repression; however, the *lac* system is under negative control, whereas the *gal* system is under positive control. Both systems are inducible.

12. RNA interference begins with a double-stranded RNA being processed by a protein called Dicer that, in combination with RISC, generates short interfering RNA (siRNA). Unwinding of siRNA produces an antisense strand that combines with a protein to cleave mRNA complementary sequences. Short RNAs called microRNAs pair with the 3′-untranslated regions of mRNAs and block their translation.

13. (a) There is no place for the TFIID to bind.

(b) There is more transcription in the nuclear extracts. Perhaps other factors not present in the purified system are present in the nuclear extracts.

(c) There is a region, probably in the −81 to −50 area, that responds to a component in the nuclear extract to bring about high efficiency transcription.

14.

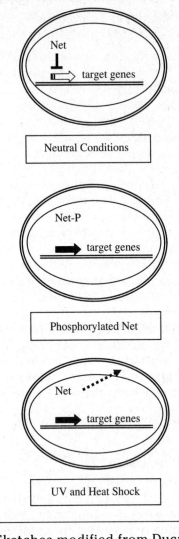

Sketches modified from Ducret et al. *Molecular and Cellular Biology* 1999 19:7076–7087

15. While the mechanism of enhancer action over long distances is unknown, supercoiling may bring about the pattern below.

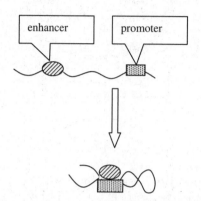

16. Given that DNA methylation plays a role in gene expression in mammals, any change in DNA methylation, plus or minus, can potentially have a negative impact on progeny development. In addition, since m^{5}C >>> thymine, transitions are likely to cause mutations in coding regions of DNA, when methylation patterns change, new sites for mutation arise. Should mutations occur at a higher rate in previously unmethylated sites (genes), embryonic development is likely to be affected.

17. If the exon 45 deletion causes a reading frameshift leading to reduced dystrophin production and if the removal of exon 46 reestablishes the reading frame, then one would expect enhanced production of dystrophin.

18. The work of Cleveland and colleagues allowed selective changes to be made in the *met-arg-glu-lys* sequence. Only the engineered mRNA sequences that caused an amino acid substitution negated the autoregulation, indicating that it is the sequence of the amino acids, not the mRNA, that is critical in the process of autoregulation. Notice that code degeneracy allows for changes in mRNA sequence without changes in the amino acid sequence. Therefore, the model that depicts binding of factors to the nascent polypeptide chain is supported. A variety of experiments could be used to substantiate such a model. One might stabilize the proposed MREI-protein complex with "crosslinkers," treat with RNAse to digest mRNA and to break up polysomes, and then isolate individual ribosomes. One may use some specific antibody or other method to determine whether tubulin subunits contaminate the ribosome population.

19. (a) Mutations within promoters alter transcription efficiencies while deletions alter the initiation point of transcription. Enhancers (and silencers) are chromosomal elements that negatively influence transcription when deleted or altered by mutation. Insertion of an enhancer by recombinant technology increases transcription.

(b) Transcription factors possess a DNA-binding domain that binds to DNA sequences and provides *cis*-regulation. Structural motifs, such as helix-turn-helix, enable DNA binding, and deletions of promoters and surrounding regions suppress such binding.

(c) Scientists determined that injection of certain short double-stranded RNAs in roundworm cells led to the degradation of specific mRNA. This process is called RNA interference (RNAi).

20. Since multiple routes lead to cancer, one would expect complex regulatory systems to be involved. More specifically, while in some cases, downregulation of a gene, such as an oncogene, may be a reasonable cancer therapy, downregulation of a tumor-suppressor gene would be undesirable in therapy.

21. Because gene amplification leads to differential gene output, it would be reasonable to classify gene amplification as a form of genetic regulation. Given the host of other regulatory schemes in eukaryotes, and the tissue specificity of gene amplification, its inclusion would seem reasonable.

22. Below is a sketch of several RNA polymerase molecules (filled circles) in what might be a transcription factory. This diagram shows eight RNA pol II molecules involved in transcription. Nascent transcripts are shown extending from the black circles (RNA polymerase). For simplicity, only one promoter (heavy line) and one structural gene (gray line) are shown.

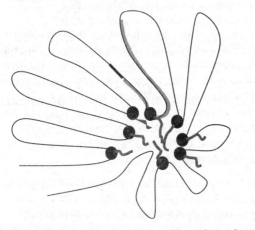

23. 5-azactidine is an analog of cytidine, but it cannot be methylated. When incorporated into DNA, it stimulates the expression of genes. Scientists have determined that cells exposed to 5-azacytidine increase their production of γ chain hemoglobin, which effectively associates with α chains. It is thought that individuals with severe β-thalassemia might benefit from its use; however, because 5-azacytidine is not gene specific, its widespread influence on the genome constitutes a considerable health hazard.

24. Since mRNA stability is directly related to the likelihood of translation, one could use a number of different constructs as shown below and test for luciferase activity in the assay system described in the problem.

5'-cap	3'-tail	mRNA (no cap, no tail)
−	−	+
+	−	+
−	+	+
+	−	−
−	+	−

25. Methylation of CpGs causes a reduction in luciferase expression, which is somewhat proportional to the amount of methylation and patch size. Methylation within the transcription unit more drastically reduces luciferase expression compared with methylation outside the transcription unit. A high degree of methylation outside the transcription unit (593 CpGs) has as great an impact on depressing transcription as the same degree of methylation within the transcription unit.

26. If mRNA transport is achieved by diffusion, then regulation could be achieved by the positioning of different concentrations of ribosomes. The closer a ribosome pool is to the source of a particular mRNA source, the higher the likelihood that a given mRNA will be translated. In addition, certain territories in cells may be less hostile to traveling mRNAs, which would also favor the translation of certain mRNAs. If nuclear territories purge their RNAs at different locations around the nucleus, then even if diffusion is the mode of mRNA transport, different cellular domains would receive different types of mRNAs. If such domains have different translation efficiencies, then genetic regulation is achieved.

27. The inherent flaw is that the genome in all nonlymphoid cells is the same, so how would DNA folding vary in such a way as to trigger specific gene-expression patterns in different cells? However, the same can be said for any form of eukaryotic genetic regulation. Highly differentiated cells have the same genetic material, so how are different genes expressed in different cells? In support of differential folding of chromatin contributing to genetic regulation, the same principles that apply to regulating gene activity as we presently view it (cell-specific factors, proteins) could also be applied to the 3D organization within the nucleus.

28. Criteria for determining the conservation of alternative splicing patterns would likely include the following:

(1) Similar mRNA length
(2) Conservation of splice junctions
(3) Positioning of homologous introns
(4) Size of homologous introns
(5) Exon nucleotide sequence homology
(6) Predicted amino acid physico-chemical similarity
(7) Same 5'-3' orientation
(8) Conserved use of alternative stop codons in frameshift splicing events
(9) Conserved use of alternative frames of translation

29. The ratio of MAG isoforms with and without exon 12 differs in an age-related manner between *+/qk* and *qk/qk* mice. Young mutant mice include exon 12 more frequently than do heterozygous mice. There is little, if any, difference in RNA splicing in adult mice, each retaining the abnormal pattern (inclusion of exon 12).

Apparently, exon 12 inclusion in mutant mice occurs preferentially in young mice and likely contributes to myelination alterations in the brain, which leads to the altered phenotype.

30. When splice specificity is lost, one might observe several classes of altered RNAs: (1) a variety of nonspecific variants producing RNA pools with many lengths and combinations of exons and introns, (2) incomplete splicing where introns and exons are erroneously included or excluded in the mRNA product, and (3) a variety of nonsense products, which result in premature RNA decay or truncated protein products. It is presently unknown as to whether cancer-specific splices initiate or result from tumorigenesis. Given the complexity of cancer induction and the maintenance of the transformed cellular state, gene products that are significant in regulating the cell cycle may certainly be influenced by alternative splicing and thus contribute to cancer.

Chapter 19: Developmental Genetics of Model Organisms

Concept Areas	Corresponding Problems
Developmental Concepts	1, 2, 3, 21, 24, 27
Variable Gene Activity Theory	3
Differential Transcription in Development	10, 11, 29
Genetics of Embryonic Development	4, 17, 19, 22, 29
Maternal-effect Genes and Body Plans	5, 6, 9, 17, 19
Zygotic Genes and Segment Formation	7, 8, 9, 20
Homeotic and Hox Genes	12, 13, 14, 15, 16, 17, 23
Vertebrate Developmental Genes	30
Arabidopsis Development	18, 25
Cell-cell Interactions in C. elegans	26, 28

Vocabulary: Organization and Listing of Terms and Concepts

Structures and Substances

Zygote

Development

  differentiated state

  variable gene activity hypothesis

Drosophila

  maternal-effect genes

    anterior

    posterior

  zygotic genes

  segmentation genes

  gap genes

  pair-rule genes

  segment polarity genes

Homeotic genes

  homeobox

  homeodomain

    Hox gene clusters

    Hox genes

    transcription factors

Arabidopsis

  MADS box proteins

Notch signaling pathway

  Delta

  Alagille syndrome (AGS)

  spondylocostal dysotosis (SD)

Caenorhabditis elegans

  male, hermaphrodite

    lin, let, etc.

      vulva

Molecular gradients

  anterior-posterior axis

  maternal-effect genes

Maternal cytoplasm

Blastoderm

cis-regulatory module

Processes/Methods

Development

  cytoplasmic localization

variable gene activity

determination

   selective expression

   regulatory events

   patterns of gene activity

     cascades

   multistep

   progressive restriction

differentiation

   genetic and morphological

cell-cell interaction

   intercellular communication

   vulval formation

Analyses

  C. elegans

  Drosophila

   oogenesis

   syncytial cellular blastoderm

   imaginal disks

   metamorphosis

   molecular gradients

     anterior-posterior

     dorsal-ventral

   segmentation

   homeotic mutants

Transcriptional network

Concepts

Development (F19.1)

   genomic equivalence

   variable gene activity (F19.1)
eukaryotes

     determination

     differentiation

     cell-cell interaction

     developmental cascades

     totipotent

     progressive restriction

       homology

       cascades

   transcriptional events

     different cells

     different times

   cell and tissue interactions

   cytoplasmic localization

Maternal influences

   anterior-posterior gradient

Cytoplasmic influences

Homeotic genes

Homeodomains

Transcriptional networks

F19.1 Illustration of the relationship between determination and differentiation. Determination sets the program that will later be revealed by differentiation. The variable gene activity hypothesis suggests that different sets of genes are transcriptionally active in differentiated cells.

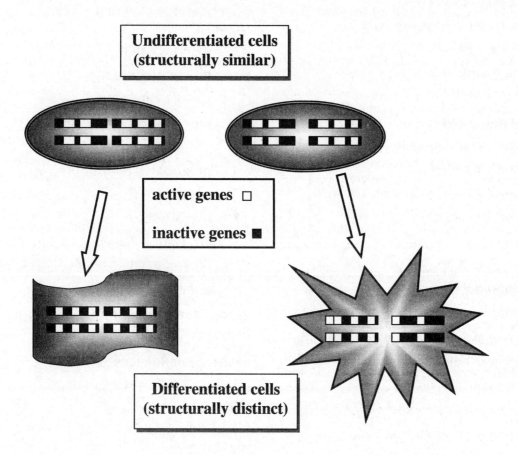

Solutions to Problems and Discussion Questions

1. *Determination* refers to early developmental and regulatory events that set eventual patterns of gene activity. Determination is not the end result of the regulatory activity; rather, it is the process by which the developmental fate of a particular cell type is fixed. *Differentiation*, on the other hand, follows determination and is the manifestation, in terms of genetic, physiological, and morphological changes, of the determined state.

2. The fact that nuclei from almost any source remain transcriptionally and translationally active substantiates the fact that the genetic code and the ancillary processes of transcription and translation are compatible throughout the animal and plant kingdoms. Because the egg represents an isolated, "closed" system that can be mechanically, environmentally, and to some extent biochemically manipulated, various conditions may be developed that allow one to study facets of gene regulation. For instance, the influence of transcriptional enhancers and suppressors may be studied along with factors that impact translational and post-translational processes. Combinations of injected nuclei may reveal nuclear-nuclear interactions, which could not normally be studied by other methods.

3. Evidence from maternal-effect examples in this chapter indicate that the egg is not an unorganized collection of molecules from which life springs after fertilization. It is a highly organized structure, "preformed" in the sense that maternal informational molecules are oriented to provide an anterior-posterior and dorsal-ventral pattern from which nuclei receive positional cues. Such positional cues lead to the "determined" state, from which cells later reveal their adult form (differentiation).

Indeed, in *Drosophila* and many other organisms, embryonic fate maps may be constructed, thereby attesting to the maternally derived "prepattern" present in the egg. The egg therefore is preformed, not in the sense that a miniature individual resides, but in a molecular prepattern upon which development depends. However, work by Spemann, Briggs and King, and Gurdon indicates that there is plasticity in the programming of nuclei and that even nuclei from somewhat specialized cells often have the potential to direct the development of the entire adult individual. Such *totipotent* behavior of cells indicates that development arises as a result of a series of progressive steps in which cells acquire new structures and functions as development progresses.

4. The syncytial blastoderm is formed as nuclei migrate to the egg's outer margin or cortex, where additional divisions take place. Plasma membranes organize around each of the nuclei at the cortex, thus creating the cellular blastoderm.

5. (a) Genes that control early development are often dependent on the deposition of their products (mRNA, transcription factors, various structural proteins, etc.) in the egg by the mother.

(b) They are made in the early oocyte or nurse cells during oogenesis.

(c) Such maternal-effect genes control early developmental events such as defining anterior-posterior polarity. Such products are placed in eggs during oogenesis and are activated immediately after fertilization.

(d) A variety of phenotypes are possible, and they are often revealed in the offspring of females.

6. It is possible that your screen was more inclusive; that is, it identified more subtle alterations than the screen of Wieschaus and Schupbach. In addition, your screen may have included some zygotic effect mutations, which were dependent on the action of maternal-effect genes. You may have identified several different mutations in some of the same genes.

7. (a, b) Zygotic genes are activated or repressed depending on their response to maternal-effect gene products. Three subsets of zygotic genes divide the embryo into segments. These segmentation genes are normally transcribed in the developing embryo, and their mutations have embryonic lethal phenotypes. The maternal genotype contains zygotic genes; these are passed to the embryo as with any other gene.

8. The three main classes of zygotic genes are (1) *gap* genes, which specify adjacent segments, (2) *pair-rule* genes, which specify every other segment and a part of each segment, and (3) *segment polarity* genes, which specify homologous parts of each segment.

9. Because the polar cytoplasm contains information to form germ cells, one would expect such a transplantation procedure to generate germ cells in the anterior region. Work done by Illmensee and Mahowald in 1974 verified this expectation.

10. There are several somewhat indirect methods for determining transcriptional activity of a given gene in different cell types. First, if protein products of a given gene are present in different cell types, it can be assumed that the responsible gene is being transcribed. Second, if one is able to actually observe, microscopically, gene activity, as is the case in some specialized chromosomes (polytene chromosomes), gene activity can be inferred by the presence of localized chromosomal puffs. A more direct and common practice to assess transcription of particular genes is to use labeled probes. If a labeled probe can be obtained that contains base sequences that are complementary to the transcribed RNA, then such probes will hybridize to that RNA if present in different tissues. This technique is called *in situ* hybridization and is a powerful tool in the study of gene activity during development.

11. A variety of approaches can be used to determine the level of control of a particular gene. First, one may determine whether levels of hnRNA are consistent among various cell types of interest. This is often accomplished by either direct isolation of the RNA and assessment by northern blotting or by use of *in situ* hybridization. If the hnRNA pools for a given gene are consistent in various cell types, then transcriptional control can be eliminated as a possibility. Support for translational control can be achieved directly by determining, in different cell types, the presence of a variety of mRNA species with common sequences. This can be accomplished only in cases where sufficient knowledge exists for specific mRNA trapping or labeling. Clues as to translational control via alternative splicing can sometimes be achieved by examining the amino acid sequence of proteins. Similarities in certain structural/functional motifs may indicate alternative RNA processing.

12. *Hox* genes in the *Drosophila* genome can be found in two clusters on chromosome 3: Antp-C and BX-C. They have two properties in common: encoding of transcription factors and colinear gene expression. A *homeotic gene* alters the identity of a segment or field within a segment. Not all homeotic genes are *Hox* genes.

13. A dominant gain-of-function mutation is one that changes the specificity or expression pattern of a gene or gene product. The "gain-of-function" *Antp* mutation causes the wild-type *Antennapedia* gene to be expressed in the eye-antenna disc, and mutant flies have legs on the head in place of antenna.

14. Many of the appendages of the head, including the mouth parts and the antennae, are evolutionary derivatives of ancestral leg structures. In *spineless aristapedia*, the distal portion of the antenna is replaced by its ancestral counterpart, the distal portion of the leg (tarsal segments). Because the replacement of the arista (end of the antenna) can occur by a mutation in a single gene, one would consider that one "selector" gene distinguishes aristal from tarsal structures. Notice that a "one-step" change is involved in the interchange of leg and antennal structures.

15. Because of the regulatory nature of *homeotic* genes in the fundamental cellular activities of determination and differentiation, it would be difficult to ignore their possible impact on oncogenesis. Homeotic genes encode DNA binding domains, which influence gene expression; any factor that influences gene expression may, under some circumstances, influence cell-cycle control.

However attractive this model, no homeotic transformations have been noted in mammary glands, so the typical expression of mutant homeotic genes in insects is not revealed in mammary tissue according to Lewis (2000). A substantial number of experiments will be needed to establish a functional link between homeotic gene mutation and cancer induction. Mutagenesis and transgenesis experiments are likely to be most productive in establishing a cause-effect relationship.

16. Because the engrailed product is absent in *ftz/ftz* embryos and *ftz* expression is normal in *en/en* embryos, one can conclude that the *ftz* gene product regulates, either directly or indirectly, *en*. Because the *ftz* gene is expressed normally in *en/en* embryos, the product of the *engrailed* gene does not regulate expression of *ftz*.

17. Two coupled approaches might be used. First, one could make transgenic flies that contain a series of deletions spanning all segments of the *bicoid* mRNA: the coding region and 5' and 3' untranslated regions. Comparison of stabilities of individual, deleted mRNAs with controls would indicate whether a particular segment of the mRNA contains a degradation signal sequence. If a degradation-sensitive region or signal sequence is located by deletion, that same intact region, when ligated to a noninvolved, nondegraded mRNA (like a ribosomal protein or tubulin mRNA) should foster degradation in a manner similar to the *bicoid* mRNA. If the mRNA from the anterior end of the egg is placed in the posterior of another egg, one could ask if the degradation process is comparable.

18. Three classes of flower *homeotic* genes are known that are activated in an overlapping pattern to specify various floral organs. Class *A* genes give rise to sepals. Expression of *A* and *B* class genes specifies petals, *B* and *C* genes control stamen formation, and expression of *C* genes gives rise to carpels.

19. First, it would be interesting to know whether inhibitors of mitochondrial-ribosomal translation would interfere with germ-cell formation. Second, one should know what types of mRNAs are being translated with these ribosomes.

20.

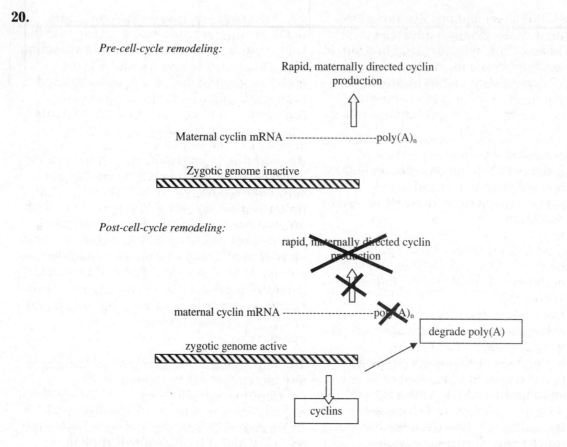

21. (a) In general, mutations provide the window for looking at the structure and function of genes. A number of mutant screens have identified hundreds of genes that influence development. Saturational mutagenesis provides an estimate of the lower limit of genes regulating a particular aspect of development.

(b) Our initial understanding of molecular gradients was based on the discovery of mutations that upset those gradients and alter development. Using a variety of labeling techniques, scientists have described egg gradients at the molecular level.

(c) Homeotic genes influence clusters of other genes involved in the specification of body parts. Mutations in these genes alter the developmental program in very specific and dramatic ways.

(d) Both the *Notch* and *anchor cell* signaling pathways in *Drosophila* and *Caenorhabditis*, respectively, provide genetic evidence, through mutation analysis, that cell-cell contact and communication are necessary for normal development.

(e) *C. elegans* and other multicellular organisms use both direct cell-cell interaction and distance signaling during development. In *C. elegans,* specific genes are known to function specifically in vulval development. Mutations in these genes only influence neighboring cells involved in vulval development.

22. The typical developmental sequence for axis and segment formation in *Drosophila* proceeds from the gap genes to the pair-rule genes to the segment polarity genes. The fact that *fushi-tarazu* (*ftz*) is affected by early (anterior-posterior determining genes) and gap genes indicates that *ftz* functions after those genes. That segment polarity genes are influenced by *ftz* indicates that *ftz* functions earlier, thus placing *ftz* before the segment-polarity genes or in the pair-rule group of genes.

23. Given the information in the problem, it is likely that this gene normally controls the expression of *BX-C* genes in all body segments. The wild-type product of *esc* stored in the egg may be required to interpret the information correctly stored in the egg cortex.

24. (a) The term *rescued* is often used when the introduction of genes from an outside source (within or among species) restores the wild-type phenotype from a mutant organism.

(b) Results such as these, and there are many like them, indicate the extreme conservation of protein structure and function across phylogenetically distant organisms. Such results attest to the conservation from a distant common ancestor of fundamental molecular species during development. Failure to adhere to a common developmental theme is rewarded by death.

25. The *Polycomb* gene family induces changes in chromatin that influence *Hox* gene expression. A gene in *Arabidopsis* has significant homology to the *Polycomb* gene family and also works by altering chromatin structure. The cross reactivity is thus related to the Polycomb product's effect on chromatin. Such parallel functions indicate that mechanisms of regulation are conserved over vast evolutionary distances.

26. Because signal-receptor interactions depend on membrane-bound structures, the pathway can only work with adjacent cells. The advantage of such a system is that only cells in a certain location will be influenced—those in contact. A disadvantage would occur if large groups of cells are to be induced into a particular developmental pathway or if cells not in contact need to be induced.

27. Since *her-1⁻* mutations cause males to develop into hermaphrodites, and *tra-1⁻* mutations cause hermaphrodites to develop into males, one may hypothesize that the *her-1⁺* gene produces a product that suppresses hermaphrodite development, while the *tra-1⁺* gene product is needed for hermaphrodite development.

28. If the *her-1⁺* product acts as a negative regulator, then when the gene is mutant, suppression over *tra-1⁺* is lost and hermaphroditism would be the result. This hypothesis fits the information provided. The double mutant should be male because even though there is no suppression from *her-1⁻*, there is no *tra-1⁺* product to support hermaphrodite development.

29. (a) The patterns somewhat follow expectations in that genes involved in photosynthesis appear to be most active in the leaf and flower. In addition, high levels of protein synthesis in the root are expected. Since pollen and seeds would be called upon early in development, it would seem reasonable to have such tissues show strong expression of transcriptional regulators.

(b) Two factors may be driving the expression of photosynthetic gene expression in flowers and seeds. First, since development in plants is more continuous or sequential, genes may not necessarily be shut off when their products are not in demand. Second, perhaps various posttranscriptional modifications redirect the function of photosynthetic gene products. In other words, alternative uses for such gene products may have evolved in plants much like that observed in some animal tissues.

(c) Having a global view of gene expression in an organism and its various tissues and organs allows one to estimate the relative contribution a particular gene may have in development. Since developmental and transcriptional networks are common in development, it is helpful to know the

213

context in which a particular gene may function. Lastly, the only way in which development will be understood at the molecular level is to have a broad view of classes and clusters of gene activity.

30. (a, b) A number of studies indicate that genes in *Drosophila* have evolutionary counterparts (orthologs) in other organisms, including humans. A number of similar genes influence eye development in both insects and vertebrates. Genes that produce eyes are part of a complex network of at least seven genes that constitute the master regulators of eye development. Each gene functions in coordination with others in a conserved network that is used by broad evolutionary groups. Such genes, descended from common ancestral genes that have the same function in different species, are called orthologs.

(c) Since development is dependent on the coordinated output of numerous genes, genetic networks are probably the rule rather than the exception. The fact that a single genetic change (in the case of the mouse homolog of the fly *eyeless* gene) can trigger the formation of ectopic eyes in *Drosophila* shows that major components of developmental networks may be evolutionarily conserved. Another example of a regulatory network involves vulval development in *C. elegans*.

Chapter 20: Cancer and Regulation of the Cell Cycle

Concept Areas	Corresponding Problems
Inherited Cancer	1, 5, 29
Cell-Cycle Mechanisms	2, 3, 4, 9, 12, 26
Cancer and the Environment	5, 6, 16, 20, 21
Apoptosis	7
Tumor Suppressors and Oncogenes	1, 4, 6, 8, 9, 11, 13, 14, 22, 23, 27, 28
Chromosome Structure	15, 17
Viruses and Cancer	10, 19
Cancer Biology	18, 22, 23, 25, 26, 27, 29, 30

Vocabulary: Organization and Listing of Terms and Concepts

Structures and Substances

Tumor

  benign

  malignant

  carcinoma *in situ*

  chronic myelogenous leukemia (CML)

    BCR-ABL

  Philadelphia chromosome

    protein kinase

  hereditary nonpolyposis colorectal cancer (HNPCC)

Burkitt's lymphoma

Carcinogen

Mutator phenotype

Cell-cycle components

  cyclins

  cyclin-dependent kinases (CDKs)

  cyclin/CDK complexes

  caspases

Bcl2, Bcl2-BAX

p53

  Mdm2

RB1

  pRB

  E2F

Proto-oncogene

  cyclin D1, cyclin E

  ras

Transcription factors

Oncogene

Tumor-suppressor gene

Cellular components

  extracellular matrix

  basal lamina

  metalloproteinases

  inhibitors of metalloproteinases (TIMPS)

Familial adenomatous polyposis (FAP)

  polyp

Chapter 20 Cancer and Regulation of the Cell Cycle

Viruses

    retrovirus

    acute transforming virus

    Rous sarcoma virus (RSV)

    reverse transcriptase

    provirus

    c-onc

    v-onc

    papillomavirus (HPV)

    human T-cell leukemia virus (HTLV-1)

Environmental agents

    tobacco smoke

      ras, p53

    X rays

Processes/Methods

Cell proliferation

    metastasis

Tumorigenesis

Cell cycle

    signal transduction

    G1, G0, S, G2, M

    checkpoints

      G1/S, G2/M, M

    apoptosis

Cell-cell contact

Loss of heterozygosity

Cell transformation

Concepts

Genetic basis of cancer

Loss of heterozygosity

Predisposition to some cancers

Viral involvement in cancer

Environmental agents and cancer

Solutions to Problems and Discussion Questions

1. Familial retinoblastoma (RB) is inherited as an autosomal dominant gene with 90 percent penetrance; that is, 90 percent of the individuals who inherit the gene will develop eye tumors. The gene usually expresses itself in youngsters. Because the husband's sister has RB, one of the husband's parents has the gene for RB and the husband has a 50:50 chance of inheriting that gene. However, because the husband is past the usual age of onset, it is quite likely that he was lucky and did not receive the RB gene. In that case, the chance that a child born to this couple having RB is no higher than the frequency of sporadic occurrence. However, because the gene is 90 percent penetrant, there is a chance that the husband has the gene but does not express it. The probability of that occurrence would be 0.50 (of inheriting the gene) × 0.10 (not expressing the gene) = 0.05. The chance of the husband then passing this nonexpressed gene to his child would again be 0.5, so 0.50 × 0.05 = 0.025 for the child inheriting this gene. If the child inherits the RB gene, he/she has a 90 percent chance of expressing it. Therefore, the overall probability of the child having RB (using this logic) would be 0.025 × 0.9 = 0.0225, or just over 2 percent (or about 1 in 50).

To test the presence of the RB gene in the husband, it is possible in some forms of RB to identify (by molecular probes) a defective or missing DNA segment. Otherwise, one might attempt to assay the RB product in cells to see if it is present and functional at normal levels.

2. The major regulatory points of the cell cycle include the following:

(1) late G1 (G1/S)

(2) the border between G2 and mitosis (G2/M)

(3) in mitosis (M)

3. Kinases regulate other proteins by adding phosphate groups. Cyclins bind to the kinases, switching them on and off. CDK4 binds to cyclin D, moving cells from G1 to S. At the G2/mitosis border, a CDK1 (cyclin-dependent kinase) combines with another cyclin (cyclin B). Phosphorylation occurs, bringing about a series of changes in the nuclear membrane via caldesmon, cytoskeleton, and histone H1.

4. The retinoblastoma gene (*RB1*), located on chromosome 13, encodes a protein designated pRB. Cells progress through the G1/S transition when pRB is phosphorylated and CDK4 binds to cyclin D. In the absence of phosphorylation of pRB, it binds to members of the E2F family of transcription factors, which controls the expression of genes required to move the cell from G1 to S. When E2F and other regulators are released by pRB, they are free to induce the expression of over 30 genes whose products are required for the transition from G1 into S phase. After cells traverse S, G2, and M phases, pRB reverts to a nonphosphorylated state, binds to regulatory proteins such as E2F, and keeps them sequestered until required for the next cell cycle.

5. To say that a particular trait is inherited conveys the assumption that when a particular genetic circumstance is present, it will be revealed in the phenotype. For instance, albinism is inherited in such a way that individuals who are homozygous recessive express albinism. When one discusses an inherited predisposition, one usually refers to situations in which a particular phenotype is expressed in families in some consistent pattern. However, the phenotype may not always be expressed or may manifest itself in different ways. In retinoblastoma, the gene is inherited as an autosomal dominant, and those that inherit the mutant *RB* allele are predisposed to develop eye tumors. However, approximately 10 percent of the people known to inherit the gene do not actually express it, and in some cases expression involves only one eye rather than two.

6. Cancer is a complex alteration in normal cell-cycle controls. Even if a major "cancer-causing" gene is transmitted, other genes, often new mutations, are usually necessary in order to drive a cell toward tumor formation. Full expression of the cancer phenotype is likely to be the result of an interplay among a variety of genes and therefore show variable penetrance and expressivity.

7. Apoptosis, or programmed cell death, is a genetically controlled process that leads to death of a cell. It is a natural process involved in morphogenesis and a protective mechanism against cancer formation. During apoptosis, nuclear DNA becomes fragmented, cellular structures are disrupted, and the cells are dissolved. Caspases are involved in the initiation and progress of apoptosis.

8. A tumor-suppressor gene is a gene that normally functions to suppress cell division. Since tumors and cancers represent a significant threat to survival and therefore Darwinian fitness, strong evolutionary forces would favor a variety of coevolved and perhaps complex conditions in which mutations in these suppressor genes would be recessive. Looking at it in another way, we find that if a tumor-suppressor gene makes a product that regulates the cell cycle favorably, cellular conditions have evolved in such a way that sufficient quantities of this gene product are made from just one gene (of the two present in each diploid individual) to provide normal function.

9. The nonphosphorylated form of pRB binds to transcription factors such as E2F, causing inactivation and suppression of the cell cycle. Phosphorylation of pRB activates the cell cycle by releasing transcription factors (E2F) to advance the cell cycle. With the phosphorylation site inactivated in the PSM-RB form, phosphorylation cannot occur, thereby leaving the cell cycle in a suppressed state.

10. There are a number of ways in which proto-oncogenes are converted to oncogenes: point mutations in which a mutant gene acts as a positive "switch" in the cell cycle, translocations where a hybrid gene might be formed, and overexpression where a gene might acquire a new promoter and/or enhancer. In the case of RSV, an oncogene (*c-src*) was captured from the chicken genome.

11. Embedded in the plasma membrane, Ras proteins act as molecular switches that transmit molecular signals from outside to inside the cell. Activated Ras proteins transduce a signal, which activates the transcription of genes that start cell division. Mutant Ras proteins are locked into the "on" position, continually signaling cell division.

12. Various kinases can be activated by breaks in DNA. One kinase called ATM and/or a kinase called Chk2 phosphorylates BRCA1 and p53. The activated p53 arrests replication during the S phase to facilitate DNA repair. The activated BRCA1 protein, in conjunction with BRCA2, mRAD51, and other nuclear proteins, is involved in repairing the DNA.

13. Oncogenes are genes that induce or maintain uncontrolled cellular proliferation associated with cancer. They are mutant forms of proto-oncogenes, which normally function to regulate cell division. Oncogenes may be formed through point mutations, gene amplification, translocations, repositioning of regulatory sequences, and so on.

14. Mutations that produce oncogenes alter gene expression either directly or indirectly and act in a dominant capacity. Proto-oncogenes are those that normally function to promote or maintain cell division. In the mutant state (oncogenes), they induce or maintain uncontrolled cell division; that is, there is a gain-of-function. Generally this gain-of-function takes the form of increased or abnormally continuous gene output. On the other hand, loss-of-function is generally attributed to tumor-suppressor genes, which function to halt passage through the cell cycle. When such genes are mutant, they have lost their capacity to halt the cell cycle. Such genes are generally recessive.

15. A translocation involving exchange of genetic material between chromosomes 9 and 22 is responsible for the generation of the "Philadelphia chromosome." Genetic mapping established that certain genes were combined to form a hybrid oncogene (*BCR/ABL*), which encodes a 200 kDa protein that has been implicated in the formation of chronic myelogenous leukemia.

16. Unfortunately, it is common to spend enormous amounts of money on dealing with diseases after they occur rather than concentrating on disease prevention. Too often pressure from special interest groups or lack of political stimulus retards advances in education and prevention. Obviously, it is less expensive, both in terms of human suffering and money, to seek preventive measures for as many diseases as possible. However, having gained some understanding of the mechanisms of disease, in this case cancer, it must also be stated that no matter what preventive measures are taken it will be impossible to completely eliminate disease from the human population. It is extremely important, however, that we increase efforts to educate and protect the human population from as many hazardous environmental agents as possible.

17. Several approaches are used to combat CML. One includes the use of a tyrosine kinase inhibitor that binds competitively to the ATP binding site of ABL kinase, thereby inhibiting phosphorylation of BCR-ABL and preventing the activation of additional signaling pathways. In addition, real-time quantitative reverse transcription-polymerase chain reaction (Q-RT-PCR) allows one to monitor drug responses of cell populations in patients so that less toxic and more effective treatments are possible. Being able to distinguish leukemic cells from healthy cells allows one not only to target therapy to specific cell populations, but also to quantify responses to therapy. Because such cells produce a hybrid protein, it may be possible to develop a therapy, perhaps an immunotherapy, based on the uniqueness of the BCR/ABL protein.

18. Normal cells are often capable of withstanding mutational insult because they have checkpoints and DNA repair mechanisms in place. When such mechanisms fail, cancer may be a result. Through mutation, such protective mechanisms are compromised in cancer cells. As a result, they show higher than normal rates of mutation, chromosomal abnormalities, and genomic instability.

19. An acute transforming virus is a retrovirus that carries an oncogene(s), while a nonacute virus can induce the activity of cellular genes that bring about tumor formation.

20. Certain environmental agents such as chemicals and X rays cause mutations. Since genes control the cell cycle, mutations in cell-cycle control genes, or those that impact cell-cycle control, can lead to cancer.

21. Radiotherapy is often administered externally or internally to damage the cell-cycle machinery, thus shrinking the cancer or killing the cancer cells. It may be completely or partially effective. Because cells have natural defenses against mutagenic insult, drugs that increase a cell's sensitivity to radiation may be administered. Radiosensitizers and radioprotectors are chemicals that alter a cell's response to radiotherapy. Radiosensitizers make cells more sensitive to therapy, whereas radioprotectors are drugs that protect normal cells from the damage caused by radiation therapy. Radiotherapy kills cells; therefore, side effects are expected.

22. No, she will still have the general population risk of about 10 percent. In addition, it is possible that genetic tests will not detect all breast cancer mutations.

23. p53 is a tumor-suppressor gene that protects cells from multiplying with damaged DNA. It is present in its mutant state in more than 50 percent of all tumors. Since the immediate control of a critical and universal cell-cycle checkpoint is mediated by p53, mutation will influence a wide range of cell types. p53's action is not limited to specific cell types.

24. Since multiple routes may lead to cancer, one would expect complex regulatory systems to be involved. More specifically, while in some cases, downregulation of a gene, such as an oncogene, may be a reasonable cancer therapy, downregulation of a tumor-suppressor gene would be undesirable in therapy. Various levels of methylation (hypermethylation and hypomethylation) influence gene activity and can therefore cause cancer.

25. (a) The clonal origin of cancer cells in a given cancer is supported by findings that mutations, chromosomal or otherwise, are of the same type in all cancerous cells. In addition, the X-chromosome inactivation patterns support the clonal origin of cancer.

(b) The progressive, time, and age-dependent development of tumorigenesis, coupled with the relatively low cancer rate compared to the mutation rate, argue for a multistep mutational model for cancer.

(c) The mutator phenotype, thought by some to be caused by defective DNA repair mechanisms, is characteristic of cancer cells. Numerous cancers, exemplified by xeroderma pigmentosum and hereditary nonpolyposis colorectal cancer, are caused by defective DNA repair systems.

26. Proteases, in general, and serine proteases, specifically, are considered tumor-promoting agents because they degrade proteins, especially those in the extracellular matrix. When such proteolysis occurs, cellular invasion and metastasis is encouraged. Consistent with this observation are numerous observations that metastatic tumor cells are associated with higher than normal amounts of protease expression. Inhibitors of serine proteases are often tested for their anticancer efficacy.

27. Various alterations in gene activity related to hyper- and hypomethylation have been associated with numerous cancers. Hypermethylation usually leads to a suppression of gene activity. *Hormonal response genes* often synthesize receptors that respond to a variety of hormones such as androgens, retinoic acid, and estrogens. For example, prostate cancer is often associated with suppressed *ESR1* and *ESR2* activity, both of which are estrogen receptors.

Cell-cycle control genes are involved in both upregulation and downregulation of the cell cycle as they influence cyclins and cyclin-dependent kinases. The cyclin-dependent kinase inhibitor *CDKN2A*, when hypermethylated, fails to inhibit cyclin-dependent kinase and thereby contributes to cancer progression. A number of *tumor cell invasion genes* have been described, some of which interfere with intercellular adhesion. When such genes are suppressed through hypermethylation, cadherin–catenin adherence mechanisms are compromised, which can influence cell-to-cell contacts.

One of the most common causes of cancer is a breakdown in *DNA repair* mechanisms. Hypermethylation suppresses the genes that normally supply DNA repair components. Proper *signal transduction* is required to maintain cell-cell adherence and response to extracellular signals. For example, when *CD44*, an integral membrane protein that is involved in matrix adhesion and signal transduction, is hypermethylated, cells cannot maintain proper cell-cell contact and communication, without which cell-cycle control is compromised.

28. (a) Because one is working with somatic cells, the usual tests for heterozygosity through crosses are not available. Therefore, one must rely on chemical/physical approaches to answer the question. A genomic library could be constructed of both osteosarcoma cell DNA and noncancerous cells from the same organism. You could then screen the library using labeled probes from the clones carrying the *RB1* gene available to you as stated in the problem. At this point, some indications might emerge because if there is a significant alteration in mutant *RB1* genes, probes may not successfully hybridize to any clones in the cancerous cell DNA library. Assuming that control hybridization occurs in the noncancerous cells, lack of hybridization in the library derived from the osteosarcoma cell line might indicate deletions. However, assuming that hybridization does allow one to identify clones containing putative *RB1* alleles, subcloning into appropriate vectors would allow sequencing to reveal sequence changes in the *RB1* alleles when compared with nonmutant genes. A second approach combines an immunoassay described in part (b) of this problem. Assuming that one can successfully make antibodies to the normal *RB1* gene product (pRB), lack of cross-reactivity of the pRB antibodies to proteins from the cancerous cell line would indicate that both *RB1* alleles are mutant.

(b) As indicated in the last portion of part (a), one can make antibodies to pRB from the noncancerous cells and test these antibodies for reactivity against proteins from the cancerous cell lines. A pRB-antibody reaction would indicate that the pRB protein is made.

(c) To determine whether addition of a normal *RB1* gene will change the cancer-causing potential of osteosarcoma cells, one could transfer the cloned normal *RB1* gene into the cells by transformation or transfection (often by electroporation or ultrasound). Transformed cells would then be introduced into the cancer-prone mice to determine whether their cancer-causing potential had been altered.

29. (a) The mRNA triplet for Gln is CAG(A). The mRNA triplet that specifies a stop is one of three: UAA, UAG, or UGA. The strand of DNA that codes for the CAG(A) would be the following: 3′-GTC(T)-5′. Therefore, if the G mutated to an A (transition), then the DNA strand would be 3′-ATC(T)-5′, which would cause a UAG(A) triplet to be produced; this would cause the stop.

(b) It is likely to be a tumor-suppressor gene because loss-of-function causes predisposition to cancer.

(c) Some women may carry genes (perhaps mutant) that "spare" for the *BRCA1* gene product. Some women may have immune systems that recognize and destroy precancerous cells, or they may have mutations in breast signal transduction genes so that cell division suppression occurs in the absence of *BRCA1*.

30. (a, b) Even though there are changes in the *BRCA1* gene, they do not always have physiological consequences. Such neutral polymorphisms make screening difficult in that one cannot always be certain that a mutation will cause problems for the patient.

(c) The polymorphism in *PM2* is probably a silent mutation because the third base of the codon is involved.

(d) The polymorphism in *PM3* is probably a neutral missense mutation because the first base is involved.

Chapter 21: Genomics, Bioinformatics, and Proteomics

Concept Areas	Corresponding Problems
Genomics Overview	1, 4, 7, 15, 16, 19, 27, 32
Sequencing	2, 6, 13, 16, 19, 28
Genomic Organization	3, 10, 11, 12, 21, 22, 28, 29, 31
Bioinformatics	5, 8, 16, 28, 32, 33
Essential Genes, Pseudogenes	4, 9, 25, 26, 29
Proteomics	7, 34
Annotation	14, 18, 20, 21, 23, 24, 30
Microarrays	17

Vocabulary: Organization and Listing of Terms and Concepts

Structures and Substances

Genome

  RFLP

  SNP

  CNV

  restriction enzymes

    partial digest

    contiguous fragments

      "contig"

    capillary gel

    3.1 billion nucleotides

  BAC

  YAC

    cosmid

  Haemophilus influenzae

  Drosophila, etc.

  Pseudomonas aeruginosa

  Homo neanderthalensis

  GenBank

    NCBI

      accession number

    BLAST

similarity score

E value

annotation

  exon

  intron

  promoter sequences

    TATA, GC, CAAT

  open reading frame (ORF)

    codon bias

intergenic DNA spacers

homologous gene

ortholog

paralog

protein domain

  motif

Transcriptome

Proteome

Encyclopedia of DNA Elements (ENCODE)

Bacterial chromosomes

  DNA

    double-stranded

    circular, linear

plasmids

  high density

    approximately one gene/kb

  operons

polycistronic transcription units

Eukaryote

 variable gene density

 introns

 repetitive sequences

 yeast

   12.1 Mb

   16 chromosomes

   approximately 6000 genes

 Arabidopsis thaliana

   1 gene/5 kb

   dynamic genome

   duplications

   intergenic spacer DNA

   gene clusters

 rice

 black cottonwood

Mycoplasma genitalium

Comparative genomics

Drosophila melanogaster

Canis familiaris

 FISH

 IGF1

 Pan troglodytes

 indel

  Alu

 synteny

Macaca mulatta

 Rh

about 20,000 genes

  repeat elements

   transposons, LINES, SINES

 phenylketonuria

 MHC

Strongylocentrus purpuratus

  pseudogene

  defensome

Multigene families

 superfamily

  globin

 paralog

  α-globin

  pseudogene

  β-globin

  intergenic regions

  epsilon, gamma (Gγ, Aγ)

  delta

Metagenomics

 environment

 microbial samples

 GOS (Global Ocean Sampling)

  Venn diagram

 transcriptome analysis

  gene expression

  microarray analysis

 gene chip

  cDNA

  PCR

  cluster algorithm

   circadian rhythm

 proteome analysis

  protein microarray

collagen

    Tyrannosaurus rex

    Mammut americanum

  isoform

  post-translationally modified product

Interactome

network map

Processes/Methods

Positional cloning

Transcriptome analysis

Proteomics

Human Genome Project

  shotgun sequencing

  high-throughput sequencing

  compiling the sequence

  clone-by-clone approach

    map-based cloning

Bioinformatics

  contig alignment

Annotation

  codon bias

Functional genomics

  similarity search

  homologous genes

Human Genome Project (HGP)

  20,000 protein-coding genes

  100,000 proteins

    alternative splicing

ELSI (ethical, legal, and social implications)

Proteomics

Metabolomics

Glycomics

Toxicogenomics

Metagenomics

Pharmacogenomics

Transcriptomics

Nutrigenomics

Comparative genomics

  in situ hybridization

  nonhuman model organisms

DNA microarray analysis

Polymerase chain reaction

Proteome analysis

  alternative splicing

  editing of pre-mRNA

  Protein Structure Initiative

  two-dimensional gel electrophoresis

  isoelectric focusing

  SDS-PAGE

  mass spectrometry

  m/z ratio

  MALDI

  time of flight (TOF)

  liquid chromatography

  protein microarray

Systems biology

Genome evolution

Genome duplication

Gene duplication

Sequence conservation

Concepts

Genomics

  structural

functional

comparative

metagenomics

"Omics" revolution

Transcriptome analysis

Proteomics

Annotation

Genome organization comparisons

Genome evolution

Minimum genome size

Comparative genomics

Systems biology

interactome

network map

Sequence conservation

Solutions to Problems and Discussion Questions

1. Functional genomics seeks to understand functional components within the genome and similarities of genomes across phylogenetic and evolutionary distances. Comparative genomics analyzes the arrangement and organization of families of genes within and among genomes.

2. Whole-genome shotgun sequencing involves randomly cutting the genome into numerous smaller segments. Overlapping sequences are used to identify segments that were once contiguous, eventually producing the entire sequence. Difficulties in alignment often occur in repetitive regions of the genome. Map-based sequencing relies on known landmarks (genes, nucleotide polymorphisms, etc.) to orient the alignment of cloned fragments that have been sequenced. Compared to whole-genome sequencing, the map-based approach is somewhat cumbersome and time consuming. Whole-genome sequencing has become the most common method for assembling genomes, with map-based cloning being used to resolve the problems often encountered during whole-genome sequencing.

3. Genomes of both types of organisms are composed of double-stranded DNA (larger in eukaryotes) associated with proteins (more transient in prokaryotes). Both contain open reading frames, but those of prokaryotes are more densely packed. Both have some genes in clusters, but are much more pronounced in prokaryotes (operons). There are a few repetitive sequences in prokaryotes, but this trend is much more common in eukaryotes. Both contain informational sequences, but those of eukaryotes are often interrupted (introns). Almost all genomes contain transposable elements.

4. The question as to how to define an organism's genome is complicated by a variety of symbiotic relationships that are known to exist in virtually all organisms. Plasmids are capable of carrying both essential and nonessential genes of the host. To complicate the matter, it is likely that all cells contain nonessential genes. An organism's genome will probably come to encompass all genetic elements that can be shown to be stable cellular inhabitants.

5. Understanding the genome is dependent on the field of bioinformatics, in which computer and mathematics applications are used to organize, share, and analyze data generated by sequencing data. World access to such data is dependent on the ability to store, efficiently share, and obtain the maximum amount of information from protein and DNA sequences. As genomics emerged, bioinformatics became a significant player and today occupies an intellectual enterprise that fuses biological data with information technology, mathematics, and statistical analysis. Most applications, such as the identification of informational content in the genome and DNA sequencing, rely on sequence alignments in nucleic acids and proteins.

6. The main goals of the Human Genome Project are to establish, categorize, and analyze functions for human genes. As stated in the text, the goals are:

• To analyze genetic variations between humans, including the identification of single-nucleotide polymorphisms (SNPs).

• To map and sequence the genomes of several model organisms used in experimental genetics, including *E. coli, S. cerevisiae, C. elegans, D. melanogaster,* and *M. musculus* (the mouse).

• To develop new sequencing technologies, such as high-throughput computer-automated sequencers in order to facilitate genome analysis.

• To disseminate genome information among both scientists and the general public.

7. High-throughput technologies allow comprehensive analyses of a number of labor-intensive tasks that would normally take days or weeks to be reduced to half-day activities. By shortening sequencing times for examples, numerous organisms can be sequenced to yield highly informative comparative sequences (comparative genomics). Applied to both genomics and proteomics, high-throughput technologies allow rapid analyses and deployment of genomic information.

8. One initial approach to annotating a sequence is to compare the newly sequenced genomic DNA to the known sequences already stored in various databases. The National Center for Biotechnology Information (NCBI) provides access to BLAST (Basic Local Alignment Search Tool) software that directs searches through databanks of DNA and protein sequences. A segment of DNA can be compared to sequences in major databases such as GenBank to identify matches that align in whole or in part. One might seek similarities of a sequence on chromosome 11 in a mouse and find that or similar sequences in a number of taxa. BLAST will compute a similarity score or identity value to indicate the degree to which two sequences are similar. BLAST is one of many sequence alignment algorithms (RNA-RNA, protein-protein, etc.) that may sacrifice sensitivity for speed.

9. Pseudogenes are nonfunctional versions of genes that resemble gene sequences but contain significant nucleotide changes, which prevent their expression. They are formed by gene duplication and subsequent mutation.

10. The human genome is composed of over 3 billion nucleotides in which about 2 percent code for genes. Genes are unevenly distributed over chromosomes with clusters of gene-rich ones separated by gene-poor ones (deserts). Human genes tend to be larger and contain more and larger introns than those in invertebrates such as *Drosophila*. It is estimated that at least half of the genes generate products by alternative splicing. Hundreds of genes have been transferred from bacteria into vertebrates. Duplicated regions are common, which may facilitate chromosomal rearrangement. The human genome appears to contain approximately 20,000 protein-coding genes; however, the total number remains uncertain.

11. While greater DNA content per cell is associated with eukaryotes, one cannot universally equate genomic size with an increase in organismic complexity. There are numerous examples in which DNA content per cell varies considerably among closely related species. Because of the diverse cell types of multicellular eukaryotes, a variety of gene products are required, which may be related to the increase in DNA content per cell. In addition, the advantage of diploidy automatically increases DNA content per cell. When we view the question in another way, however, it is likely that a much higher *percentage* of the genome of a prokaryote is actually involved in phenotype production than in a eukaryote. Eukaryotes have evolved the capacity to obtain and maintain what appears to be large amounts of "extra," perhaps "junk," DNA. Prokaryotes, on the other hand, with their relatively short life cycle, are extremely efficient in their accumulation and use of their genome. Given the larger amount of DNA per cell in eukaryotes and the requirement that the DNA be partitioned in an orderly fashion to daughter cells during cell division, certain mechanisms and structures (mitosis, nucleosomes, centromeres, etc.) have evolved for *packaging* the DNA.

In addition, the genome is divided into separate entities (chromosomes) to perhaps facilitate the partitioning process in mitosis and meiosis. Eukaryotic chromosomes characteristically contain a variety of noncoding regions that were once thought to be "junk" in a sense that no function was expected. Recent evidence indicates that such regions, even regions known as introns, often have function.

12. Bacterial genes are densely packed in the chromosome. The protein-coding genes are mostly organized in polycistronic transcription units without introns. Eukaryotic genes are less densely packed in chromosomes, and protein-coding genes are mostly organized as single transcription units with introns.

13. Because many repetitive regions of the genome are not directly involved in production of a phenotype, they tend to be isolated from selection and show considerable variation in redundancy. Length variation in such repeats is unique among individuals (except for identical twins) and, with various detection methods, provides the basis for DNA fingerprinting. Single-nucleotide polymorphisms also occur frequently in the genome and can be used to distinguish individuals.

14. One usually begins to annotate a sequence by comparing it, often using BLAST, to the known sequences already stored in various databases. Similarity to other annotated sequences often provides insight as to a sequences function. Hallmarks to annotation include the identification of gene-regulatory sequences found upstream of genes (promoters, enhancers, and silencers), downstream elements (termination sequences), and triplet nucleotides that are part of the coding region of the gene. In addition, 5′ and 3′ splice sites that are used to distinguish exons from introns, as well as polyadenylation sites, are also used in annotation. Similar hallmarks are used to annotate prokaryotic genes, but because prokaryotic genes do not contain introns, their annotation is sometimes less complicated. Annotation is an ongoing process and community effort involving scientists worldwide.

15. A number of new subdisciplines of molecular biology will provide the infrastructure for major advances in our understanding of living systems. The following terms identify specific areas within that infrastructure:

proteomics—proteins in a cell or tissue

metabolomics—enzymatic pathways

glycomics—carbohydrates of a cell or tissue

toxicogenomics—toxic chemicals

metagenomics—environmental issues

pharmacogenomics—customized medicine

transcriptomics—expressed genes

Many other "-omics" are likely in the future.

16. Metagenomics is a relatively new discipline that examines the genomes from entire communities of microbes in environmental samples of water, air, and soil. Virtually every environment on Earth is being sampled in metagenomics projects. A major initiative is a global expedition called the *Sorcerer II* Global Ocean Sampling (GOS) in which researchers travel the globe by yacht and sample as many microbes as possible. Metagenomics is teaching us more about millions of species of microbes, of which only a few thousand have been well characterized. According to the text,

> Metagenomics is providing important new information about genetic diversity in microbes that is key to understanding complex interactions between microbial communities and their environment, as well as allowing phylogenetic classification of newly identified microbes. Metagenomics also has great potential for identifying genes with novel functions, some of which have potentially valuable applications in medicine and biotechnology.

17. Most microarrays, known also as gene chips, consist of a glass slide that is coated, using a robotic system, with single-stranded DNA molecules. Some microarrays are coated with single-stranded sequences of expressed sequenced tags or DNA sequences that are complementary to gene transcripts. A single microarray can have as many as 20,000 different spots of DNA, each containing a unique sequence. Researchers use microarrays to compare patterns of gene expression in tissues under different conditions or to compare gene expression patterns in normal and diseased tissues. In addition, microarrays can be used to identify pathogens. Microarray databases allow investigators to compare any given pattern to others worldwide.

18. $0.8^5 = 33\%$

19. Knowing the sequence of DNA in an organism is only the beginning. Annotating the DNA is a significant challenge. Even at that, knowing how gene products interact in time and space (proteomics) will take additional rounds of technological advances that are as yet unconsidered. The work of Haas et al. identified variation in intron/exon splice sites, micro-exons, and alternative transcription start sites. Correlating various transcriptional and translational schemes with the phenotype will be an interesting adventure.

20. Aneuploidy in humans occurs for the sex chromosomes (X and Y) and three of the autosomes (13, 18, and 21). Other aneuploids are apparently not compatible with survival. Extra or missing X chromosomes are apparently tolerated because of dosage compensation, while Y chromosome aneuploids are most likely compatible with survival because of the general paucity of Y-linked genes. Notice that the number of genes on chromosomes 13, 18, and 21 are the lowest for the autosomes. It is probably not coincidental that chromosomes with the fewest genes and no known mechanism for dosage compensation are the only ones that survive as human aneuploids.

21. **(a)** Assuming an average gene size of 5000 base pairs, there would be about 6.7×10^7 base pairs comprising genes. Subtracting this value from 116.8 Mb gives 49.8 Mb between genes. Dividing 49.8 Mb by 13,379 genes gives about 3700 bases between genes.

(b) 54,934/13,379 = 4.11 exons

(c) 48,257/13,379 = 3.61 introns

(d) There is a marked increase in the number of genes involved in alternative transcripts.

(e) Alternative transcripts are RNAs that are variable in sequence due to different splicing of introns or other processes such as use of alternative promoters (13 percent) and alternative polyadenylation sites (6 percent).

22. Accurate annotation of genomes will not be a simple, straightforward process. Limitations on interpretation of sequence data will mean that new, uncharted levels of genomic, transcriptomic, and proteomic complications will be discovered. Since computer programs can only identify what is already predicted, manual verification and examination will be needed to bridge the gap between what we think we know and what has actually evolved over a few billion years. All the information will be highly significant in terms of understanding how organisms go about daily living and how we manage our relationships among them. For instance, one clinical application of genome sequence information is based on the development of antisense DNA to nullify the function of harmful RNAs and proteins within a cell. Opposite-strand RNA transcription overlap generates the possibility of natural antisense interactions for gene regulation *in vivo* and may provide insight into the development of antisense therapies presently being developed.

23. Open reading frames are identified by computer programs based on identification of start (ATG) and stop (TAA, TGA, TAG) codons. Notice that the percentage of GC pairs compared with AT pairs is quite low in such punctuation triplets. Therefore, when scanning DNA sequences for ORFs with high AT content, many short sequences are obtained that are clearly not likely to be involved in protein production. However, when DNA is GC rich, the likelihood of long ORFs similar to protein-coding size is increased. Therefore, the likelihood of falsely considering a sequence "protein-coding" increases with increasing GC content, as indicated in the figure.

24. Increased protein production from approximately 20,000 genes is probably related to alternative splicing and various post-translational processing schemes. In addition, a particular DNA segment may be read in a variety of ways and in two directions.

25. The issue here is whether the organism under consideration is independent and self-reproducing. It appears that the minimum number of genes for a free-living organism is in the 250–350 range. Symbionts can have much smaller genomes and exist with fewer genes because of materials supplied by the host cell. As long as one defines the lifestyle (free-living or symbiont) of the organism in question, it is informative to consider how many genes are needed to accomplish the task of "living."

26. Assuming that the APS strain is the ancestral strain, the remaining strains appear to have smaller genome sizes indicating genome reduction. The smallest *Buchnera* genome is approximately 448 kb compared with the genome size of *M. genitalium* of about 600 kb with about 480 protein-coding genes. The APS genome codes for about 564 genes in its 641 kb genome. A gene is coded every 1136 bp (641,000/564) for the APS strain and every 1250 bp (600,000/480) for *M. genitalium*. Given these data, the CCE species should code for approximately:

$$(448,000/1193) = 375.5$$

genes. (*Note*: 1193 was obtained as the average gene spacing of the two bacterial species mentioned above.) Using these calculations, the CCE strain would contain fewer genes than *M. genitalium*. Other possible approaches to determine minimum genome size to sustain life include computational studies whereby one might estimate the number of essential chemical reactions that are needed for life. Another would be to take an organism with a small number of genes and then systematically mutate genes to see if elimination of genes caused reduced survival. By eliminating individual and groups of genes by mutation, the minimum number might be obtainable.

27. (a) Generally, contigs are suspected to be part of the same chromosome in that their end sequences overlap.

(b) Identification of a protein-coding region is suspected if similar sequences are conserved in other species and various upstream, downstream, splicing, and punctuation sequences are present and are appropriately in the proper reading frames.

(c) Comparisons of base sequence data with other organisms indicates conservation of a considerable number of sequences. Because of such conservation, functional relationships are strongly supported. Comparative mutation analyses indicating similar function add more support.

(d) Proteomics is the identification and analysis of proteins in cells, tissues, and organisms. Genome annotation provides an estimate of the number of protein-coding genes, while a number of sophisticated techniques including electrophoresis, chromatography, spectrophotometry, and microarrays indicate the number of proteins actually produced. The finding that there are many more types of proteins than genes in the genome has generated a number of explanations.

(e) By comparing the amino acid sequences of proteins, the base sequences of genes, and intron/exon architecture, researchers have determined that many genes originated by duplication. Sequence divergence often alters duplicated genes, thus providing the raw material for the evolution of new genes.

(f) Microarrays provide a method for identifying active genes by the hybridization of complementary gene products to stretches of DNA. Different hybridization patterns indicate that while some genes are expressed in almost all cells, others show cell- and tissue-specific expression.

28. In general, one would expect certain factors (such as heat or salt) to favor evolution and increase protein stability: distribution of ionic interactions on the surface, density of hydrophobic residues and interactions, and number of hydrogen and disulfide bonds. By examining the codon table, a high GC ratio would favor the amino acids Ala, Gly, Pro, Arg, and Trp and minimize the use of Ile, Phe, Lys, Asn, and Tyr. How codon bias influences actual protein stability is not yet understood. Most genomic sequences change through relatively gradual responses to mild selection over long periods of time. These sequences strongly resemble patterns of common descent; that is, they are conserved. Although the same can be said for organisms adapted to extreme environments, extraordinary physiological demands may dictate unexpected sequence bias.

29. While the β-globin gene family is a relatively large (60 kb) sequence and restriction analyses show that it is composed of six genes, one is a pseudogene and therefore does not produce a product. Each of the five functional genes contains two similar-sized introns, which, when included with noncoding flanking regions (5′ and 3′) and spacer DNA between genes, account for the 95 percent mentioned in the question.

30. Since structural and chemical factors determine the function of a protein, it is likely to have several proteins share a considerable amino acid sequence identity, but not be functionally identical. Since the *in vivo* function of such a protein is determined by secondary and tertiary structures, as well as local surface chemistries in active or functional sites, the nonidentical sequences may have considerable influence on function. Note that the query matches to different site positions within the target proteins. A number of other factors suggesting different functions include: associations with other molecules (cytoplasmic, membrane, or extracellular), chemical nature and position of binding domains, post-translational modification, and signal sequences.

31. (a) To annotate a gene, one identifies gene-regulatory sequences found upstream of genes (promoters, enhancers, and silencers), downstream elements (termination sequences), and in-frame triplet nucleotides that are part of the coding region of the gene. In addition, 5′ and 3′ splice sites that are used to distinguish exons from introns as well as polyadenylation sites are also used in annotation.

(b) Similarity to other annotated sequences often provides insight into a sequence's function and may serve to substantiate a particular genetic assignment. Direct sequencing of cDNAs from various tissues and developmental stages aid in verification.

(c) Taking an average of 22,500 for the estimated number of genes in the human genome and computing the percentage represented by 3141 gives 13.96 percent. It might be safe to say that chromosome 1 is gene rich.

32. Whenever a DNA sequence is conserved in other species, that sequence likely has an influence on similar phenotypes. The higher the number of species that conserve the sequence, the higher the likelihood of determining its function. Coupled with mutation analysis and physical mapping, comparative genomics provides a powerful method for linking DNA sequences with complex human diseases.

33. Two factors may be significant in causing a similar gene to function one way in one species and another way in a closely related species. First, despite the fact that humans and chimps share significant sequence overlap, there are still approximately 35 million single-base differences and about 5 million deletion/addition differences. Such changes influence the molecular environment in which a gene is expressed.

Second, the external environment, especially in terms of carbohydrate availability and metabolism, has been different during the evolution of these two species. Such environmental differences may engage a different genetic background (therefore proteome) in which a particular gene is expressed. A protein functioning in one molecular environment may function quite differently in a slightly different environment. Such complexities in gene expression must be addressed when therapies are developed using model organisms.

34. First, because blood is relatively easy to obtain in a pure state, its components can be analyzed without fear of tissue-site contamination. Second, blood is intimately exposed to virtually all cells of the body and may therefore carry chemical markers to certain abnormal cells; it represents, theoretically, an ideal probe into the human body. However, when blood is removed from the body, its proteome changes, and those changes are dependent on a number of environmental factors. Thus, what might be a valid diagnostic under one condition might not be so under others. In addition, the serum proteome is subject to change depending on the genetic, physiologic, and environmental state of the patient. Age and sex are additional variables that must be considered.

Validation of a plasma proteome for a particular cancer can be strengthened by demonstrating that the stage of development of the cancer correlates with a commensurate change in the proteome in a relatively large, statistically significant pool of patients. The types of changes in the proteome should be reproducible and, at least until complexities are clarified, should involve tumorigenic proteins. It would be helpful to have comparisons with archived samples of each individual at a disease-free time.

Chapter 22: Genome Dynamics: Transposons, Immunogenetics, and Eukaryotic Viruses

Concept Areas	Corresponding Problems
Transposable Elements, Overview	1, 23
Transposition	2, 6, 25
Jumping Genes	3
Evolution of Transposons	4
Ds, Ac	5, 27
Copia	7, 24
IS Elements	8
P Elements	9, 26
Immune System, Overview	10, 12, 13, 28
Immune System, Diversity	11, 28
Immunodeficiency	14
DNA Viruses, RNA Viruses, Retroviruses	15, 16, 17, 18, 19, 20, 21, 22, 29, 30

Vocabulary: Organization and Listing of Terms and Concepts

Structures and Substances

Transposable element, transposon

  jumping gene

  junk DNA

Insertion sequences, IS elements

  transposase

  terminal repeats

   ITRs

Bacterial transposon

  Tn element

   heteroduplex

Ac-Ds (Activator, Dissociation)

  maize

  transposase

Mobile elements in peas

  starch-branching enzyme I (SBEI)

Drosophila

  copia

  direct terminal repeat (DTR)

P elements

  hybrid dysgenesis

Humans

  long interspersed elements (LINES)

  short interspersed elements (SINES)

  Alu elements

DNA transposons

  repeated DNA sequences

   target-site duplications

DNA viruses

  lytic infection

  latent infection

  herpesvirus 8 (HHV-8)

Kaposi's sarcoma herpes virus (KSHV)

Kaposi's sarcoma

v-cyclin

cyclin D2

pRB

Retrotransposons

reverse transcriptase

long terminal repeat (LTR)

RNA intermediate

Provirus

viral envelope

receptors

gag, pol, env

RNA viruses

RNA-dependent RNA polymerases

RdRps

genomic variability

severe acute respiratory syndrome

SARS

Coronaviruses

SARS-associated coronavirus

Transducing virus

Transforming retrovirus

replication defective

helper virus

Immunoglobulins

antigen

antibody

humoral immunity

cellular immunity

T lymphocyte (T cell)

T cell receptor

structure

heavy chain

light chain

constant region

variable region

kappa chains

lambda chains

IgM, IgD, IgE, IgG, IgA

plasma cells

V, J, C regions

Processes/Methods

Hybrid dysgenesis

Transposition

nonreplicative

replicative

Transposon silencing

cytosine methylation

Exon shuffling

Template switching

Apoptosis

Immunoglobulin class switching

hypermutation

RAG1, RAG2

Horizontal gene transfer

Concepts

Hybrid dysgenesis

germ-line transformation

Chapter 22 Genome Dynamics: Transposons, Immunogenetics, and Eukaryotic Viruses

Transposition
    evolutionary implications
        selfish DNA
        exon shuffling
Horizontal gene transfer
Genome rearrangement

Transposon silencing
Insertional mutagenesis
Antibody diversity
    clonal selection theory
    hypermutability
    class switching

Solutions to Problems and Discussion Questions

1. Each organism possesses a variety of transposable elements. Bacteria possess insertion sequences (about 800 to 1500 base pairs in length) as well as transposons, which are larger. Both are mobile in bacterial, viral, and plasmid DNAs, and both have repeated base sequences at their ends. Barbara McClintock described the genetic behavior of mobile elements (*Ds* and *Ac*) in maize. *Ds* can move if *Ac* is present; thus, *transposable controlling elements* exist. An *Ac* element is 4563 base pairs long and is similar in structure to some bacterial transposons. Transposons often code for transposase enzymes, which are essential for transposition. *Copia* elements in *Drosophila* may be present in numerous copies in the genome and contain direct and inverted terminal repeats. *P* elements, also in *Drosophila,* are responsible for a phenomenon called hybrid dysgenesis. Humans possess a variety of transposable elements, including the *Alu* family of short interspersed elements (SINES), which are between 200 and 300 base pairs long and may exist in 300,000 copies per genome. Long interspersed elements (LINES) also occur in the human genome and seem to be capable of movement. Such elements share common structural features, are often mobile, and may influence gene activity.

2. It is likely that the reverse transcriptase, in making DNA, provides a DNA segment that is capable of integrating into the yeast chromosome, as other types of DNA are known to do.

3. When one thinks of "jumping," the jumper leaves one place and comes to rest in another. The site where the jumper left is unaltered. Transposons move by two schemes, nonreplicative and replicative. In nonreplicative transposition, the transposon leaves its original site and inserts itself in a new location, much like a jumper would do.

In some cases, however, the original site can be altered in the process. In replicative transposition, the transposon is copied, leaving the original transposon in the original location. The copied element is inserted into a new location. If transposition is nonreplicative and the site of origin is not altered, then the term *jumping genes* is descriptive.

4. Some transposons contain genes (*reverse transcriptase, integrase,* structural genes) and structural elements (terminal repeats, polyadenylation signals, etc.) common to proviral forms of retroviruses. If, after entering the genome as retroviruses do, they lost the ability to continue through the infective state but retained their ability to transpose, a transposon has evolved. Some transposons encode RNA and proteins that form virus-like particles inside the cell, but are not able to leave the cell.

5. The *Ac* element is structurally similar to that of bacterial transposons and *Ds-a* is almost identical to *Ac* except for a 194-bp deletion within the transposase gene. Because of this deletion, transposition of *Ds* is dependent on the presence of *Ac*. Other *Ds* elements that have been sequenced contain even larger deletions in the transposase gene, but all retain the inverted terminal repeats like *Ac*. *Ds* transposition is dependent on *Ac* because of a deletion in its transposase gene. *Ac* supplies the needed transposase activity for *Ds* movement.

6. One way in which a transposon can move genes within the genome is by read-through transcription, producing a chimeric transcript containing a downstream gene(s). When this chimeric transcript is reverse transcribed and inserted into the genome, it can include the downstream gene(s). When two or more identical genetic elements exist in a genome an opportunity exists for unequal homologous recombination. The result can be a variety of chromosomal aberrations: duplications, deletions, inversions, and/or translocations.

7. Below is a representation of the transposon positions mentioned in the question. Various pairing possibilities provide opportunities for generating chromosomal aberrations.

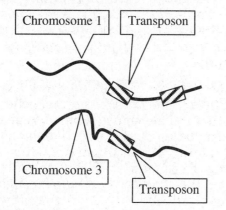

For chromosome 1, looping and pairing of homologous segments provides an opportunity to create an inversion.

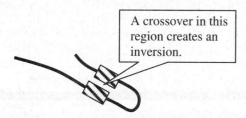

If homologous segments from chromosomes 1 and 3 pair, crossing over would produce a translocation. Depending on the positions of the transposons, chromosomes can be created that have two centromeres or no centromere at all.

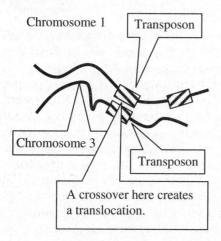

8. In the presence of a "helper element," a defective element may be able to transpose. Within a single bacterium, the transposase gene works in *trans* because a cytoplasmic transposase enzyme is produced. Therefore, the intact element may compensate for the loss of the deletion-defective transposase, assuming that the transposase function is compatible.

9. Hybrid dysgenesis occurs in the offspring of some crosses when the protein that represses transposition is absent. If a female carries the repressor and she passes it through her egg cytoplasm to her offspring, dysgenic offspring are not produced. In a reciprocal cross, the egg cytoplasm may not carry the repressors. Offspring from such a mating may show dysgenesis because *P* elements are mobilized, not repressed.

10. During the maturation of millions of lymphocytes, each produces one type of immunoglobulin or T-cell receptor capable of recognizing and binding to one particular antigen. When a foreign antigen interacts with a "matching" lymphocyte, a chemical signal stimulates proliferation of that lymphocyte. A pool of such stimulated lymphocytes represents a selected clone of cells.

11. While random recombination of different LV regions to different J regions accounts for considerable antibody diversity, additional diversity is achieved by imprecise joining and can occur anywhere within a region containing several base pairs. Such imprecision alters amino acid sequences in the resulting variable region.

12. Assuming that you can identify chromosomes 4 and 10, it should be possible to determine their intimate association and subsequent recombination microscopically. Since formation of a complete heavy chain is dependent on recombination, if such chromosomes are intimately associated, the creature is likely to be at least 13 years old. If the chromosomes are not associated, the creature is probably less than 13 years of age.

13. The IgM immunoglobulin differs from IgG and IgE by the composition of the constant regions of their heavy chains. IgM contains a μ region, IgG contains a γ region, and IgE contains an ε region. Because of the sequential organization of the heavy chain exons, μ, δ, γ, ε, α, once the μ, δ, and γ sequences are eliminated by recombination to make an IgE molecule, no opportunity remains to make an IgG molecule because the exon making the γ chain is no longer available.

14. B cells synthesize antibodies, whereas T cells directly recognize and mark infected cells for destruction. Immunoglobulin gene rearrangement brought about by somatic recombination is dependent on the *RAG1* and *RAG2* genes. They produce two proteins that create double-stranded breaks at the junctions of the V, D, J, and C regions. Without such recombination, immunoglobulin diversity is not possible in either the T or B lymphocytes.

15. Although direct recombination between a viral DNA and nuclear DNA occurs, sequence evidence suggests that an RNA intermediate is involved. Using reverse transcriptase from simultaneous infection by a retrovirus, a cDNA is made from a cellular RNA. The resulting cDNA can integrate into the viral DNA by recombination.

16. The sequence of the proviral DNA would be as follows:

3'-TTATCGATCGATTCCGCTACGCGCTA

5'-AATAGCTAGCTAAGGCGATGCGCGAT

Notice that regardless of the reading frame, one encounters a termination codon (underlined). Since the *gag* gene produces a protein necessary for viral maturation and infection, it is highly unlikely that the sequence would produce new infectious

retroviruses unless the stop codons were at the 3' end of the mRNA and truncation of the C terminal portion of the peptide did not influence gag function.

5'-AA<u>UAG</u>C<u>UAG</u>C<u>UAA</u>GGCGAUGCGCGAU

17. If the new virus is a retrovirus, drugs that inhibit reverse transcriptase, such as AZT (zidovudine), could be administered. If the viral infection stops or is hindered, then the new virus is probably a retrovirus.

Isolation and chemical analysis could also be used to characterize the new virus. The RNA within a retrovirus would be sensitive to RNase, whereas DNA would be insensitive. The genome of a DNA virus could be cleaved with DNase to which RNA would be insensitive. Another method would employ a northern blot with a reverse transcriptase probe.

18. Retroviruses are relatively small RNA viruses that generate double-stranded DNA that is integrated into the host's genome. With proper genetic engineering that disables transposition, a modified virus can become an endogenous provirus and, under ideal conditions, produce desired gene products at the appropriate time and place. Unfortunately, it is difficult to regulate the output of introduced genes. In addition, the host may mount an immune response to the vector and because the site(s) of integration is uncertain at present, insertional mutagenesis of host genes may occur. The provirus may also contain enhancers that cause aberrant expression of nearby genes.

19. Retroviruses undergo rapid evolution because reverse transcriptase is highly error-prone and is not able to proofread replication errors. In addition, the retroviral genome is capable of a variety of genomic rearrangements that further increase genetic variability. Resistance is achieved when the AZT binding site is altered by one to five amino acid substitutions. The higher the number of amino acid substitutions, the greater the resistance to AZT.

20. Both a bacterial prophage and retroviral provirus are integrated as double-stranded DNAs that replicate with the host chromosomes. Though different processes, each can produce progeny viruses, and each can acquire and transfer host genes. Bacteriophage engage in transduction where the generation of a defective phage provides for the acquisition of host DNA. For a retrovirus, occurrence of a deletion between a provirus and a cellular gene can result in a retroviral RNA that is missing some of its own genes and gained cellular DNA. This defective RNA can be packaged into a new virus particle if another viral RNA genome is present in the cell transcribed from another copy of the provirus. Template switching during the next round of reverse transcription creates a viral genome that contains host DNA.

21. There are several paths by which a virus may alter the normal regulatory machinery of a cell and cause a tumor. First, when retroviruses insert their DNA into the host's genome (via reverse transcriptase and integrase), mutations can occur. Should a mutation occur in a tumor-suppressor gene, a tumor might result, especially if the mutation has become homozygous. Second, some retroviruses introduce elements (promoters, enhancers) that alter the expression of host genes. Should such an introduction alter normal regulatory mechanisms, a tumor may result. Third, some retroviruses introduce genes acquired from other host cells. Such transforming retroviruses may bring in oncogenes that may lead to tumors.

22. Host shifting can occur when the S protein changes its specificity. Both its high mutation rate and high recombination frequency generate a variety of sequences. The high mutation rate is caused by error-prone RNA polymerases and lack of proofreading that copy the RNA genome. In addition RNA genomes can recombine during RNA synthesis by strand switching.

23. (a) Certain mutations in the *gal* operon of *E. coli* were shown to be caused by insertion sequence (IS) elements. The mutations were caused by the addition of several hundred base pairs of extra DNA inserted at the beginning of the operon. Other work in prokaryotes and eukaryotes (corn) showed that phenotypic changes occurred when transposable elements were present and in some cases mobilized in the genome.

(b) Direct sequencing of viral genomes has revealed a number of homologies to both prokaryotic and eukaryotic genomes. Comparative genomics has revealed that viruses can not only carry host DNA sequences, but they can also account for the movement of genes between genomes (horizontal or lateral gene transfer).

(c) The mobility and mutagenic effects of transposons have been documented as a cause of hemophilia (loss of blood-clotting factor VII). A number of diseases, including Duchenne muscular dystrophy, colon and breast cancers, and hemophilia B, contain common transposons that are suspected as causative agents.

24. The original insertion of a *copia* transposon within the normal allele of the *rg* eye color gene can directly disrupt function by altering coding and/or splicing, or by causing termination of transcription or translation. Although suppression of the *rg* mutation by a nonallelic gene may explain the origin of a few red-eyed flies in the mutant cell line, a more likely origin is the excision of the *copia* element. Because sizable terminal repeats are found at each end of *copia* elements, loop formation and synapsis of these elements followed by crossing over can lead to excision. If the excision is precise, the original wild-type gene may be restored. In addition, once the mutant line was established, there was an opportunity for unequal synapsis of homologous chromosomes to occur at terminal repeats. If followed by crossing over, a chromosome somewhat free of the *copia* element can be generated. If deletions or duplications are not generated in either of the above processes, then wild-type function of the *rg* eye color gene may be restored. A replication error that causes a deletion of the *copia* element may also occur.

25. By having a transposase generate a staggered cut at the target site, terminal duplications of identical sequence are generated for each target. Because transposases are responsible for the insertion of a number of mobile elements, repeated sequences in relatively close proximity may be used to identify the location of such elements. Open reading frames with sequences typical of transposon genes between such repeats would support the identification of a transposon and be helpful in determining the location and number of transposons in the human genome.

26. To introduce a gene into a strain of *Drosophila*, the gene of interest is cloned into the middle of a *P* element that also contains a gene that produces a visible marker. The *P* elements are injected into embryos along with a helper plasmid that carries the *transposase* gene. If the *P* element inserts into the germ-line genome of the embryo, resulting progeny can be identified by the visible marker and are likely to carry the gene of interest (transgene).

27. If a transposable element moves, it may move precisely or imprecisely to another location in the genome, or it may move nearby, even within the same gene or its regulatory apparatus. Such an intragenic move of a transposon, even if precisely excised from its original location, may produce a more severe phenotype. If the removal of the original transposon is imprecise and still intragenic, then a more severe phenotype may result. Imprecise excision of mobile elements like *Ac* and *Ds* often leaves small rearrangements or stretches of DNA called transposition footprints at sites where they excise. In many cases, each excision footprint is unique, varying in size and sequence. Depending on the size and location of such footprints, significant alterations in gene function and regulation may occur. In addition, such footprints may sponsor an array of chromosomal aberrations.

28. The type of Burkitt's lymphoma described in the question is caused by the translocation of elements from chromosome 8 to within the H chain immunoglobulin gene of chromosome 14. Formation of the translocated chromosome misregulates the expression of *c-myc* by combining enhancer elements in chromosome 14 with *c-myc*, leading to high levels of a C-MYC transcription factor. In addition, some negative regulatory elements within c-*myc* are often removed or altered as a result of the translocation, thereby contributing to increased c-*myc* activity. This C-MYC transcription factor plays a central role in the control of a diverse set of cellular processes, including cell-cycle progression and programmed cell death (apoptosis). Because chromosome 14 contains the only location for production of the heavy immunoglobulin chain in humans, and the translocation disrupts the region, usually in the joining (J) sites, production of heavy chains and therefore normal immunoglobulins from a t(8:14) chromosome is unlikely. However, because human cells are diploid, H chains can be synthesized from a nontranslocated chromosome 14 within a cell.

Studies reveal that in the majority of cases, H chain synthesis is drastically reduced in cells containing a t(8:14) chromosome. The translocation probably occurs during attempted V(D)J recombination under the influence of RAG1 and RAG2. However, sequencing studies have shown no homologies between c-myc and V(D)J. Therefore, translocations are probably common in the normal process of immunoglobulin chain recombination. Burkitt's lymphoma is but one example of the activation of an oncogene by an interrupted immunoglobulin gene.

29. In a genome scan, one could identify both proviral and retrotranspons by the presence of terminally repeated elements (LTR) and certain genes usually in common (*gag* and *pol*). To distinguish between the two sequences, one would look for differences that influence infectivity. Retrotransposons lack sequences that enable completion of the infectious cycle, whereas proviral sequences should have them. The *env* gene is present in proviral sequences and absent or altered in retrotransposons.

30. Replication of an RNA virus like the influenza virus is dependent on the viral RNA-dependent RNA polymerases that, like reverse transcriptases, can sponsor recombination between cellular RNAs. Since a large abundance of 28s ribosomal RNA is present in a cell, template switching could occur during RNA replication and enable the incorporation of a 28s-specifying segment in the viral genomic RNA. Changing the conformation of the HA glycoprotein alters the interaction of the virus with host receptors. In this way, host shifting can occur by shifting HA glycoproteins.

Chapter 23: Genomic Analysis—Dissection of Gene Function

Concept Areas	Corresponding Problems
Traits of Model Organisms	2, 11, 12, 18, 24, 25, 29
Genetic Analyses	1, 4, 5, 13, 15, 17, 19, 25, 26, 30
Gene Targeting	4, 17
Screening and Selecting for Mutants	3, 5, 6, 7, 8, 9, 10, 16, 17, 20
Functional Genomics	14, 27, 28, 29
RNAi	22, 23

Vocabulary: Organization and Listing of Terms and Concepts

Structures and Substances

Model organisms

Saccharomyces cerevisiae (budding yeast)

Saccharomyces pombe (fission yeast)

Drosophila melanogaster (fruit fly)

Caenorhabditis elegans (nematode)

Arabidopsis thaliana (mustard plant)

Mus musculus (mouse)

transgene

 SRY

Mutation analysis

radiation

ultraviolet light

ethyl methane sulfonate (EMS)

nitrosoguanidine

 conditional mutation

Transposons

ORF (open reading frame)

P-element

Suppressor mutations

Complementation group

Genetic network

Suppressor mutation

Enhancer mutation

Sequence motif

CDC2, Cdc2

Database

 SwissProt

Northern blot

Embryonic stem cell

Targeting vector

Chimeric organism

M13 bacteriophage

RNAi (interference)

Microarray

 formaldehyde

Processes/Methods

Model organism

 vast genetic knowledge

 DNA and protein sequence databases

host of strains with mutations

advantageous life cycle features

 ease of laboratory culture

short generation time

 abundance of progeny

 readily mutagenized

 readily crossed

Saccharomyces cerevisiae, budding yeast

 haploid (1*n*) diploid (2*n*)

 mating types (a and α)

 approximately 6,600 genes

 deletions in each ORF

Drosophila melanogaster, fruit fly

 about 13,000 genes

 four chromosomes

 1-day generation time

 body plan

  embryo

  larva

  adult

 no crossing over in males

 available balancer chromosomes

 P-element transposons

Mus musculus, mouse

 short generation time

 relevant to human diseases

 about 30,000 genes

 genome about 2.6 billion base pairs

 2*n* = 40

 gene homologies with human genes

 gene organization similar to humans

 relative ease of genetic manipulation

large scale screens difficult

 transgenic organisms

  pseudopregnant female

  Southern blot

  polymerase chain reaction (PCR)

Gene targeting

 gene knockout

 targeted gene replacement

 site-directed mutagenesis

Forward genetics

 saturation mutagenesis

  radiation

  ultraviolet light

  ethyl methane sulfonate (EMS)

  nitrosoguanidine

  conditional mutation

   permissive condition

   restrictive condition

  transposons

  P-element

Screening for mutants

 advantages of haploid organisms

 ClB technique

Selecting for mutants

Complementation analysis

Recombination analysis

Genetic networks

 epistasis and pathways

 suppressors and enhancers

  rescue

Reverse genetics

 hemophilia A

Functional genomics

Sequence alignment

Gene expression

In situ hybridization

Northern blot

Mitotic recombination

Gene silencing

High-throughput technologies

  microarrays

Concepts

Traits of model organisms

Genetic analyses

  forward

  reverse

Gene targeting

Screening and selecting for mutants

Functional genomics

Solutions to Problems and Discussion Questions

1. A suppressor mutation is a mutation that maps to another site in the genome and can rescue the phenotype of another mutation. For instance, if a given gene causes a bristle mutation in *Drosophila*, as *forked bristles* would do, a second mutation, *suppressor-of-forked* would mask the original *forked* mutation. The double mutant (original plus suppressor) would have normal bristles. If a gene has a deleterious phenotype, it is often possible to use a suppressor mutation to suppress the deleterious phenotype so that the organism can survive and reproduce. If information exists as to the nature of suppression, then the molecular nature of an original mutation can often be inferred by its response to a suppressor mutation.

2. (a) *Control of kidney development* can be studied most directly in humans and/or mice because both are similar. Since mice, rather than humans, can be genetically manipulated, the study of the genetics of kidney development in mice would probably be more productive. While *Drosophila* has excretory organs (Malpighian tubules), they are not closely related to the mammalian kidney. Yeast do not have excretory organs; however, both yeast and *Drosophila* engage in membrane transport processes, and the genetics of such processes will be fundamental and most likely apply to all organisms.

(b) Cancer can be studied in virtually all model organisms because it involves fundamentals of cell-cycle control. However, much of what we know about cell-cycle control derives from work in yeast, and given that cell-cycle systems are highly conserved processes, information obtained from any organism is often universally applicable. Yeast are well understood genetically, and they can be more easily manipulated (genetically and environmentally) than the other organisms listed. Mammalian cell lines are often used

to discover regulatory elements homologous to those seen in yeast.

(c) Cystic fibrosis is caused by mutations in the cystic fibrosis transmembrane conductance regulator gene, which normally funnels chloride ions out of a cell, leading to a saltier cellular external environment, which in turn draws water out of the cell by osmosis. The human *CFTR* gene has been cloned and expressed in yeast, so a viable way to look at the gene, its regulation, and product is available in a yeast model. In addition, *Drosophila* cell lines have been developed to study vertebrate expression systems for anion channel proteins. Using these transgenic systems, one could expand knowledge of the transport systems in general.

Seemingly, the most appropriate system to study human cystic fibrosis from a genetic standpoint would be the mouse. However, while strains have been generated with numerous mutations in the *CRTR* gene, mice do not develop the most serious symptom of human cystic fibrosis, namely, chronic lung infections by *Pseudomonas aeruginosa*. Recently, this problem has been overcome by the development of a mouse strain that is hypersusceptible to this bacterium (Coleman et al. 2003) and holds promise as a model organism for CF. Depending on the experimental approach, either human cell lines, transgenic *Drosophila* or yeast, or new mouse models may be most appropriate.

(d) Molecular aspects of purine metabolism are highly conserved throughout the animal and plant kingdom. To study the genetics of purine metabolism, it might be easiest to take advantage of the ease of mutant screens in yeast. In addition, certain strains of *Drosophila* respond differently to purine nutritional supplements. Therefore, one might use *Drosophila* to screen or select strains with altered purine metabolism.

(e) Genetic analyses of vertebrate immune function could be studied most directly in mouse models where genetic manipulation is possible. However, a relatively large number of forkhead-box (FOX) transcription factors have been found and characterized in *Drosophila melanogaster*. These transcription factors are members of a broader FOX family and have crucial roles in various aspects of immune regulation ranging from lymphocyte survival to thymic development. It would be possible, therefore, to study the immune system in a variety of organisms, taking advantage of the peculiarities of each.

(f) Like the study of cancer, the genetics of cell division might be most directly studied using yeast. The vast genetic understanding coupled with the relative ease of genetic manipulation has already greatly enhanced our understanding of cell division processes. Because cell-cycle mutations hamper the proliferation of the organism, conditional mutants are often successfully employed. Although cultured mouse and human cells are also useful for studying specific aspects of cell division, their genetic manipulation is more difficult than that of yeast cells. In most cases, knockout/rescue strategies are useful.

3. In general, use of a Southern blot or PCR analysis is used to verify that a gene of interest in ES cells has been effectively disrupted by the targeting vector DNA. In addition, northern blots and immunostaining may be used to verify the absence of gene products; however, these techniques are more laborious and indirect than those mentioned above.

4. The basic procedure in oligonucleotide site-directed mutagenesis is to synthesize an appropriate oligonucleotide that is homologous to the gene or portion of gene of interest. The oligonucleotide contains a desired mutation that may involve one or more nucleotides. The oligonucleotide is hybridized to M13 DNA, which contains a cloned gene (or gene fragment) of interest and anneals to a homologous region. DNA polymerase is added along with other *in vitro* DNA polymerizing components to yield a double-stranded M13 molecule, which is then transformed into *E. coli* where replication occurs. Semiconservative replication provides mutant molecules, which are then screened or selected using a variety of standard techniques.

5. (a) In general, spontaneous mutations are quite rare compared with EMS mutagenesis. However, given that EMS and spontaneous mutations are generally created by single base-pair changes or small deletions and insertions, it would be very difficult to distinguish between the two causes with absolute certainty.

(b) Segregation analysis could help determine whether the suppressor mutation occurred at a second site. Since true reversion would occur in the original mutant gene, a second site mutation could be separated from the original mutation by recombination. Such recombination would then expose the original mutant phenotype.

(c) Classical mapping could be used to determine the map location of the suppressor mutation. If the suppressor gene could be cloned and sequenced, its location could be determined by hybridization to polytene chromosomes in *Drosophila* larval salivary glands. In addition, it could be located by searching the *Drosophila* sequence database.

(d) There are many examples of intragenic suppression that are not the result of true reversion to the original base sequence of the gene of interest. In general, amino acid substitutions may alter the higher-level structure of a protein and thus partly or completely restore the wild-type phenotype.

6. Balancer chromosomes contain multiple overlapping inversions that greatly reduce the recovery of crossover chromatids. By using such chromosomes, the mutagenized chromosome(s) remains intact. Such balancer chromosomes are most useful when they contain dominant marker genes such as wing or eye shape or eye color. Balancer chromosomes usually contain a recessive lethal gene so that the balancer chromosome cannot exist in the homozygous state.

7. Transposons represent a powerful and dependable tool for generating mutations. *P*-elements, for example, are mobile elements in *Drosophila* that can move into and out of the genome. When such elements insert into genes, they usually mutate those genes because large insertions are generated that disrupt gene function.

8. Coat color markers are useful in generating knockout mice because when embryonic stem cells are injected into blastocysts, the resulting chimeras will have patches of different fur colors, making them easy to recognize. Theoretically, any other surface marker (hair or hairless, etc.) would be usable as long as expressivity and penetrance of the dominant marker are high. Any test, molecular, biochemical, or visible, that allows one to determine the presence of a gene in an organism would be usable; however, clearly visible tests are much more efficient. One could imagine using a gene that provided some needed substance for survival that circulates through body fluids. If the blastocyst is deficient for this vital substance, only the chimeras would survive.

9. The basic strategy for selecting *pro-1* suppressor strains of yeast would involve growing prol-1 yeast on a medium containing proline plus a mutagen (preferably one that causes relatively mild changes in DNA). If one replica plates colonies onto a prolineless medium, those that grow will either have undergone true reversion or suppression. Mapping can be used to identify intergenically suppressed strains. More detailed mapping and sequencing methods would be needed to identify strains suppressed intragenically.

10. (a) Although autosomal and dominant mutations may be detected with the *ClB* technique, it is specifically designed to detect recessive mutations, especially, but not exclusively, lethals that are X-linked.

(b) The recessive, X-linked *l* gene is used to exclude hemizygous *ClB*/Y flies (males) in the F2 generation. If no males appear in the F2, then one (or more) X-linked recessive lethal was introduced on the mutagenized male.

(c) The multiple-inverted X chromosome (*C*) suppresses the recovery of crossing over products on the X, thereby leaving the mutagenized X chromosome intact.

(d) *C* is a balancer chromosome that contains multiple overlapping inversions to greatly reduce the recovery of crossover products (chromatids).

11. (a) Due to a variety of advantages, yeast are extremely useful as experimental organisms. First, their life cycle has both haploid and diploid phases, and there are mating types that can be influenced by simple environmental shifts. Mating produces diploid cells. Because of haploidy, mutations can be easily selected and because of diploidy, a gene's mode of action (complementation) can be studied. The DNA sequence is known, and a vast collection of mutations and deletions is available. About 5700 of the 6600 genes have known function. Yeast are easy to grow and manipulate in the laboratory. However, the study of yeast does not offer the possibility of studying multicellularity and development.

(b) The advantage of the haploid life cycle in yeast is the ease with which recessive mutations can be studied. Because of haploidy, recessive mutations are expressed.

12. Temperature-sensitive mutations allow one to collect mutations that impact the vital functions of cells. To select such mutations, one conducts a mutagenesis experiment in which the yeast cells are grown at 23°C, for example. In general, the mutagen selected is one that causes minor changes in DNA, such as base analogs, ultraviolet light, or nitrosoguanidine. The resulting colonies are then replica plated at the permissive temperature (23°C, for example), and one is incubated at the restrictive temperature (36°C, for example). Colonies that do not grow at the restrictive temperature are likely to contain temperature-sensitive lethal mutations. Returning to the original plate (permissive temperature) allows one to select cells for further analysis.

Since yeast cells produce buds, the size of which characterizes the stage of the cell cycle, it is possible to isolate cell division cycle (*cdc*) defects by the morphology of the cells. In addition, if a gene is controlling a specific point in the cell cycle, a uniform morphology is likely.

13. (a) Given that you have the protein suspected to be involved in cell wall synthesis, you can determine the amino acid sequence of that protein. From that sequence you can deduce its corresponding DNA sequence (several sequences because of the degenerate code) and synthesize various combinations of labeled oligonucleotides that likely correspond to all codon combinations. Probing genomic or cDNA libraries with the labeled oligonucleotides, one can select a clone that contains the gene(s).

(b) Often, rescue experiments are used to determine the significance of a cloned gene to a particular process if mutations exist. In addition, since the gene has been cloned, it can be used to generate altered genes by site-directed mutagenesis. Once the mutagenized genes are incorporated into the yeast genome, their influence on cell wall construction can be studied.

14. Tissue-specific and/or temporal-specific patterns of gene expression are often studied by *in situ* hybridization, which may reveal the mRNA pattern in an organism. A labeled cDNA is used as a probe to hydrogen bond with the RNA. One may also use the northern blot technique that involves purification of mRNA from a tissue(s) of interest. Lastly, immunostaining may be used to generate a protein's expression profile.

15. DNA microarrays contain microscopic droplets of specific DNA samples in specific positions on a chip. Theoretically, all the genes of an organism can be placed on a microarray. Since microarrays can be both tissue- and temporal-specific, they are lauded as powerful tools in gene expression studies. However, various studies (Kothapalli et al. 2002) indicate that inconsistent results are likely: variation in DNA sequences on microarrays, variation in microarray probes, and failure of probes to bind to different isoforms of a gene. Given that complete genes are not usually present on a microarray, only partial "truth in binding" is possible.

Messenger RNAs are often highly processed, and probes generated from mRNAs probably represent a small portion of the transient pool of potentially significant RNA in a cell. In addition, calibration of the detection device will determine which genes are viewed as being expressed and which are not. In other words, relative expression is assayed, and in some cases a very low level of gene expression may have more actual influence than high expression. Since a genomic DNA profile is contained on the microarray, many genes of unknown function can be analyzed, making interpretation of data difficult. With genomics and transcriptomics coupled through microarray analyses, a new field of bioinformatics is evolving to interpret such data. At present, microarray technologies are somewhat expensive and out of reach of some researchers.

It is feared that public access to commercial microarray databases will be limited. Many of these limitations will be overcome as the technology improves and as costs for such analyses drop. In addition, as chips become more customized for individual applications, problems with DNA content and probe specificity will lessen.

16. *P*-elements containing a visible marker in the host fly are modified to contain a gene of interest. The recombinant *P*-element is then injected into *Drosophila* eggs along with a helper plasmid that contains the transposase gene, which is transcribed and translated in the embryo, thus enabling the *P*-element to insert into the embryo's DNA. Recombinant adult flies can be identified by expression of the visible marker. Offspring from such a fly may contain the gene of interest.

To generate a transgenic mouse, DNA is injected into the haploid nucleus of the egg (or the blastocyst), which is then placed into the oviduct of a pseudopregnant female mouse. Next resulting offspring are screened for evidence of transgenesis. The difference between the two techniques resides in the type of DNA used and the cell in which the DNA is injected.

17. Null experiments are extremely useful for a variety of reasons. First, by examining the phenotype of a null mutant, one can often gain insight into the function of the missing gene. In addition, null mutations can be used in rescue experiments, where various genetic elements are tested for their ability to restore wild-type function by functional complementation. Assume that one wished to study the influence of a free radical scavenger gene on longevity in *Drosophila*. By having null mutations for the superoxide dismutase gene, for example, one could generate strains with zero, one, two, or more genes for superoxide dismutase. One might even be lucky enough to observe a dose response between the number of genes present and a particular phenotype. Another approach might be to determine whether genes from one organism (developmental genes in humans or cell-cycle genes in yeast, for example) have homologous functions in flies. Using fly null mutants transformed with suspected homologs, one could test for functional overlap.

18. If transgenesis occurs in a vital gene, the organism may not survive, and that could seriously complicate a study. In addition, genes are often influenced by position effects whereby their function is altered by their neighbors or broad chromosomal location (in heterochromatin, for example). If such position effects occur, accurate interpretation of gene action will be compromised.

19. Forward genetic analysis of *Drosophila* can be accomplished without the use of a mutagen. However, unless the gene of interest already exists in a mutant state in an accessible fly, there may be a long wait ahead.

One may screen and/or select mutants from natural populations where the mutation might be enriched in frequency for some reason. Depending on the goals of a particular study, one may be more interested in studying naturally occurring genes than those induced by mutagens.

20. Selecting for mutants occurs when one creates conditions that remove irrelevant organisms, leaving only the mutants of interest. Screening for mutants is often very labor intensive and involves visual examination of organisms.

21. The general scheme will involve reverse genetics. From the sequence given, one can deduce its corresponding DNA sequence (several sequences because of the degenerate code) and synthesize various combinations of labeled oligonucleotides that likely correspond to all codon combinations. Probing genomic or cDNA libraries with the labeled oligonucleotides, a clone can be selected that contains the gene that produces the amino acid sequence of interest. A variety of methods could be used to suggest that the gene you isolated actually produces a protein involved in blood clotting. By transforming cells with the gene and isolating purified proteins from the transformed cells, various fractions could be tested for their ability to function in a blood-clotting cascade.

Fortunately, a number of mouse models exist for examining mammalian blood-clotting pathways. Given that you have a cloned gene suspected to be involved in blood clotting, site-directed mutagenesis or knockouts could be used to generate mice with alterations of your cloned gene. Alteration of blood clotting in the presence of a mutant or knocked-out gene would indicate a functional relationship between the gene you cloned and the blood-clotting cascade.

22. RNAi (RNA interference) provides a new technology that allows researchers to create single-gene defects without creating heritable mutations. Short double-stranded RNA molecules are introduced into cells that trigger RNA-degradation pathways. To introduce RNAi into cells, researchers may transform cells with vectors that express RNA hairpin structures that may integrate into a cell's genome. Alternatively, an inducible promoter may be used to drive the expression of the RNAi gene. Often, heat-shock gene promoters are effective.

23. Although it is true that the "knockout" of a gene usually results in no genetic output, RNAi-mediated gene silencing relies on the uptake, expression, and hybridization of the RNAi vehicle as well as association of the RNAi to its target(s). At all three levels, uptake, expression, and association, opportunities for target escape exist. Therefore, it is often possible to reduce the output of a gene (knockdown), but not completely. In addition, if a protein has a long half-life, its function may continue after RNA degradation.

24. (a) The overall biochemical and physiological mechanisms that characterize living systems are highly conserved. Such conservation allows for considerable extrapolation of findings from one taxon to another. Direct evidence for such conservation comes from complementation and rescue studies where DNA sequences that have function in yeast, *Drosophila*, and humans are highly conserved and can often rescue or complement function when transgenic organisms are produced.

(b) Multiple steps in pathways provide multiple metabolites and multiple points for regulation. Often, complementation and mutation analyses indicate that more than one gene is operating in a given pathway. Such genetic networks are often revealed by studying the genetic and phenotypic relationships by epistasis.

(c) Pioneering work done in yeast demonstrated that multiple genes were involved in the regulation of the cell cycle in yeast and that homologs of these genes can be found in virtually all eukaryotic organisms. In addition, transgenesis experiments demonstrated complementation among a variety of organisms.

25. The process of tanning and hardening the insect cuticle is complex, involving numerous gene products and many activities other than cuticle tanning and hardening. Basically, dopa, catecholamines, and serotonin biosynthetic pathways are involved, in addition to a variety of brain hormones. The process of hardening the cuticle involves crosslinking cuticular proteins with phenols, a process that takes about six hours and is under the control of the hormone bursicon. The teneral condition exists if the fly has just emerged from the pupal case, and the pharate condition exists if the fly is within the pupal case. Given this background, many different mutations will likely be involved in cuticular tanning and hardening; some will be embryonic lethals, others will generate pharate organisms, and yet others will produce teneral organisms.

(a) Since many genes involved in cuticular tanning and hardening are likely to be lethal or at least have severe effects on the phenotype, one would most likely select a mutagen that causes minor alterations in base sequences: EMS, base analogs, or nitrosogranidine. Use of these mutagens will increase the likelihood of causing potentially useful conditional mutations as well.

(b, c) Many of the mutations will be lethal or generate pharate pupae that can be identified visually. Teneral adults may die shortly after emergence; therefore, care must be taken to aggressively examine mutagenized cultures. Using a series of balancer chromosomes covering the three major chromosome pairs in *Drosophila* (because the fourth chromosome is small, it is often ignored in general mutant screens), one can identify lethal genes when no nonbalancer offspring are produced in crosses among mutagenized, heterozygously balanced stocks.

(d) Assuming that larvae and pupae are carefully examined, if no mutations are discovered that influence cuticular tanning and hardening in adults, it is likely that they are early (embryonic) lethals. As stated above, using a series of balancer chromosomes covering the three major chromosome pairs in *Drosophila* (because the fourth chromosome is small it is often ignored in general mutant screens), lethal genes are identified when no nonbalancer offspring are produced in crosses among mutagenized, heterozygous balanced stocks. One would have to look at the eggs laid by the mutagenized, backcrossed flies that produced no nonbalancer homozygotes and inspect any unhatched eggs for evidence of embryonic lethals.

26. It is possible that yeast may process the candidate gene in a form that is similar to that seen in humans. Because abnormal accumulation of a protein is involved, yeast may accumulate the same protein if transformed with the candidate gene. It would be worth the effort to examine this possibility. For instance, Dr. Susan Lindquist at the Whitehead Institute has discovered a yeast protein that forms amyloid fibers similar to those found in Alzheimer's patients. Perhaps transforming yeast with the human gene would provide a gene product that, ideally, would be the same as that seen in humans, or at least, give some idea of the gene's behavior.

27. Since null mutations are desired, it would probably be most efficient to attempt the targeted knockout procedure taking advantage of the high levels of mitotic recombination in yeast. Generally, an antibiotic resistance gene is inserted into the gene of interest, leaving sufficient DNA sequences on either side that are homologous to the gene of interest. Linear pieces of the recombinant DNA (gene of interest with antibiotic resistance gene insert) are then transformed into yeast cells. Homologous recombination with the gene of interest generates the desired null mutant, and as the cells sporulate, they are grown on medium containing the antibiotic. The surviving haploid cells most likely contain a null mutation for the gene of interest.

28. The first step in gaining insight into the possible functionality of a DNA sequence is to annotate that sequence. Given that an interesting motif may be produced, we have a suggestion, but not proof, that the sequence is not "junk" DNA. Annotating the sequence involves the use of a variety of annotation tools that scan the sequence in search of open reading frames (ORFs), which begin with an initiation sequence and end with a termination sequence. In addition, other landmarks are typically present in genes: intron/exon topology, intron/exon junction sequences, codon bias, upstream regulatory sequences, a 3' polyadenylation signal, and, in some cases, CpG islands.

Once a sequence is identified as a likely gene, a second step often involves comparisons with other known, well-studied genes that may provide clues as to function. From a DNA sequence, the amino acid sequences can be predicted that can be compared with amino acid sequences in databases such as SwissProt or BLAST. From such searches, one may discover homologies to other proteins with known function. It is possible that additional significant motifs may be found to provide clues to function.

A third step often involves the analysis of tissue-specific and temporal-specific patterns of gene expression using any number of techniques such as *in situ* hybridization, northern blots, immunostaining, or microarray technology.

29. Transgenic mice that contain different mutations in the CF transmembrane conductance regulator gene mostly show abnormalities in ion transport that are similar to the intestinal maladies of CF in humans. However, the most serious manifestation of human CF is chronic lung infection caused by *Pseudomonas aeruginosa*, which, until recently has not been common in mice. This shortcoming as a mouse CF model organism has hampered CF research until recently when hypersusceptibility of transgenic mice to chronic lung infection was developed (Coleman et al. 2003). Others have developed a mouse model of lung disease using genetic manipulation to increase sodium channels. This system led to the decreased airway hydration and mucus plugs typically seen in CF patients. This model will be useful in testing whether therapies that improve airway hydration will be effective in CF and other lung diseases.

30. Consider the following diagram when answering this question:

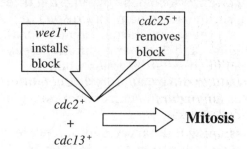

Mutations	Progress to mitosis?
cdc25	No, block not removed
wee1	Yes, no block installed
cdc25 wee1	Yes, no block installed
cdc13 wee1	No, no cyclin
cdc2 wee1	No, no cyclin-dependent kinase
cdc25 cdc13	No, no cyclin

Chapter 24: Applications and Ethics of Genetic Engineering and Biotechnology

Concept Areas	Corresponding Problems
Genetically Modified Organisms	1, 2, 8, 10, 22, 26, 30
Use of Genetically Engineered Products	5, 11, 12
Genetic Engineering	4, 9, 15, 22, 30
Diagnosing and Screening Genetic Disorders	7, 18, 20, 21, 25, 26, 27
Gene Therapy	3, 13, 14, 15, 16, 23
Genome Analysis	17, 19
DNA Profiling	6, 26, 28
Ethical Issues	1, 2, 24, 26

Vocabulary: Organization and Listing of Terms and Concepts

Structures and Substances

Genetically modified organisms (GMOs)

  biopharmaceuticals

    insulin

    transgenic organisms

      bioreactors

      biofactories

      E. coli lac Z

      baculovirus

    α1-antitrypsin

    antithrombin

    Pompe disease

    human growth hormone

    EnviroPig

  transgenic plants

    edible vaccine

    inactivated vaccine

    subunit vaccine

human papillomavirus (HPV)

  Gardasil

herbicide resistance

  glyphosate

pest resistance

T1 plasmid

  Bt crops

golden rice

Food and Drug Administration (FDA)

Biotechnology

RFLP

  sickle-cell anemia

  cystic fibrosis

    CFTR

Genomic scan

  microarray

    field

    genotyping

  single-nucleotide polymorphism

Gene therapy

   adenovirus

   RNAi

   siRNA

   RISC

DNA profile

   minisatellite

   VNTR

   microsatellite

   STR

     CODIS

   cold case

Processes/Methods

Genetic engineering

   selective breeding

Biopharming

   insulin production

Medical diagnostics

RFLP analysis

Amniocentesis

Chorionic villus sampling

Polymerase chain reaction (PCR)

Preimplantation genetic diagnosis

Microarray analysis

   transcriptome analysis

     gene expression

Targeted medical therapy

   rational drug design

Gene therapy

   somatic

     severe combined immunodeficiency

     adenosine deaminase

germ-line

   enhancement

   ELSI

RNA interference

DNA profiling

   fingerprinting

   capillary gel electrophoresis

   forensic applications

Concepts

Genetic engineering

Animal and plant applications

Genomics

Medical diagnostics

   genetic diagnosis

   genomic scan

   genotyping

   gene-expression analysis

Targeted medical therapy

   rational drug design

Gene therapy

DNA profiling

   forensic applications

Emerging technologies

   terrorism

   natural disasters

Ethical issues

   genetically modified foods

   genetic testing

   legal protections

     health insurance

     employment

   ELSI

Solutions to Problems and Discussion Questions

1. There are concerns about proper testing of GM crops and foods for allergenicity, environmental impact, and the possibility of cross-pollination leading to the contamination of native species. If certain crops become the standard and under the control of a few manufacturers, it is likely that the world's supply of genetic variability might be reduced. Concern would increase if such crops routinely contained antibiotic-resistant genetic markers and genes conferring toxicity to pests. A broader concern is that the design and patenting of crops might allow domination of the world food supply by a few companies.

2. Because of the recent rise in food sensitivities (allergies and adverse reactions), the public should probably have access to the contents of all foods. GMOs have the potential for possessing suites of gene products that might be atypical for a given food, and unless consumers know of that possibility, harm could result. Some argue that consumers have a right to know about GMOs as a matter of principle regardless of potential health risks.

3. Although some success has been achieved using gene therapy, major questions remain. First, the vectors that deliver the desired gene must not trigger adverse reactions. Second, at present, the integration of some vectors is dependent on DNA replication in the host. Therefore, not all cells in the body are available to integration of some vectors. Third, precise target integration must be achieved to reduce the introduction of new mutations. Fourth, most human genes are large, whereas many vectors in use today can carry only small inserts. Large cargos will be needed to achieve a broad range of therapies. Finally, the desired products of the vector should have long-lasting effects, and the vectors themselves must remain incapable of reverting to an infectious virus.

4. Glyphosate (a herbicide) inhibits EPSP, a chloroplast enzyme involved in the synthesis of the amino acids phenylalanine, tyrosine, and tryptophan. To generate glyphosate resistance in crop plants, a fusion gene was created that introduced a viral promoter to control the EPSP synthetase gene. The fusion product was placed into the Ti vector and transferred to *A. tumifaciens*, which was used to infect crop cells. Calluses were selected on the basis of their resistance to glyphosate. Resistant calluses were later developed into transgenic plants. There is a remote possibility that such an "accident" can occur as suggested in the question. However, in retracing the steps to generate the resistant plant in the first place, it seems more likely that the trait will not "escape" from the plant. Rather, the engineered *A. tumifaciens* may escape, infect, and transfer glyphosate resistance to pest species.

5. The nature of the digestion process is the breakdown of foodstuffs for eventual absorption by the small intestine. Antigens are usually quite large molecules, and in the process of digestion, they are sometimes broken down into smaller molecules, thus becoming ineffective in stimulating the immune system. Some individuals are allergic to the food they eat, demonstrating that not all antigens are completely degraded or modified by digestion. In some cases, ingested antigens do indeed stimulate the immune system (oral polio vaccine) and provide a route for immunization. Localized (intestinal) immunity can sometimes be stimulated by oral introduction of antigens, and in some cases this can offer immunity to ingested pathogens.

6. Short tandem repeats are very similar to VNTRs, but the repeat motif is much shorter (2–9 base pairs). STRs have been used to generate a marker panel for DNA profiling. STR typing is less expensive, less labor intensive, and quicker to perform than traditional DNA typing.

7. Even though you have developed a method for screening seven of the mutations described, it is possible that negative results can occur when the person carries the gene for CF. In other words, the specific probes (or allele-specific oligonucleotides) that have been developed will not necessarily be useful for screening all mutant alleles. In addition, the cost-effectiveness of such a screening proposal would need to be considered.

8. Kleter and Peijnenburg used the BLAST tool from the *http://www.ncbi.nlm.nih.gov/BLAST* Web site to conduct a series of alignment comparisons of transgenic sequences with sequences of known allergenic proteins. Of 33 transgenic proteins screened for the identities of at least six contiguous amino acids found in allergenic proteins, 22 gave positive results.

9. In general, bacteria do not process eukaryotic proteins in the same manner as eukaryotes. Transgenic eukaryotes are more likely to correctly process eukaryotic proteins, thus increasing the likelihood of their normal biological activity.

10. From a purely scientific viewpoint, there will be no added danger to consuming cow's milk from cloned animals. However, some individuals may have an aversion to organismic cloning, and supporting such activities through consumption of products of cloned organisms may be viewed negatively on moral grounds. Public sentiment will likely pressure for labeling of "cloned products" on the grounds that consumers should be able to make an informed choice as to the origin of such products.

11. (a) Both the saline and column extracts of Lkt50 appear to be capable of inducing at least 50 percent neutralization of toxicity when injected into rabbits.

(b) In order for a successful edible vaccine to be developed, numerous hurdles must be overcome. First, the immunogen must be stably incorporated into the host plant hereditary material, and the host must express only that immunogen. During feeding, the immunogen must be transported across the intestinal wall unaltered, or altered in such a way as to stimulate the desired immune response. There must be guarantees that potentially harmful by-products of transgenesis have not been produced. In other words, broad ecological and environmental issues must be addressed to prevent a transgenic plant from becoming an unintended vector for harm to the environment or any organisms feeding on the plant (directly or indirectly).

12. As with all therapies, the cure must be less hazardous than the disease. In the case of viral-mediated gene therapy, the antigenicity of the virus must not interfere with the delivery system; such antigenicity can cause inflammation or more severe immunologic responses. Combating the host immune response may involve the use of immunosuppressive drugs or modification of the vector. The duration of desired gene expression at the diseased site is an issue. Short-period expression may require repeated exposure to the vehicle, which may present undesired responses. For some diseases, local gene therapy through inhalation or injection may produce fewer side effects than systemic exposure. Adenoviruses appear to be particularly useful for gene therapy because they can infect nondividing cells and they can accept relatively large amounts of additional DNA (30 kb or more).

13. Somatic gene therapy involves attempts to alter the genetic material in non-germ-line cells. Clinical trials are currently underway.

Germ-line therapy, while being more efficient (though perhaps more difficult technically), alters the germ line and is transmitted to offspring. Considerable ethical problems are associated with germ-line therapy. It recalls previous attempts of the eugenics movements of past decades, which involved the use of selective breeding to purify the human stock. Some present-day biologists have said publicly that germ-line gene therapy will *not* be conducted.

Enhancement gene therapy raises an important ethical dilemma. Should genetic techniques be used to enhance human potential? It is generally felt that enhancement gene therapy, like germ-line therapy, is unacceptable.

14. A major problem associated with engineering the capsid to specifically engage target cells is that the capsid itself is now altered. A reconfigured capsid, either by size or shape, may no longer serve its packaging and infecting roles properly. One may end up with a very specific viral-target interaction, but the virus may be incapable of replicating efficiently. A nongenetic approach is to use bispecific molecules to conjugate vectors with target cells. Such approaches often employ desired electrostatic bridges or monoclonal antibody conjugates. Although such approaches often work in the test tube, their application *in vivo* is often limited owing to instability.

15. p53 and pRB are tumor-suppressor proteins and are required by the cell to effectively monitor the cell cycle. Reduction in their activity would diminish normal cell-cycle controls and most likely lead to cancer. It would be especially important if such viral-vectors are intended to treat cancer where cell-cycle control is likely already compromised.

16. (a,b) One of the main problems with gene therapy is delivery of the desired virus to the target tissue in an effective manner. Several of the problems involving the use of retroviral vectors are the following: (1) Integration into the host must be cell specific so as not to damage nontarget cells. (2) Retroviral integration into host cell genomes occurs only if the host cell is replicating. (3) Insertion of the viral genome might influence nontarget, but essential, genes. (4) Retroviral genomes have a low cloning capacity and cannot carry large inserted sequences as are many human genes. (5) Host viruses may possibly produce a harmful infectious virus.

(c) The question posed here plays on the practical versus the ethical. It would certainly be more efficient (though perhaps more difficult technically) to engineer germ tissue, for once it is done in a family, the disease would be eliminated. However, germ-line therapy presents considerable ethical problems. It recalls previous attempts of the eugenics movements of past decades, which involved the use of selective breeding to purify the human stock. Some present-day biologists have said publicly that germ-line gene therapy will *not* be conducted.

17. A microarray is a solid support containing an orderly arrangement of DNA samples. A typical array contains thousands of DNA spots that may be small oligonucleotides, cDNAs, or short genomic sequences. Labeled sequences hybridize to the immobilized DNAs by standard base pairing. Such technology allows a method for monitoring RNA expression levels of thousands of genes in virtually any cell population. Using microarray technology, researchers can observe the overall behavior of the genome in cancer and normal cells and, by comparison, determine which genes are active or inactive under various circumstances. It is possible to identify the set of genes whose expression or lack thereof defines the properties of each tumor type. This application can, therefore, lead to precise diagnosis and refine possible therapies. In addition, microarray profiling can be used to determine the efficacy of particular therapies. For instance, one can monitor responses to radiation and/or chemotherapy to determine the degree to which cells are responding to a particular cancer treatment.

18. Since both mutations occur in the CF gene, children who possess both alleles will suffer from CF. With both parents heterozygous, each child born will have a 25 percent chance of developing CF.

19. In the case of haplo-insufficient mutations, gene therapy holds promise. However, in gain-of-function mutations, in all probability the mutant gene's activity or product must be compromised. RNAi strategies may apply more effectively. Addition of a normal gene probably will not help unless it can compete out the mutant gene product.

20. It will hybridize by base complementation to the normal DNA sequence.

21. The answer provided here is based on the condition that individual I-2 is a carrier and the son, II-4, has the disorder. The 3 kb fragment occurs in the normal I-1 father and the normal son II-1. The affected son, II-4, has the 4 kb fragment. One daughter, II-2, is a carrier, while the other daughter, II-3, is not a carrier.

22. One method is to use the amino acid sequence of the protein to produce the gene synthetically. Alternatively, since the introns are spliced out of the pre-mRNA during the maturation of mRNA, if mRNA can be obtained, it can be used to make DNA (cDNA) through the use of reverse transcriptase. The resulting cDNA can then be used (free of introns) to make the desired product.

23. The two major problems described here are common concerns related to genetic engineering. The first is the localization of the introduced DNA into the target tissue and target location in the genome. Inappropriate targeting may have serious consequences. In addition, it is often difficult to control the output of introduced DNA. Genetic regulation is complicated and subject to a number of factors including upstream and downstream signals as well as various posttranscriptional processing schemes. Artificial control of these factors will prove difficult.

24. At this point, there is considerable reluctance to allow the open sharing of genetic information among institutions. In general, the establishment of governmental databases containing our most intimate information is viewed with skepticism. It is likely that considerable time and discussion will elapse before such databases are established.

25. Using restriction enzyme analysis to detect point mutations in humans is a tedious trial-and-error process. Given the size of the human genome in terms of base sequences and the relatively low number of unique restriction enzymes, the likelihood of matching a specific point mutation, separate from other normal sequence variations, to a desired gene is low.

26. (a) In general, if the modified plant is not toxic or allergenic as determined in test organisms, and no other negative physiological properties have been identified, it is considered safe for human consumption. Potentially harmful agents are usually tested at mega-dose levels to detect potential problems. Protein-based allergenicity is often detected by comparing proteins of transgenic plants with amino acid sequences of known allergens.

(b) Physical evidence of gene introduction comes from various forms of analysis including PCR, RT-PCR, RFLP, Southern blotting, and DNA sequencing. Functional evidence can be obtained from microarray analysis and direct assays of the gene product.

(c) PCR, Southern blot or similar detection/blotting methods coupled with allele-specific oligonucleotide detection are standard methods to determine the presence of certain genes and their mutations (see Problem 20). Coupled with RFLP analysis using *Mst*II and *Cvn*I, it is possible to distinguish sickle-cell from normal hemoglobin DNA.

(d) Microarrays can be used as platforms on which to hybridize DNA or RNA from various tissues. RNA populations from different tissues will give different patterns of hybridization, a so-called transcriptome analysis.

(e) The results of DNA profiling, whether it be VNTR or STR analysis, is dependent on the number and frequency of alleles being typed. If the number of alleles tested is high, say above 10, and their frequencies of occurrence are low, then the product of their individual occurrence probabilities can be extremely discriminating. Such probabilities may indicate an occurrence rate as low as one in 10 billion, thereby being useful for the identification of a single individual (excluding identical twins). Sample contamination can be excluded by assays designed to determine the number of alleles present. Detecting more than two alleles for a unique polymorphism would indicate contamination.

27. The child in question is a carrier of the deletion in the β-globin gene, just as the parents are carriers. Its genotype is therefore $\beta^A\beta^o$.

28. (a) Y-linked excluded, X-linked recessive excluded, autosomal recessive is possible, but unlikely because the gene is stated as being rare; X-linked dominant is possible if heterozygous, autosomal dominant is possible.

(b) Chromosome 21 with the B1 marker probably contains the mutation.

(c) The disease gene is segregating with some certainty with the B1 RFLP marker in the family. Since the mother also has the B3 marker, the offspring could be tested. If the child carries the B3 marker, then he or she does not carry the B1 marker, which has been segregating with the defective gene. This prediction is not completely accurate because a crossover in the mother could put the undesirable gene with the B3 marker.

(d) The possibilities would include: a crossover between the restriction sites in the father giving a B1 chromosome, or a mutation eliminating either the B2 or B3 restriction site.

29. (a) Small tandem repeats are highly variable and therefore, with the exception of identical twins, represent a potentially unique DNA fingerprint among individuals. Because each DNA fingerprint can be extremely rare in a population, it is possible to say with some certainty that a particular DNA sample matches, to the exclusion of others, that of a particular individual.

(b) Because of the relatively high mutation rate (usually the result of change in repeat copy number), enough genetic variation exists to make each individual's DNA sequence unique. It is the uniqueness of DNA fingerprints that provides a powerful tool in forensics.

(c) The frequencies of STRs from different sites are multiplied together to give an overall probability of a given STR pattern.

(d) Because different populations often have different STR frequencies, each overall probability must be based on an appropriate comparison population.

30. There are numerous methods for generating transgenic mammals using retroviral vectors. One method involves

injection of an engineered retroviral RNA
into embryonic (pronuclear) cells directly.
Another scheme uses cultured embryonic
stem cells (ES) and is presented in the
following mouse example.

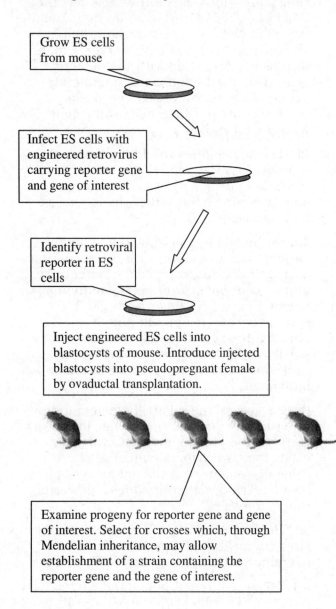

Grow ES cells from mouse

Infect ES cells with engineered retrovirus carrying reporter gene and gene of interest

Identify retroviral reporter in ES cells

Inject engineered ES cells into blastocysts of mouse. Introduce injected blastocysts into pseudopregnant female by ovaductal transplantation.

Examine progeny for reporter gene and gene of interest. Select for crosses which, through Mendelian inheritance, may allow establishment of a strain containing the reporter gene and the gene of interest.

Chapter 25: Quantitative Genetics and Multifactorial Traits

Concept Areas	Corresponding Problems
Phenotypic Expression	1, 2, 10, 22, 24, 28, 32
Continuous Variation and Polygenes	1, 2, 3, 4, 5, 6, 7, 25, 26, 27, 29, 30, 31
Heritability	2, 8, 9, 12, 13, 14, 16, 17, 18, 19, 20, 33
Mapping	2, 21, 23
Statistics	11, 15
Twin Studies	2, 8, 9

Vocabulary: Organization and Listing of Terms and Concepts

Structures and Substances

Threshold traits

Meristic traits

QTLS

RFLP

Dizygotic twin (fraternal)

Monozygotic twin (identical)

Processes/Methods

Transmission genetics

Quantitative, polygenic inheritance

Discontinuous traits

Continuous traits

    multiple-factor hypothesis

    additive (cumulative, quantitative) alleles

    nonadditive alleles

    polygenic

    $1/4^n$

Statistical analysis

    descriptive summary

    statistical inference

    statistics

parameters

    mean

        central tendency

    frequency distribution

    variance

    standard deviation

    standard error of the mean

    covariance

Heritability

    broad-sense heritability

        phenotypic variation

        environmental variance

        genetic variance

        interaction (genotype by environment)

    narrow-sense heritability

        additive variance

        dominance variance

        interactive variance

    artificial selection

        response

        selection differential

        realized heritability

twin studies

    monozygotic (identical) twins

    dizygotic (fraternal) twins

    concordant, discordant

Concepts

Transmission genetics

Quantitative inheritance

Heredity and environment

Mapping quantitative traits

restriction fragment length

polymorphism

    quantitative trait loci

Heritability

    inbred lines

    heritability index (H^2)

        broad-sense heritability

        narrow-sense heritability

Twin studies

Solutions to Problems and Discussion Questions

1. In *discontinuous* variation, the influences of each gene pair are not additive, and more typical Mendelian ratios such as 9:3:3:1 and 3:1 result. In *continuous* variation, different gene pairs interact (usually additively) to produce a phenotype that is less "stepwise" in distribution. Inheritance involving polygenic systems follows a more continuous distribution.

2. (a) *Polygenes* are those genes involved in determining continuously varying or multiple factor traits.

(b) *Additive alleles* are those alleles that account for the hereditary influence on the phenotype in an additive way.

(c) *Correlation* is a statistic that varies from -1 to $+1$ and describes the extent to which variation in one trait is associated with variation in another. It does not imply that a cause-and-effect relationship exists between two traits.

(d) *Monozygotic twins* are derived from a single fertilized egg and are thus genetically identical to each other. They provide a method for determining the influence of genetics and environment on certain traits. *Dizygotic twins* arise from two eggs fertilized by two sperm cells. They have the same genetic relationship as siblings.

The role of genetics and the role of the environment can be studied by comparing the expression of traits in monozygotic and dizygotic twins. The higher concordance value for monozygotic twins as compared with the value for dizygotic twins indicates a significant genetic component for a given trait.

(e) *Heritability* is a measure of the degree to which the phenotypic variation of a given trait is due to genetic factors. A high heritability indicates that genetic factors are major contributors to phenotypic variation, while environmental factors have little impact.

(f) QTL stands for Quantitative Trait Loci, which are situations in which multiple genes contribute to a quantitative trait.

3. (a) Since 1/256 of the F_2 plants are 20 cm and 1/256 are 40 cm, four gene pairs must be involved in determining flower size.

(b) Since there are nine size classes, one can conduct the following backcross:

$$AaBbCcDd \times AABBCCDD$$

The frequency distribution in the backcross would be:

1/16	=	40 cm
4/16	=	37.5 cm
6/16	=	35 cm
4/16	=	32.5 cm
1/16	=	30 cm

(c) The mean is the sum of the individual values divided by the number of values:

$$\text{mean} = 35.0 \text{ cm}$$

The variance is the sum of the squared differences between the individual values and the mean, divided by n-1:

$$\text{variance} = 6.67 \text{ cm}$$

The standard deviation is the square root of the variance:

$$\text{standard deviation} = 2.58 \text{ cm}$$

4. If you add the numbers given for the ratio, you obtain the value of sixteen, which is indicative of a dihybrid cross. The distribution is that of a dihybrid cross with additive effects.

(a) Because a dihybrid result has been identified, there are two loci involved in the production of color. There are two alleles at each locus for a total of four alleles.

(b,c) Because the description of red, medium red, and so on, gives us no indication of a *quantity* of color in any form of units, we would not be able to actually quantify a unit amount for each change in color. We can say that each gene (additive allele) provides an equal unit amount to the phenotype and that the colors differ from each other in multiples of that unit amount. The number of additive alleles needed to produce each phenotype is as follows:

$$1/16 = \text{dark red} \qquad\qquad = AABB$$
$$4/16 = \text{medium-dark red} = 2AABb$$
$$2AaBB$$
$$6/16 = \text{medium red} \qquad = Aabb$$
$$4AaBb$$
$$aaBB$$
$$4/16 = \text{light red} \qquad\quad = 2aaBb$$
$$2Aabb$$
$$1/16 = \text{white} \qquad\qquad = aabb$$

(d)

$$F_1 = \text{all light red}$$
$$F_2 = 1/4 \text{ medium red}$$
$$2/4 \text{ light red}$$
$$1/4 \text{ white}$$

5. (a) It is *possible* that two parents of moderate height can produce offspring that are much taller or shorter than either parent because segregation can produce a variety of gametes as illustrated in the following:

$$rrSsTtuu \times RrSsTtUu$$

(moderate) (moderate)

Offspring from this cross can range from very tall *RrSSTTUu* (14 "tall" units) to very short *rrssttuu* (8 "small" units).

(b) If the individual with a minimum height, *rrssttuu*, is married to an individual of intermediate height *RrSsTtUu*, the offspring can be no taller than the height of the tallest parent. Notice that there is no way of having more than four upper-case alleles in the offspring.

6. As you read this question, notice that the strains are inbred, therefore homozygous, and that approximately 1/250 represent the shortest and tallest groups in the F_2 generation. See the $1/4^n$ formula in the text.

(a,b) Referring to the text, see that where four gene pairs act additively, the proportion of one of the extreme phenotypes to the total number of offspring is 1/256. The same may be said for the other extreme type. The extreme types in this problem are the 12 cm and 36 cm plants. This observation suggests that four gene pairs are involved.

(c) If there are four gene pairs, there are nine $(2n + 1)$ phenotypic categories and eight increments between these categories. Since there is a difference of 24 cm between the extremes, 24 cm/8 = 3 cm for each increment (each of the additive alleles).

(d) A typical F_1 cross that produces a "typical" F_2 distribution would be where all gene pairs are heterozygous (*AaBbCcDd*), independently assorting, and additive. Many possible sets of parents would give an F_1 of this type. The limitation is that each parent has genotypes that give a height of 24 cm as stated in the problem. Because the parents are inbred, it is expected that they are fully homozygous. For example:

$$AABBccdd \times aabbCCDD$$

(e) Since the *aabbccdd* genotype gives a height of 12 cm and each upper-case allele adds 3 cm to the height, there are many possibilities for an 18 cm plant:

> *AAbbccdd*,
> *AaBbccdd*,
> *aaBbCcdd*, etc.

Any plant with seven upper-case letters will be 33 cm tall:

> *AABBCCDd*,
> *AABBCcDD*,
> *AABbCCDD*, for example.

7. (a) There is a fairly continuous range of "quantitative" phenotypes in the F_2 and an F_1 that is between the phenotypes of the two parents; therefore, one can conclude that some phenotypic blending is occurring that is probably the result of several gene pairs acting in an additive fashion. Because the extreme phenotypes (6 cm and 30 cm) each represent 1/64 of the total, it is likely that there are three gene pairs in this cross. Remember, trihybrid crosses that show independent assortment of genes have a denominator (4^3) of 64 in ratios. Also, the fact that there are seven categories of phenotypes, which, because of the relationship 2n + 1 = 7, would give the number of gene pairs (n) of 3. The genotypes of the parents would be combinations of alleles that would produce a 6 cm (*aabbcc*) tail and a 30 cm (*AABBCC*) tail, while the 18 cm offspring would have a genotype of *AaBbCc*.

(b) A mating of an *AaBbCc* (for example) pig with the 6 cm *aabbcc* pig would result in the following offspring:

Gametes (18cm tail)	Gamete (6cm tail)	Offspring
ABC		AaBbCc (18 cm)
ABc		AaBbcc (14 cm)
AbC		AabbCc (14 cm)
Abc	abc	Aabbcc (10 cm)
aBC		aaBbCc (14 cm)
aBc		aaBbcc (10 cm)
abC		aabbCc (10 cm)
abc		aabbcc (6 cm)

In this example, a 1:3:3:1 ratio is the result. However, had a different 18 cm tailed-pig been selected, a different ratio would occur:

$$AABbcc \times aabbcc$$

Gametes (18cm tail)	Gamete (6cm tail)	Offspring
ABc	abc	AaBbcc (14 cm)
Abc		Aabbcc (10 cm)

8. For height, notice that average differences between MZ twins reared together (1.7 cm) and those MZ twins reared apart (1.8 cm) are similar (meaning little environmental influence) and considerably less than differences of DZ twins (4.4 cm) or

sibs (4.5) reared together. These data indicate that genetics plays a major role in determining height.

For weight, however, notice that MZ twins reared together have a much smaller (1.9 kg) difference than MZ twins reared apart, indicating that the environment has a considerable impact on weight. By comparing the weight differences of MZ twins reared apart with DZ twins and sibs reared together, one can conclude that the environment has almost as much an influence on weight as genetics.

For ridge count, the differences between MZ twins reared together and those reared apart are small. For the data in the table, it would appear that ridge count and height have the highest heritability values.

9. Comparison of phenotypic variances between monozygotic and dizygotic traits provides an estimate of broad-sense heritability (H^2).

10. Many traits, especially those we view as quantitative, are likely to be determined by a polygenic mode with possible environmental influences. The following are some common examples: height, general body structure, skin color, and perhaps most common behavioral traits, including intelligence.

11. At first glance, this problem looks as if it will be an arithmetic headache; however, the problem can be simplified.

(a) The mean is computed by adding the measurements of all of the individuals, then dividing by the number of individuals. In this case there are 760 corn plants. To keep from having to add 760 numbers, merely multiply each height group by the number of individuals in each group. Add all the products and then divide by n (760). This gives a value for the mean of 140 cm.

(b) For the variance, use the formula given below (as in the text):

$$s^2 = V = n\Sigma f(x^2) - (\Sigma fx)^2 / n(n-1)$$

To simplify the calculations, determine the square of each height group (10 cm, for example); then multiply the value by the number in each group.

For the first group (100 cm) we would have:

$$100 \times 100 \times 20 = 200000$$

The rest of the groups are as follows:

$$110 \times 110 \times 60 \ = 726000$$
$$120 \times 120 \times 90 \ = 1296000$$
$$130 \times 130 \times 130 = 2197000$$
$$140 \times 140 \times 180 = 3528000$$
$$150 \times 150 \times 120 = 2700000$$
$$160 \times 160 \times 70 \ = 1792000$$
$$170 \times 170 \times 50 \ = 1445000$$
$$180 \times 180 \times 40 \ = 1296000$$
$$= 15180000$$

Now, the mean squared, multiplied by n, is as follows:

$$140 \times 140 \times 760 = 14896000$$

Completing the calculations gives the following:

$$(15180000 - 14896000)/759 = 284000/759$$
$$s^2 = V = 374.18$$

(c) The *standard deviation* is the square root of the variance, or 19.34.

(d) The *standard error* of the mean is the standard deviation divided by the square root of *n*, or about 0.70. The plot approximates a normal distribution. Variation is continuous.

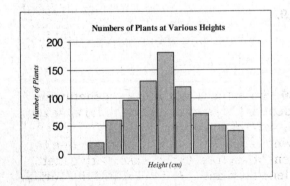

12. (a) Using the following equations, H^2 and h^2 can be calculated as follows.

For back fat:

Broad-sense heritability $= H^2 = 12.2/30.6 = 0.398$
Narrow-sense heritability $= h^2 = 8.44/30.6 = 0.276$

For body length:

Broad-sense heritability $= H^2 = 26.4/52.4 = 0.504$
Narrow-sense heritability $= h^2 = 11.7/52.4 = 0.223$

(b) For a trait that is quantitatively measured, the relative importance of genetic versus environmental factors may be formally assessed by examining the heritability index (H^2 or broad heritability). In animal and plant breeding, a measure of potential response to selection based on additive variance and dominance variance is termed narrow-sense heritability (h^2). A relatively high narrow-sense heritability is a prediction of the impact selection may have in altering an initial randomly breeding population. Therefore, of the two traits, selection for back fat would produce more response.

13. The formula for estimating heritability is

$$H^2 = V_G/V_P$$

where V_G and V_P are the genetic and phenotypic components of variation, respectively. The main issue in this question is obtaining some estimate of two components of phenotypic variation: genetic and environmental. V_P is the combination of genetic and environmental variance. Because the two parental strains are inbred, they are assumed to be homozygous and the variances of 4.2 and 3.8 are considered to be the result of environmental influences. The average of these two values is 4.0. The F_1 is also genetically homogeneous and gives us an additional estimation of the environmental factors.

By averaging with the parents

$$[(4.0 + 5.6)/2 = 4.8]$$

we obtain a relatively good idea of environmental impact on the phenotype. The phenotypic variance in the F_2 is the sum of the genetic (V_G) and environmental (V_E) components. We have estimated the environmental input as 4.8, so 10.3 (V_P) minus 4.8, gives us an estimate of (V_G), which is 5.5. Heritability then becomes 5.5/10.3, or 0.53. This value, when viewed in percentage form, indicates that about 53 percent of the variation in plant height is due to genetic influences.

14. (a)

For Vitamin A:

$$h_A^2 = V_A/V_P = V_A/(V_E + V_A + V_D) = 0.097$$

For Cholesterol:

$$h_A^2 = 0.223$$

(b) Cholesterol content should be influenced to a greater extent by selection.

15. (a) Taking the sum of the values and dividing by the number in the sample gives the following means:

> mean sheep fiber length = 7.7 cm
> mean fleece weight = 6.4 kg

The variance for each is:

> variance sheep fiber length = 6.097
> variance fleece weight = 3.12

The standard deviation is the square root of the variance:

> sheep fiber length = 2.469
> fleece weight = 1.766

(b,c) The covariance for the two traits is 30.36/7, or 4.34, while the correlation coefficient is +0.998.

(d) There is a very high correlation between fleece weight and fiber length, and it is likely that this correlation is not by chance. Even though correlation does not mean cause-and-effect, it would seem logical that as you increased fiber length, you would also

increase fleece weight. It is probably safe to say that the increase in fleece weight is directly related to an increase in fiber length.

16. Given that both narrow-sense heritability values are relatively high, it is likely that a farmer would be able to alter both milk protein content and butterfat by selection. The value of 0.91 for the correlation coefficient between protein content and butterfat suggests that if one selects for butterfat, protein content will increase. However, correlation coefficients describe the extent to which variation in one quantitative trait is associated with variation in another and does not reveal the underlying causes of such variation. Assuming that these dairy cows had been selected for high butterfat in the past and increased protein content followed that selection (for butterfat), we would find it likely that selection for butterfat would continue to correlate with increased protein content. However, there may well be a point where physiological circumstances change and selection for high butterfat may be at the expense of protein content.

17.

$$h^2 = (7.5 - 8.5/6.0 - 8.5) = 0.4$$
$$\text{(realized heritability)}$$

18. Given the realized heritability value of 0.4, it is unlikely that selection experiments would cause a rapid and/or significant response to selection. A minor response might result from intense selection.

19.

$$h^2 = 0.3 = (M_2 - 60/80 - 60)$$
$$M_2 = 66 \text{ grams}$$

20. Since the rice plants are genetically identical, V_G is zero and $H^2 = V_G/V_P =$ zero. Broad-sense heritability is a measure to which the phenotypic variance is due to genetic factors. In this case, with genetically identical plants, H^2 is zero, and the variance observed in grain yield is due to the environment. Selection would not be effective in this strain of rice.

21. (a,b) In many instances, a trait may be clustered in families; yet, traditional mapping procedures may not be applicable because the trait might be influenced by a number of genes. In general, researchers look for associations to particular DNA sequences (molecular markers). When the trait cosegregates with a particular maker and it statistically associates with that trait above chance, a likely QTL has been identified. Markers such as RFLPs, SNPs, and microsatellites are often used because they are highly variable, relatively easy to assess, and present in all individuals.

22. (a) In general, polygenic conditions involving thresholds occur if a range of expression is possible, but the trait is either expressed or not expressed. In addition, with polygenic systems (including those with thresholds) environmental factors carry considerable impact.

(b) The number of polygenes involved in a polygenic trait can often be estimated by solving for *n* in the formula if the ratio of F_2 individuals resembling either of the two extreme P_1 phenotypes can be determined.

$$1/4^n$$

It is also possible to estimate the number of polygenes using the $(2n + 1)$ rule, where $(2n + 1)$ is the number of possible phenotypes, and *n* equals the number of additive loci.

(c) The multiple allele hypothesis was originally based on experiment results involving pigmentation in wheat. Such results showed that a number of additive alleles acting in Mendelian fashion could explain continuous variation.

(d) When a number of parameters are known, environmental impact on a quantitatively inherited trait is often assessed by heritability estimates (broad and narrow sense). Highly inbred strains of

plants and animals reared under varying conditions and twin studies in humans are helpful in determining the environmental impact on traits.

23. Chromosome 2 seems to confer considerable resistance to the insecticide, somewhat in the heterozygous state and more in the homozygous state. Thus, some partial dominance is occurring.

24. (a) The most direct explanation would involve two gene pairs, with each additive gene contributing about 1.2 mm to the phenotype.

(b) The fit to this backcross supports the original hypothesis.

(c) These data do not support the simple hypothesis provided in part (a).

(d,e) With these data, one can see no distinct phenotypic classes suggesting that the environment may play a role in eye development or that there are more genes involved.

25. The best way to approach this problem is to first determine the number of gene pairs involved. Notice that all the F_1 plants are uniform and are in the middle of the extremes of 3″ and 15″; therefore, the parents must each be homozygous and at the extremes. Notice also that there are 13 classes in the F_2, so, there must be six gene pairs. See the text for an explanation of the $2n + 1$ formula.

(a) There are two ways to answer this section, a hard way and an easy way. The hard way would be to take a big sheet of paper, make the cross (*AaBbCcDdEeFf* × *AaBbCcDdEeFf*), collect the genotypes, and calculate the ratios.

This method would be very laborious and error-prone. The easy way would be to re-read the material on the binomial expansion and note the pattern preceding each expression. Notice that all numbers other than the 1's are equal to the sum of the two numbers directly above them. By enlarging the numbers to include six gene pairs, you can arrive at the 13 classes and their frequencies:

$3'' = 1$	$4'' = 12$	$5'' = 66$
$6'' = 220$	$7'' = 495$	$8'' = 792$
$9'' = 924$	$10'' = 792$	$11'' = 495$
$12'' = 220$	$13'' = 66$	$14'' = 12$
$15'' = 1$		

To check your calculations, be certain that your frequencies total 4096. You will also notice an additional shortcut in that since the distribution is symmetrical, you need only calculate to the center and the remainder will be in the reverse order.

(b) To determine the outcome of a cross of the F_1 plants in the testcross, apply the formula that allows you to calculate any set of components: $n!/(s!t!)$ where n = total number of events (6), s = number of events of outcome a and t = number of events of outcome b. For example, to determine how many $6''$ plants would be recovered from the cross $AaBbCcDdEeFf \times aabbccddeeff$, we are really asking how many will have three additive alleles (upper case) and three nonadditive alleles (lower case).

$$6!/(3!3!) = 20$$

Applying this formula throughout gives the following frequencies:

$3'' = 1$	$4'' = 6$	$5'' = 15$
$6'' = 20$	$7'' = 15$	$8'' = 6$
$9'' = 1$		

And the total is 64. You can check your logic by considering that there should be only 1/64 with no additive alleles ($3''$) and 1/64 with all additive alleles ($9''$).

26. *Monozygotic twins* are derived from a single fertilized egg and are thus genetically identical to each other. They provide a method for determining the influence of genetics and environment on certain traits. *Dizygotic twins* arise from two eggs fertilized by two sperm cells. They have the same genetic relationship as siblings. The role of genetics and the role of the environment can

be studied by comparing the expression of traits in monozygotic and dizygotic twins. The higher concordance value for monozygotic twins as compared with the value for dizygotic twins indicates a significant genetic component for a given trait. Notice that for traits including blood type, eye color, and mental retardation, there is a fairly significant difference between MZ and DZ groups. However, for measles, the difference is not as significant, indicating a greater role of the environment. Hair color has a significant genetic component, as do idiopathic epilepsy, schizophrenia, diabetes, allergies, cleft lip, and clubfoot. The genetic component to mammary cancer is present but minimal according to these data.

27. The solution to these types of problems rests on determining the ratio of individuals expressing the extreme phenotype to the total number of individuals. In this case, 8:2028 is equal to 1:253, which is close to 1:256. If there are three gene pairs, the ratio is 1:64, four gene pairs 1:256, or five gene pairs 1:1024. Therefore, these data indicate that four gene pairs influence size in these guinea pigs.

28. As with many traits that are caused by numerous loci acting additively, some genes have more influence on expression than others. In addition, environmental factors may play a role in the expression of some polygenic traits. In the case of brachydactyly, numerous modifier genes in the genome can influence brachydactyly expression. Examination of OMIM (*Online Mendelian Inheritance of Man*) through *http://www.ncbi.nlm.nih.gov/* will illustrate this point.

29. (a,b) Because there are nine phenotypic classes in the F_2, there must be four gene pairs involved. The genotypes of the parents could be symbolized as *AABBCCDD* × *aabbccdd*, and the F_1 as *AaBbCcDd*.

30. It is likely that the flies maintained in the *Drosophila* repository are more highly inbred and less heterozygous than those recently obtained from the wild. Response to selection is dependent on genetic variation. The greater the genetic variation in a species, the more likely and dramatic the response to selection. Therefore, one would expect a greater response to selection in the wild population.

31.

$$6 \times 5 \times 4 \times 3 \times 2 \times 1/(2 \times 1)(4 \times 3 \times 2 \times 1)$$
$$= 15 \text{ of a total of 64.}$$

32. Breeders attempt to "select" out this disorder by first maintaining complete and detailed breeding records of afflicted strains. Second, they avoid breeding dogs whose close relatives are afflicted. The molecular-developmental mechanism that causes the "month of birth" effect in canine hip dysplasia is unknown. However, with many, perhaps all quantitative traits, it is clear that there is a significant environmental influence on both the penetrance and/or expression of the phenotype. With many genes acting in various ways to influence a phenotype, there are opportunities for varied molecular and developmental intraorganismic microenvironments. Stated another way, the longer and more complex the molecular distance from the genome to the phenotype, the greater the likelihood for environmental factors to be involved in expression.

33. (a) The average response to selection (in mm) would be the sum of the differences between the control and offspring, divided by three: $(2.17 + 3.79 + 4.06)/3 = 3.34$ mm.

(b) One computes realized heritability by the following formula:

$$h^2 = \frac{M2 - M}{M1 - M}$$

where M represents the mean size (control), M1 represents the selected parents, and M2 represents the size in offspring.

For 1997:

$$h^2 = (32.21 - 30.04)/(34.13 - 30.04) = 0.53$$

For 1998:

$$h^2 = (31.90 - 28.11)/(31.98 - 28.11) = 0.98$$

For 1999:

$$h^2 = (33.74 - 29.68)/(31.81 - 29.68) = 1.91$$

The overall realized heritability would be the average of all three heritability values, or 1.14.

(c) A key factor in determining response to selection is the genetic variability available to respond to selection. The greater the genetic variability, the greater the response. Another key factor in rapid response to selection often relates to the number of loci involved. If there are few loci, each with large phenotypic effects controlling a trait, response to selection is usually high. Lastly, if flower size is not genetically correlated with other floral traits, size alone may not be subject to strong stabilizing selection, which would reduce genetic variation. Therefore, whereas other floral traits may show low response to selection, size alone may be more responsive.

(d) With high heritability, one expects a high genetic contribution to phenotypic variation. Genetic variability that provides rapid adjustments to changing environments is an evolutionary advantage. Therefore, in general, one would expect that high heritability would contribute to high evolutionary potential.

Chapter 26: Genetics and Behavior

Concept Areas	Corresponding Problems
Methodology of Behavior Genetics	1, 8, 11, 12
Genetic Analysis: Drosophila	2, 6, 14, 15
Genetic Analysis: Mice	3
Genetic Analysis: Caenorhabditis	8, 9, 13
Mosaic Analysis	4
Human Behavioral Genetics	5, 7, 10, 16, 17

Vocabulary: Organization and Listing of Terms and Concepts

Structures and Substances

RFLP

Alcohol dehydrogenase

Acetaldehyde dehydrogenase

Isozymes

Ethylmethanesulfonate

Attached-X chromosomes

Ring-X chromosome

Ion channels

cAMP

Trinucleotide repeats

  CAG repeat

  exons

  polyglutamine tracts

Neurotransmitters

  oligodendrocyte

Microarray

Processes/Methods

QLT analysis

Behavior

  nature-nurture controversy

Methodologies

  alcohol preference in mice

  open-field behavior in mice

    pleiotropic

    heritability analysis

  selection

    maze learning in rats

    geotaxis in *Drosophila*

      taxis: positive or negative

    polygenic control

  genetic dissection/mosaic analysis

    Drosophila courtship

      orientation

      vibration

    phototaxis

    primary focus

      ring-X chromosome

    memory-deficient mutant

  Molecular biology of behavior

    neurophysiological approaches

    potassium/sodium transport

    temperature-sensitive genes

    myelination

Human behavior genetics
   genetic basis
      bipolar disorder
         manic depression
   less-defined genetic basis
   single gene disorders
      Huntington disease
   multifactorial traits
      schizophrenia

Concepts

Behaviorist school

Nature/nurture controversy

Analytical approaches
   behavior-first approach
   gene-first approach
   QTL
   microarrays
   inbred strains
      selected lines
   mosaics
   heritability
   twin studies

Primary focus of a gene

Concordance/discordance

Solutions to Problems and Discussion Questions

1. One method, a behavior-first approach, attempts to correlate existing behavioral differences with general genetic differences. It is a comparative approach in which a particular behavior is examined among several (to many) closely related but genetically different strains of organisms. If the environment is held constant, yet the behavioral differences persist, there must be a genetic component to the behavior.

A second approach involves selection for certain behaviors. When selection and interbreeding of a behavior yields a consistent phenotype, then the genetics of the behavior can be examined.

A third approach takes advantage of the fact that some behaviors are strongly influenced by a major locus. In a genetics-first approach, mutagens can be used to induce mutations from which those behaviors of interest can be studied. If an induced mutation produces a consistent behavioral change, it is often the most useful way to analyze a behavior. The latter two approaches can only be used if the organism of interest can be genetically manipulated, which is not always the case (primates, for example). In addition, once selection and mutation approaches are applied, the natural expression of most behaviors is usually altered. On the positive side, selection and mutation analyses offer unique opportunities to examine genetic and physiological factors at the molecular levels.

2. One of the easiest ways to determine whether a genetic basis exists for a given abnormality is to cross the abnormal fly to a normal fly. If the trait is determined by a dominant gene, that trait should appear in the offspring—in probably half of them if the gene was in the heterozygous state. If the gene is recessive and homozygous, then one may not see expression in the offspring of the first cross; however, if one crosses the F_1, the trait might appear in approximately 1/4 of the offspring. Such ratios would not be expected if the trait is polygenic, which would complicate the study. Modifications of these patterns would be expected if the mode of inheritance is X-linked or shows other modifications of typical Mendelian ratios. One might hypothesize that the trait influences the nervous, cuticular, or muscular system.

Mapping the primary focus of the gene could be accomplished using the unstable ring-X-chromosome. Given that the gene is X-linked, one would use classical recombination methods to place recessive markers (*singed bristles* and/or *yellow body*) on the X chromosome with the gene causing the limp. This would help one identify the male/female boundary. One would then cross homozygous females (for the trait and markers) to ring-X-males, or the reciprocal, and examine the offspring for gynandromorphs (and marker mosaics). If one obtained a pool of gynandromorphs, one could assess the phenotype (limp or normal) with respect to exposure of the recessive gene in the male tissue. Correlating mosaic boundaries with the limp phenotype would allow one to provide an educated guess as to the primary focus of the gene causing the limp.

3. If one can select inbred strains for a certain behavior, it might be possible to analyze molecular and physiological characteristics that differ from normal mice. Like mutation analysis, inbred strains provide an opportunity for comparative studies. Differences in alcohol tolerance, metabolism, and physiology can be examined. In addition, refined studies on known factors (receptors, etc.) related to addiction are open to investigation. Once major genes are located (by QTL analysis in this case), the genes, their regulation, and products can be studied. Such a molecular approach provides an opportunity to determine the exact differences between the normal state and the addictive state. Both approaches can provide insight into the nature of behavioral traits, and because of the complexity of most behaviors, both approaches are often necessary.

4. First, when one examines cuticular markers in a gynandromorphic analysis, one is not always certain that underlying tissues and organs follow the surface mosaic pattern. The finding that flies with male/female cuticular markers had circadian activity patterns with both male and female components indicates that the brain can be genetically mosaic if cuticular markers are mosaic. The observation also suggests that the male and female oscillators function autonomously.

5. From the information provided, one can conclude that the tasting trait is determined by a dominant gene. Notice that a 3:1 ratio of tasters to nontasters is obtained in the third cross. This result strongly argues for the *TT* or *Tt* condition providing taste of PTC. Information from other crosses does not contradict the dominant nature of PTC tasting.

6. One limitation of this approach is the intensity of effort required to establish genetically uniform strains reflecting a particular behavior. Another complexity is that genes often have multiple functions or may function somewhat differently in different strains and/or environments. In addition, since geotaxis is a complex trait, selection experiments offer little indication of the number and location of selected genes. New technologies, including microarrays, have been applied to this problem and enable the analysis of the expression patterns of many genes simultaneously. Strains having high and low responses to geotaxis selection showed reproducible differences in gene expression and revealed some of the molecular and physiological characteristics of geotaxis behavior. However, it is important to state that association of a particular microarray pattern with a particular behavior may not indicate a cause-effect relationship. Some genes having little or nothing to do with geotaxis may "hitch-hike" near global regulatory genes that just happen to influence geotaxis.

7. Concordance for traits such as addictive behavior in monozygotic and dizygotic twins has been applied to many types of behaviors. Monozygotic twins are genetically identical, whereas dizygotic twins are genetically like siblings. Since members of each set of twins are likely to be reared under similar environmental conditions, it is possible to get some estimate of the genetic contribution to a given behavior. A higher rate of concordance for monozygotic twins compared with dizygotic twins often indicates a genetic component to a trait. Although such studies suggest that a genetic component exists, they do not reveal the precise genetic basis of pathological gambling.

8. Because of the rigidity of development in *Caenorhabditis* and the extensive knowledge of cellular fates and connectivity, it represents an excellent experimental organism for the study of development. In addition, because of their fixed fate, cells can be altered, physically and/or genetically, and resulting development and behavior can be studied. However, the behavioral repertoire of *C. elegans* is somewhat narrow. In addition, *C. elegans* has more protein-coding genes than *Drosophila*, another organism whose behavioral genetics has been highly studied. Such an additional number of protein-coding genes coupled with a sparse behavioral repertoire creates a disadvantage when using *C. elegans*.

9. The simplest model would place each component in a linear pathway as shown in the following:

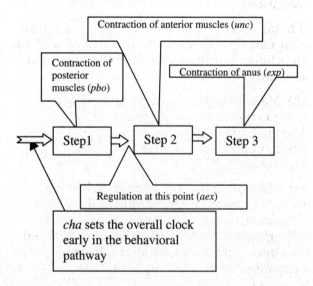

10. A number of issues limit the study of human behavior, including the following:

(1) With relatively small numbers of offspring per mating, standard genetic methods are difficult.

(2) Records on family illnesses, especially behavioral illnesses, are difficult to obtain.

(3) The long generation time makes longitudinal studies difficult.

(4) The scientist cannot direct matings.

(5) There are limits to the experimental treatments that can be applied.

(6) Traits that are interesting to study are often complex and difficult to quantify.

(7) Culture and family background may strongly influence behavior.

11. Usually, if traits that are considered to be homozygous (the pure breeds of dogs) fail to breed true, it is likely that the trait is determined by conditioning or complex genetic factors that each have minor influences. Such breeds of dogs, while being highly selected, are not homozygous for all genes. Although the dogs are considered to be pure breeds, it is likely that alleles are segregating and combining in various ways to produce the variations noted. There may also be different interactions with environmental stimuli from subtle genetic variations.

12. (a) Alcohol preference in mice is a trait that can exist in some inbred strains and not in others. Selection can alter the degree of alcohol preference.

(b) Maze behavior in rats can be learned, and certain selected lines are better at learning a maze than others. Such selected lines retain their abilities in varied environments.

(c) The behavior-first approach was used originally to establish strains of flies that responded differently in geotaxis experiments. Mutations have been isolated in a gene-first approach that influenced responses to geotaxis experiments.

(d) Mosaic analysis using unstable ring-X chromosomes allows one to map the primary focus of a gene. In doing so, the primary focus of some genes relating to behavior was identified in specific brain regions.

(e) Microarray analysis among schizophrenics identified a cluster of genes involved in myelination that had lower or higher expression levels when compared to nonschizophrenic controls.

13. Recessive mutations are typically observed only at the phenotypic level when homozygous. Self-fertilization, the ultimate form of inbreeding, greatly enhances the likelihood that recessive genes will become homozygous. Homozygous strains are of considerable advantage when studying complex traits.

14. Examine the data and notice that the magnitude of change attributed to the X chromosome is relatively small when compared to the unselected line. Notice that chromosome 2 contributes relatively strongly to negative geotaxis, while chromosome 3 contributes fairly strongly to positive geotaxis. Because this is a whole chromosome comparison, it is possible that there are strong positive geotaxis alleles and strong negative geotaxis alleles on the same chromosome that cancel each other.

15. One might compare gene expression through microarray analysis between space reared flies with a control population on Earth. By comparing behavioral (metabolic, mating, feeding, walking, flying) rituals between the two populations (space and Earth), one might be able to correlate genetic expression profiles and determine which genes are most likely to respond to which behavioral alteration. Although a number of parameters would be interesting to study in this way, one might concentrate the study on genes known to influence muscle and nerve function in flies and humans. A second study might focus on the immune system since it is known that there are surprisingly high genetic correlations between the immune response of flies and mammals (Hoffmann, 2003). Since it is known that microgravity negatively influences the human immune system (reduces the mitogenic activity of T cells), a comparison of the gene-expression profiles of the immune-response system would also be worthy of study. The behavioral side of the experiment would focus on determining whether changes in gravitational stress alter behavior (inactivity, muscle, and nerve use) to a point where the immune response is altered. Coupling the two studies, gene-expression profiles associated with behavioral and the immune response, might provide insight into a number of significant problems that humans encounter in space flight, and thereby be justifiable and relatively inexpensive.

16. Schizophrenia is a complex familial brain disorder, with relatives of schizophrenics having a higher incidence than the general population. The closer the relationship to the schizophrenic, the greater is the probability of the disorder occurring. Concordance for schizophrenia is higher in monozygotic twins (~ 50 percent) than dizygotic twins (~ 17 percent) and suggests that a genetic component exists along with shared environmental risk factors.

Recently, microarrays have been used to identify genes whose expression is altered in schizophrenia. Researchers have isolated RNA from the brains of normal and schizophrenic individuals and used the RNA to prepare cDNA for hybridization to the microarrays. The microarrays carried over 6000 probes for the human genome. Some of the identified genes have low levels of expression in schizophrenia, whereas others express at high levels. One cluster of genes involved in myelination has lower levels of expression in schizophrenics, but some other clusters have increased levels of expression, suggesting that schizophrenia is associated with functional disruption in oligodendrocytes. A variety of genome-wide microarray scans of gene expression in schizophrenia have identified candidate genes whose expression is altered in schizophrenics. Knockout mice missing a myelin-related gene are being studied in order to relate changes in gene expression with a specific behavioral phenotype.

From such studies, it is hoped that therapies can be targeted at specific genes involved in schizophrenia. However, gene-expression patterns during early development may eventually cause behavioral problems and not be detectable in adult samples regardless of their sophistication.

17. Data in the table indicate that females (*Gasterosteus aculeatus*) spend more time with males having the optimal MHC constitution than those that do not. As with other organisms, it appears that genetic diversity for the MHC is a selective advantage. Since immunological functions are associated with the MHC complex, mate selection mechanisms that support the maintenance of such diversity seem reasonable from an evolutionary viewpoint.

Chapter 27: Population Genetics

Concept Areas	Corresponding Problems
Populations and Gene Pools	4, 26
Calculating Allele Frequencies	1, 2, 3, 5, 6, 7, 8, 17
The Hardy-Weinberg Law	4, 17, 19, 27
Extensions of the Hardy-Weinberg Law	8, 9, 10, 22, 23, 30, 31
Using the Hardy-Weinberg Law	11, 12, 14, 15, 16, 18, 19, 20, 21, 23, 24, 27
Factors That Alter Allele Frequencies	8, 9, 10, 11, 12, 13, 28, 29, 30

Vocabulary: Organization and Listing of Terms and Concepts

Historical

Charles Darwin

The Origin of Species (1859)

Alfred Russell Wallace

Hardy and Weinberg

Structures and Substances

Population

Species

Gene pool

HIV-1

CC-CKR-5

chemokine

CCR5

CD4

CCR5-Δ32

major histocompatibility complex (MHC)

HLA-A and *HLA-B*

I locus

isoagglutinin

acetylcholinesterase (ACE), Ace^R

chlorpyrifos

aspartate aminotransferase 1

cystic fibrosis transmembrane conductance regulator (CFTR)

Processes/Methods

Natural selection

fitness

Gene frequencies

mutation

migration

selection

random genetic drift

ABO blood groups

Symbolism

p, q

$p + q = 1$

$p^2 + 2pq + q^2 = 1$

Multiple alleles

$p + q + r = 1$

$p^2 + 2pq + 2pr + q^2 + 2qr + r^2 = 1$

Heterozygote frequency

$\sqrt{q^2}$

$p = 1 - q$

$2pq$

Demonstrating equilibrium

  expected frequencies

  observed frequencies

  selection coefficient(s)

    directional selection

    stabilizing selection

    disruptive selection

    Drosophila

  X-linked traits

Changes in gene frequencies

  mutation (generates variability)

    recessive

    dominant

      achondroplasia

  migration

  genetic drift

    small populations

    population size

  Drosophila

    forked bristles

      isolated subpopulations

        achromatopsia

    inbreeding and heterosis

      assortative

        positive

        negative

    inbreeding

      self-fertilization

    consanguineous marriages

    inbreeding coefficient

    inbreeding depression

    hybrid vigor

      dominance theory

      overdominance

Concepts

Population genetics

Gene pool

  gene (allelic) frequencies (F27.1)

Population

Hardy-Weinberg Law

  multiple alleles

  X-linked traits

Hardy-Weinberg assumptions

  infinitely large

  no drift

  random mating

  no selection

  no mutation

  no migration

Genetic equilibrium

  genetic variability

Inbreeding and hybrid vigor (F27.2)

Fitness

F27.1 Simple illustration of the relationships among populations, individuals, alleles, and allelic frequencies (*p* and *q*).

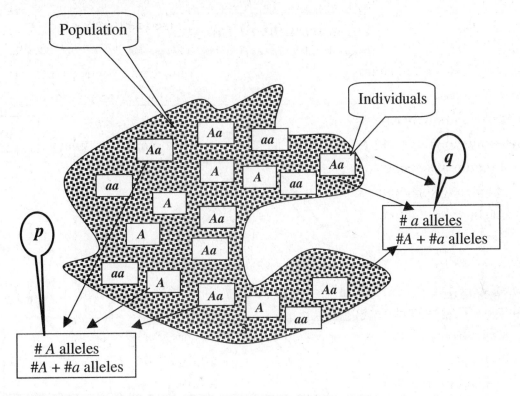

F27.2 Diagram of the relationships among inbreeding, heterosis, and homozygosity. Note that as inbreeding occurs, heterosis decreases and homozygosity increases.

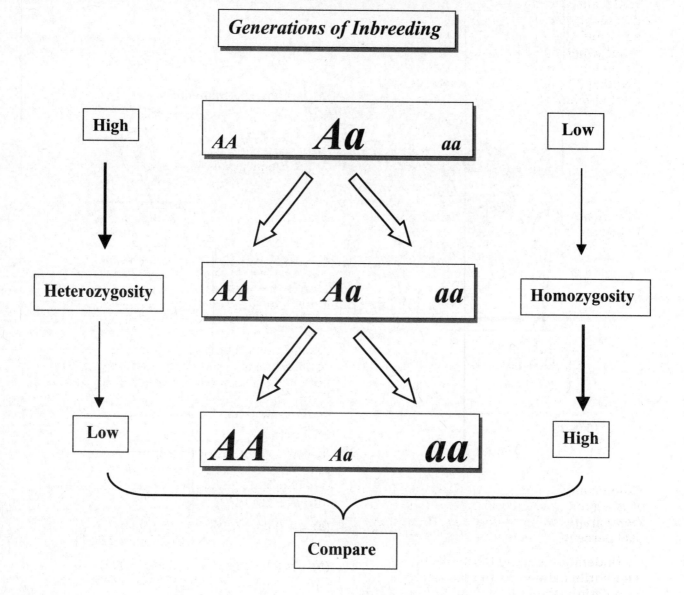

Solutions to Problems and Discussion Questions

1. Because the alleles follow a dominant/recessive mode, one can use the equation $\sqrt{q^2}$ to calculate q from which all other aspects of the answer depend. The frequency of aa types is determined by dividing 37 (number of nontasters) by the total number of individuals (125).

$$q^2 = 37/125 = 0.296$$
$$q = 0.544$$
$$p = 1 - q$$
$$p = 0.456$$

The frequencies of the genotypes are determined by applying the formula $p^2 + 2pq + q^2$ as follows:

Frequency of $AA = p^2$
$$= (0.456)^2$$
$$= 0.208 \text{ or } 20.8\%$$

Frequency of $Aa = 2pq$
$$= 2(0.456)(0.544)$$
$$= 0.496 \text{ or } 49.6\%$$

Frequency of $aa = q^2$
$$= (0.544)^2$$
$$= 0.296 \text{ or } 29.6\%$$

When completing such a set of calculations, it is a good practice to add the final percentages to be certain that they total 100 percent.

2. Understanding the Hardy-Weinberg equilibrium allows us to state that if a population is in equilibrium, the genotypic frequencies will not shift from one generation to the next unless there are factors such as selection and migration, which alter gene frequencies. Since none of these factors are stated in the problem, we need only to determine whether the initial population is in equilibrium. Calculate p and q, then apply the equation $p^2 + 2pq + q^2$ to determine genotypic frequencies in the next generation.

p = frequency of A
$$= 0.2 + 0.3$$
$$= 0.5$$
$$q = 1 \quad p = 0.5$$

Frequency of $AA = p^2$
$$= (0.5)^2$$
$$= 0.25 \text{ or } 25\%$$

Frequency of $Aa = 2pq$
$$= 2(0.5)(0.5)$$
$$= 0.5 \text{ or } 50\%$$

Frequency of $aa = q^2$
$$= (0.5)^2$$
$$= 0.25 \text{ or } 25\%$$

The initial population was not in equilibrium, however, after one generation of mating under the Hardy-Weinberg assumptions. The population is in equilibrium and will continue to be so (and not change) until one or more of the Hardy-Weinberg assumptions is not met. Note that *equilibrium* does not necessarily mean p and q equal 0.5.

3. For each of these values, one merely takes the square root to determine q; then one computes p, and one "plugs" the values into the $2pq$ expression.

(a) $q = 0.08$; $2pq = 2(0.92)(0.08)$
$$= 0.1472 \text{ or } 14.72\%$$

(b) $q = 0.009$; $2pq = 2(0.991)(0.009)$
$$= 0.01784 \text{ or } 1.78\%$$

(c) $q = 0.3$; $2pq = 2(0.7)(0.3)$
$$= 0.42 \text{ or } 42\%$$

(d) $q = 0.1$; $2pq = 2(0.9)(0.1)$
$$= 0.18 \text{ or } 18\%$$

(e) $q = 0.316$; $2pq = 2(0.684)(0.316)$
$$= 0.4323 \text{ or } 43.23\%$$

(Depending on how one rounds off the decimals, slightly different answers will occur.)

4. In order for the Hardy-Weinberg equations to apply, the population must be in equilibrium.

5. If one has the frequency of individuals with the dominant phenotype, the remainder will have the recessive phenotype (q^2). With q^2 one can calculate q, and from this value one can arrive at p. Applying the expression $p^2 + 2pq + q^2$ will allow a solution to the question.

6. (a) For the CCR5 analysis, first determine p and q. Since one has the frequencies of all the genotypes, one can add

0.6 and 0.351/2 to provide p (= 0.7755)

q will be

$1 - 0.7755$ or 0.2245

The equilibrium values will be as follows:

Frequency of $l/l =$ $p^2 = (0.7755)^2$
$= 0.6014$ or 60.14%

Frequency of $l/\Delta32$ $= 2pq$
$= 2(0.7755)(0.2245)$
$= 0.3482$ or 34.82%

Frequency of $\Delta32/\Delta32 = q^2 = (0.2245)^2$
$= 0.0504$ or 5.04%

Comparing these equilibrium values with the observed values strongly suggests that the observed values are drawn from a population in equilibrium.

(b) For the AS analysis, first determine p and q. Since one has the frequencies of all the genotypes, one can add

0.756 and 0.242/2 to provide p (= 0.877)

q will be

$1 - 0.877$ or 0.123

The equilibrium values will be as follows:

Frequency of $AA = p^2 = (0.877)^2$
$= 0.7691$ or 76.91%

Frequency of $AS = 2pq = 2(0.877)(0.123)$
$= 0.2157$ or 21.57%

Frequency of $SS = q^2 = (0.123)^2$
$= 0.0151$ or 1.51%

Comparing these equilibrium values with the observed values suggests that the observed values may be drawn from a population that is not in equilibrium. Notice that there are more heterozygotes than predicted and fewer SS types.

To test for a Hardy-Weinberg equilibrium, apply the chi-square test as follows.

$$\chi^2 = \frac{\Sigma(o - e)^2}{e}$$

$(75.6 - 76.9)^2/76.9 +$
$(24.2 - 21.6)^2/21.6 +$
$(0.2 - 1.51)^2/1.5 = 1.47$

In calculating degrees of freedom in a test of gene frequencies, the "free variables" are reduced by an additional degree of freedom because one estimated a parameter (p or q) used in determining the expected values. Therefore, there is one degree of freedom, even though there are three classes. Checking the χ^2 table with 1 degree of freedom gives a value of 3.84 at the 0.05 probability level. Since the χ^2 value calculated here is smaller, the null hypothesis (the observed values fluctuate from the equilibrium values by chance and chance alone) should not be rejected. Thus, the frequencies of AA, AS, and SS sampled a population that is probably in equilibrium.

7. Given that $q^2 = 0.04$, then $q = 0.2$, $2pq = 0.32$, and $p^2 = 0.64$. Of those not expressing the trait, only a mating between heterozygotes can produce an offspring that expresses the trait, and then only at a frequency of 1/4. The different types of matings possible (those without the trait) in the population, with their frequencies, are as follows:

$AA \times AA = 0.64 \times 0.64 = 0.4096$
$AA \times Aa = 0.64 \times 0.32 = 0.2048$
$Aa \times AA = 0.64 \times 0.32 = 0.2048$
$Aa \times Aa = 0.32 \times 0.32 = 0.1024$
$Aa \times Aa = 0.32 \times 0.32 = 0.1024$

Notice that of the matings of the individuals who do not express the trait, only the last two (about 20 percent) are capable of producing offspring with the trait. Therefore, one would arrive at a final likelihood of $1/4 \times 20\%$, or 5 percent of the offspring with the trait.

8. The following formula calculates the frequency of an allele in the next generation for any selection scenario, given the frequencies of a and A in this generation and the fitness of all three genotypes.

$$q_{g+1} = [w_{Aa}p_gq_g + w_{aa}q_g^2]/$$

$$[w_{AA}p_g^2 + w_{Aa}2p_gq_g + w_{aa}q_g^2]$$

where q_{g+1} is the frequency of the a allele in the next generation, q_g is the frequency of the a allele in this generation, p_g is the frequency of the A allele in this generation, and each "w" represents the fitness of its respective genotype.

(a) $q_{g+1} =$

$[.9(.7)(.3)+.8(.3)^2/[1(.7)^2+.9(2)(.7)(.3)+.8(.3)^2]$

$q_{g+1} = 0.278 \qquad p_{g+1} = 0.722$

(b) $q_{g+1} = 0.289 \qquad p_{g+1} = 0.711$

(c) $q_{g+1} = 0.298 \qquad p_{g+1} = 0.702$

(d) $q_{g+1} = 0.319 \qquad p_{g+1} = 0.681$

9. The general equation for responding to this question is

$$q_n = q_0/(1 + nq_0)$$

where n = the number of generations, q_0 = the initial gene frequency, and q_n = the new gene frequency.

(a) n = 1

$$q_n = q_0/(1 + nq_0)$$
$$q_n = 0.5/[1 + (1 \times 0.5)]$$
$$q_n = 0.33 \qquad p_n = 0.67$$

(b) n = 5

$$q_n = q_0/(1 + nq_0)$$
$$q_n = 0.5/[1 + (5 \times 0.5)]$$
$$q_n = 0.143 \qquad p_n = 0.857$$

(c) n = 10

$$q_n = q_0/(1 + nq_0)$$
$$q_n = 0.5/[1 + (10 \times 0.5)]$$
$$q_n = 0.083 \qquad p_n = 0.917$$

(d) n = 25

$$q_n = q_0/(1 + nq_0)$$
$$q_n = 0.5/[1 + (25 \times 0.5)]$$
$$q_n = 0.037 \qquad p_n = 0.963$$

(e) n = 100

$$q_n = q_0/(1 + nq_0)$$
$$q_n = 0.5/[1 + (100 \times 0.5)]$$
$$q_n = 0.0098 \qquad p_n = 0.9902$$

(f) n = 1000

$$q_n = q_0/(1 + nq_0)$$
$$q_n = 0.5/[1 + (1000 \times 0.5)]$$
$$q_n = 0.00099 \qquad p_n = 0.99901$$

10. Since a dominant lethal gene is highly selected against, it is unlikely that it will exist at too high of a frequency, if at all. However, if the gene shows incomplete penetrance or late age of onset (after reproductive age), it may remain in a population.

11. For this question, apply the equations

$$\Delta p = m(p_m - p)$$

$$\text{and} \quad p_1 = p + \Delta p$$

Substituting, $p_1 = p + m(p_m - p)$.

(a) $p_1 = 0.6 + 0.2(0.1 - 0.6) = 0.5$

(b) $p_1 = 0.2 + 0.3(0.7 - 0.2) = 0.35$

(c) $p_1 = 0.1 + 0.1(0.2 - 0.1) = 0.11$

12. What one must do is predict the probability of one of the grandparents being heterozygous in this problem. Given the frequency of the disorder in the population as 1 in 10,000 individuals (0.0001), then $q^2 = 0.0001$ and $q = 0.01$. The frequency of heterozygosity is $2pq$ or approximately 0.02 as also stated in the problem. The

283

probability for one of the grandparents to be heterozygous would therefore be 0.02 + 0.02 or 0.04 or 1/25. If one of the grandparents is a carrier, then the probability of the offspring from a first-cousin mating being homozygous for the recessive gene is 1/16. Multiplying the two probabilities together gives $1/16 \times 1/25 = 1/400$.

Following the same analysis for the second-cousin mating gives $1/64 \times 1/25 = 1/1600$. Notice that the population at large has a frequency of homozygotes of 1/10,000; therefore, one can easily see how inbreeding increases the likelihood of homozygosity.

13. *Inbreeding depression* refers to the reduction in fitness observed in populations that are inbred. With inbreeding comes an increase in the number of homozygous individuals (see F27.2 in this book) and a decrease in genetic variability. Genetic variability is necessary for a genetic response to environmental change. As deleterious genes become homozygous, more individuals are less fit in the population.

14. Because heterozygosity tends to mask expression of recessive genes that may be desirable in a domesticated animal or plant, inbreeding schemes are often used to render strains homozygous so that such recessive genes can be expressed. In addition, assume that a particularly desirable trait occurs in a domesticated plant or animal. The best way to increase the frequency of individuals with that trait is by self-fertilization (not often possible) or by matings to blood relatives (inbreeding). In theory, one increases the likelihood of a gene "meeting itself" by various inbreeding schemes. There are disadvantages to increasing the degree of homozygosity by inbreeding. *Inbreeding depression* is a reduction in fitness often associated with an increase in homozygosity.

15. While inbreeding increases the frequency of homozygous individuals in a population, it does not change the *gene* frequencies. There will be fewer heterozygotes in the population to compensate for the additional homozygotes. See F27.2 in this book.

16. The quickest way to generate a homozygous line of an organism is to *self-fertilize* that organism. Because this is not always possible, brother-sister matings are often used.

17. Given that the recessive gene *a* is present in the homozygous state (q^2) at a frequency of 0.0001, the value of *q* is 0.01 and *p* = 0.99.

(a) *q* is 0.01

(b) $p = 1 - q$ or 0.99

(c) $2pq = 2(0.01)(0.99)$
$= 0.0198$ (or about 1/50)

(d) $2pq \times 2pq$
$= 0.0198 \times 0.0198$
$= 0.000392$ or about 1/255

18. If there were two males with hemophilia, $q = 2/2000$ or 1/1000 and $p = 1998/2000$. The frequency of heterozygous females would be $2pq$ or $2(1998/2000 \times 2/2000) = 0.001998$. The number of heterozygous females would be 3.996, or approximately 4.

19. The frequency of a gene is determined by a number of factors including the fitness it confers, mutation rate, and input from migration. There is no tendency for a gene to reach any artificial frequency such as 0.5. In fact, you have seen that rare alleles tend to remain rare even when they are dominant—unless there is very strong selection for the allele. The distribution of a gene among individuals is determined by mating (population size, inbreeding, etc.) and environmental factors (selection, etc.). A population is in equilibrium when the distribution of genotypes occurs at or around the $p^2 + 2pq + q^2$ expression. Equilibrium does not mean 25 percent *AA*, 50 percent *Aa*, and 25 percent *aa*. This confusion often stems from the 1:2:1 (or 3:1) ratio seen in Mendelian crosses.

20. Because three of the affected infants had affected parents, only two "new" genes, from mutation, enter into the problem. The gene is dominant; therefore, each new case of achondroplasia arose from a single new mutation. There are 50,000 births; therefore, 100,000 gametes (genes) are involved. The frequency of mutation is therefore given as follows: $2/100,000$ or 2×10^{-5}.

21. The probability that the woman (with no family history of CF) is heterozygous is $2pq$ or $2(1/50)(49/50)$. The probability that the man is heterozygous is 2/3. The probability that a child with CF will be produced by two heterozygotes is 1/4. Therefore, the overall probability of the couple producing a CF child is $98/2500 \times 2/3 \times 1/4$.

22. Since $r1 = 0.81$ and $r2 = 0.19$, the expected frequency of heterozygotes would be $2pq \times 125$ or $2(0.81 \times 0.19) \times 125 = 38.475$. Given the following equation and substituting the values:

$$F = (H_e - H_o)/H_e$$
$$F = (38.475 - 20)/38.475 = 0.48$$

23. Given that only 10 percent of the sensitive (bb) corn borer larvae feeding on Bt corn plants survive, the selection coefficient against them would be 0.9. The B allele for resistance exists at an initial frequency of 0.02 (represented as p); therefore, $q = 0.98$. The frequency of the b allele after one generation of corn borers fed on Bt corn would be computed as follows:

$$q' = q(1 - sq)/1 - sq^2$$
$$q' = 0.98[1 - (0.9)(0.98)]/1 - [(0.9)(0.98)(0.98)]$$
$$q' = 0.852 \text{ and } p' = 0.148$$

24. The following distribution of genotypes occurs among the 50 desert bighorn sheep in which the normal dominant C allele produces straight coats.

$$CC = 29 = \text{straight coats}$$
$$Cc = 17 = \text{straight coats}$$
$$cc = 4 = \text{curled coats}$$

Computing, $p = 0.75$ and $q = 0.25$ and $2pq = 0.375$ for the expected frequency of heterozygotes. Since 17/50 or (0.34) are observed as heterozygotes, the following equation applies:

$$F = (H_e - H_o)/H_e$$
$$F = (0.375 - 0.34)/0.375 = 0.093$$

This problem could also be solved using the actual numbers of sheep in each category where there would be 18.75 heterozygotes expected $(2pq)(50)$:

$$F = (18.75 - 17)/18.75 = 0.093$$

25. The equation for determining the impact of immigration on the gene pool of an existing population is estimated by

$$p_i' = (1 - m)p_i + mp_m$$

Substituting in the appropriate values, one obtains the following expression. Note that the value of 0.2 comes from the fact that 10 sheep out of 50, or 20 percent, are being introduced and there are no cc alleles in the introduced population, so $p_m = 1.0$.

$$p_i' = (1 - 0.2)(0.75) + (0.2)(1.0)$$
$$p_i' = 0.8$$

26. (a, b) Different alleles in organisms can often be detected visually (coat colors and other visible markers) or by some physiological or molecular assay. Often, starch gel electrophoresis identifies variations in proteins, while agarose or polyacrylamide electrophoresis provides information on variations of genotypes. RFLPs, SNPs, minisatellites, and microsatellites along with direct sequencing of nucleic acids are also used to detect genetic variation.

27. (a) The gene is most likely recessive because all affected individuals have unaffected parents and the condition clearly runs in families. For the population, since $q^2 = 0.002$, then $q = 0.045$, $p = 0.955$, and $2(pq) = 0.086$. For the community, since $q^2 = 0.005$, then $q = 0.07$, $p = 0.93$, and $2(pq) = 0.13$.

(b) The "founder effect" is probably operating here. Relatively small, local populations that are relatively isolated in a reproductive sense tend to show differences in gene frequencies when compared with larger populations. In such small populations, homozygosity is increased as a gene has a higher probability of "meeting itself."

28. Given small populations and very similar environmental conditions, it is more likely that "sampling error" or genetic drift is operating. Under such conditions (small population sizes), large fluctuations in gene frequency are likely, regardless of selection pressures. Since the same gene is behaving differently under similar environmental conditions, selection is an unlikely explanation.

29. In small populations, large fluctuations in gene frequency occur because random gametic sampling may not include all the genetic variation in the parents. The same phenomenon occurs in molecular populations. Two factors can cause the extinction of a particular mutation in small populations. First, sampling error may allow fixation of one form to the elimination of others. If an advantageous mutation occurs, it must be included in the next replicative round in order to be maintained in subsequent generations. If the founding population is small, it is possible that the advantageous mutation might not be represented. Second, while the above statements also hold for deleterious mutations, if a deleterious mutation becomes fixed, it can lead to extinction of that population.

30. When a population bottleneck occurs and the number of effective breeders is reduced in a population, two phenomena usually follow. First, because the population is small, wide fluctuations in genotypic frequencies occur, thereby revealing deleterious alleles by chance. Second, inbreeding often occurs in small populations, thereby increasing the chance for homozygosity. With increased homozygosity comes an increased likelihood that recessive alleles will be expressed. Since many disease-producing genes are recessive, an increase in genetic diseases is a likely aftermath to a population bottleneck.

31. (a) The symbol F represents the inbreeding coefficient, a value that quantifies the probability that the two alleles of a given gene are identical because of common descent.

(b) In general, inbred lines in organisms are those that show the least amount of hybrid vigor, and in the case of commercially significant organisms, those that are the smallest. Therefore, strains 33 and 55 are probably the inbred lines, while strains 35 and 53 are likely to be the hybrid lines.

(c) If hybrid vigor is operating there, it may be caused by dominance (masking of deleterious recessive genes) or overdominance (benefits achieved by heterozygote superiority). The phenomenon of hybrid vigor is not well understood at the molecular level; however, molecular diversity achieved through heterozygosity appears to be beneficial to an organism's survival.

Chapter 28: Evolutionary Genetics

Concept Areas	Corresponding Problems
Evolution and Speciation	1, 2, 3, 4, 13, 14, 21
Chromosomal Polymorphism	7, 8
Models of Speciation	4, 5, 9, 16, 28
Measuring Genetic Variation	6, 10, 12, 22, 23, 24, 25, 27, 30
Formation of Species	2, 5, 17, 18, 19, 28, 31
Molecular Techniques	10, 11, 15, 22, 23, 24, 25, 26, 27, 30
Human Evolution	20, 22, 23, 25, 29

Vocabulary: Organization and Listing of Terms and Concepts

Structures and Substances

Origin of Species (1859)
Species
Allozyme
  alcohol dehydrogenase
  cystic fibrosis transmembrane
  conductance regulator (CFTR)
Cytochrome c
Polymorphism
Polytene chromosome
Drosophila pseudoobscura
Fundulus heteroclitus (mummichog)
  lactate dehydrogenase
  ectotherm
Clade
Arabidopsis thaliana
  MADS-box homeotic genes
Mitochondrial DNA
Molecular clock

Processes/Methods

Evolutionary divergence (F28.1)
  variation
  overpopulation
  struggle for survival
  differential survival

species formation
Artificial selection
Genetic divergence
Genetic diversity
  heterozygosity
    protein polymorphism
    allozymes (F28.1)
      molecular phylogenetic trees
  amino acid sequence homology
    cytochrome c
  chromosomal polymorphism
    inversions
    translocations
  DNA sequence polymorphism
    mitochondrial DNA
Ecological diversity
  niche
Speciation
  stasis
  phyletic evolution (anagenesis)
  cladogenesis
  neutralist theory
  selectionist theory
  reproductive barriers
    physiological
    behavioral
    mechanical

isolating mechanisms
  reproductive
    prezygotic
    postzygotic
      MADS-box genes
Gel electrophoresis
  protein polymorphism
  nucleic acid sequence variation
UPGMA
  neanderthal genomics

Concepts

Microevolution
Macroevolution
Cladogenesis
Neo-Darwinism
Neutral theory
Evolutionary divergence

molecular clock
minimal mutational distance
minimal genetic divergence
rates of speciation
divergence dendrograms
evolutionary trees
Artificial selection
Species formation (speciation)
  isolating mechanisms
    prezygotic
    postzygotic
Biological species concept
Phylogenetic reconstruction
Sequence homology
  amino acid, nucleic acid
Sequence conservation
Parsimony
Maximum likelihood
Mutation and speciation

F28.1 The following diagram is meant to illustrate the meaning of the term *allozyme*. Notice that alleles A^1 and A^2 produce protein products that differ electrophoretically, but that accomplish the same function.

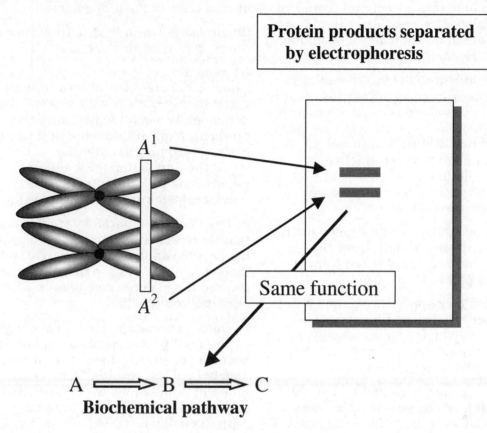

Solutions to Problems and Discussion Questions

1. Neo-Darwinism is defined as the explanation of natural selection in terms of changes in allelic frequencies or the combining of Darwin's theory of evolution with that of Mendelian genetics.

2. A species is a group of interbreeding or potentially interbreeding populations that is reproductively isolated from all other such groups. Speciation is the process that leads to the formation of species. It usually involves some form of reproductive isolation. Evolution is the change in a population over time. Speciation is one of many results of evolution.

3. Darwin and Wallace could explain neither the origin of species variation nor the manner in which such variations were passed from parent to offspring.

4. Organisms may appear to be similar but be reproductively isolated for a sufficient period to justify their species identity. If significant genetic differences occur, they can be considered separate species.

5. Natural selection is viewed as a gradual process that leads to genetic differences over time. However, more dramatic forms of speciation may involve more rapid genomic changes in the form of transposable elements or polyploidy. New species can be formed by hybridization and chromosome doubling.

6. The subterranean niche is less broad and less dynamic than above ground. The underground microhabitat consists of a narrower range of climatic changes; thus, genetic polymorphism is not selected for. This conclusion has been supported by additional studies indicating that genetic diversity is positively correlated with niche-width.

7. Assume that a chromosome in the "standard arrangement" undergoes an inversion (*pericentric* or *paracentric*). The following are possible consequences of such an inversion:

(a) change in gene order with possible introduction of position effects,

(b) breakage within a structural gene or other functional element, and

(c) reduction in the recovery of crossover gametes in heterokaryotypes (those that carry an inversion as well as a standard homolog). While (c) may reduce the production of variation, the first two (a and b) may introduce variation.

At the population level, different populations with different inversion polymorphisms are genetically distinct.

8. Results from laboratory studies indicated that there was a selective advantage in having the two inversions present, rather than either one. Thus, natural selection favored the maintenance of both inversions over the loss of either.

9. During speciation, individuals or groups of potentially interbreeding organisms become genetically distinct from other members of the species. Members of different populations with substantial genetic divergence are, at first, not reproductively isolated from each other, although gene flow may be restricted. The distinction between such groups is not absolute in that one group may blend with other groups of the species. Any process that favors changes in gene frequencies has the potential of generating substantial genetic differences.

Factors such as selection, migration, genetic drift, or even mutation may be important in generating significant genetic change. One would certainly include geographic isolation as a major barrier to gene flow and thus an important process in such formation.

Natural selection occurs when there is nonrandom elimination of individuals from a population. Since such selection is a strong force in changing gene frequencies, it should also be considered a significant factor in subspecies formation.

10. (a) Missense mutations cause amino acid changes.

(b) Horizontal transfer refers to the process of passing genetic information from one organism to another without producing offspring. In bacteria, plasmid transfer is an example of horizontal transfer.

(c) The fact that none of the isolates shared identical nucleotide changes indicates that there is little genetic exchange among different strains. Each alteration is unique, most likely originating in an ancestral strain and maintained in descendants of that strain only.

11. Because of degeneracy in the code, there are some nucleotide substitutions, especially in the third base, that do not change amino acids. In addition, if there is no change in the overall charge of the protein, it is likely that electrophoresis will not separate the variants. If a positively charged amino acid is replaced by an amino acid of like charge, then the overall charge on the protein is unchanged. The same may be said for other negatively charged and neutral amino acid substitutions.

12. The approximate similarity of mutation rates among genes and lineages should provide more credible estimates of divergence times of species and allow for broader interpretations of sequence comparisons. It also provides for increased understanding of the mutational processes that govern evolution among mammalian genomes. For instance, if the rate of mutation is fairly constant among lineages or cells that have a more rapid turnover, it indicates that replication-related errors do not make a significant contribution to mutation rates.

13. The text lists several cornerstones of the *neutral mutation theory:*

(a) there is a relatively uniform rate of amino acid substitution in different organisms (under different types of selection);

(b) there is no particular pattern to the substitutions, indicating that selection is not eliminating some variations;

(c) the rate of mutation is relatively high and has remained relatively constant for millions of years, even though environments have fluctuated greatly over that period of time;

(d) certain regions of molecules and certain functions of those molecules should logically be less likely to have amino acid substitutions influence the phenotype;

(e) the rate of amino acid substitution in some proteins is much too high to have been produced by selection. The *selectionists* suggest that even though amino acid substitutions *appear* to be neutral, it is more likely that their influence has just not been determined. In addition, they point out that many polymorphisms are clearly maintained in the population by selection. Thus, the issues listed above do not really challenge present views of genetic variation.

Like many other debates that surround the nature of evolution, it is important to see that debate is a natural component of scientific understanding. It is likely that some genes (like histone genes) will not tolerate nucleotide substitutions to a significant degree and the neutral mutation theory will not hold. However, other genes produce quite variable products and provide support for the neutral mutation theory. Usually, controversy is resolved as one dives deeper into the problem and seeks to define the variables and complexities of the process. It is controversy that stimulates a desire to seek answers.

14. In general, speciation involves the gradual accumulation of genetic changes to a point where reproductive isolation occurs. Depending on environmental or geographic conditions, genetic changes may occur slowly or rapidly. They can involve point or chromosomal changes.

15. The *Ldh-B^b* allele is more efficient in cold waters, while the *Ldh-B^a* allele is more efficient in warm waters. There is a correlation between allele frequency and water temperature. Catalytic efficiency of the *Ldh-B^b* allele is higher in cold water; the transcriptional rate of *Ldh-B^b* is also higher than the *Ldh-B^a* allele.

16. Reproductive isolating mechanisms are grouped into prezygotic and postzygotic and include the following:

- geographic or ecological
- seasonal or temporal
- behavioral
- mechanical
- physiological
- hybrid inviability or weakness
- developmental hybrid sterility
- segregational hybrid sterility
- F$_2$ breakdown

17. Reproductive isolating mechanisms are grouped into prezygotic and postzygotic. Prezygotic mechanisms are most efficient because they occur before resources are expended in the processes of mating.

18. Polyploid plants that result from the hybridization of two species would be expected to be more heterozygous than the diploid parental species because two distinct genomes are combined. Generally, genetic variation is an advantage unless a significant degree of that variation is outside acceptable physiological tolerance.

19. With some exceptions, plants tolerate departures from diploidy more successfully than animals. Some vertebrate exceptions include amphibians. It is possible that such genomic restrictions in animals are the result of narrow physiological limits on development of a complex nervous system and the resulting characteristics of that system.

20. Somatic gene therapy, like any therapy, allows some individuals to live more normal lives than those not receiving therapy. As such, the ability of such individuals to contribute to the gene pool increases the likelihood that less fit genes will enter and be maintained in the gene pool. This is a normal consequence of therapy, genetic or not, and in the face of disease control and prevention, societies have generally accepted this consequence. Germ-line therapy could, if successful, lead to limited, isolated, and infrequent removal of a gene from a gene lineage. However, given the present state of the science, its impact on the course of human evolution will be diluted and negated by a host of other factors that afflict humankind.

21. (a) Different alleles in organisms can often be detected visually (coat colors and other visible markers) or by some physiological or molecular assay. Often, starch gel electrophoresis identifies variations in proteins, while agarose or polyacrylamide electrophoresis provides information on variations of genotypes. RFLPs, SNPs, minisatellites, and microsatellites, along with direct sequencing of nucleic acids, are also used to detect genetic variation.

(b) Artificial selection occurring over thousands of years (dogs and cats) and short-term intensive selection experiments have provided ample evidence that similar selective forces in nature could account for genetic differences in natural populations. While mutation is the original source of genetic variation, studies on a variety of natural populations (*Drosophila, Biston*) support natural selection as a primary cause of genetic differences in populations across time and space.

(c) Closely related species can be compared for a number of morphological and/or molecular markers. In addition, DNA sequence comparisons can reveal how much genetic variation has occurred. In some cases, only a few gene changes appear to be sufficient for speciation.

(d) The last common ancestor of two divergent species is the most recent branch on a phylogenetic tree. Such trees are developed using a variety of methods including UPGMA as illustrated in the text.

22. All of the amino acid substitutions

(Ala – Gly, Val – Leu, Asp – Asn, Met – Leu)

require only one nucleotide change. The last change from

Pro (CC-) – Lys (AAA,G)

requires two changes (the minimal mutational distance).

23. Approach this problem by writing the possible codons for all the amino acids (except Arg and Asp, which show no change) in the human cytochrome c chain. Then determine the minimum number of nucleotide substitutions required for each changed amino acid in the various organisms. Once listed, count up the numbers for each organism: horse, 3; pig, 2; dog, 3; chicken, 3; bullfrog, 2; fungus, 6.

24. Construct a chart similar to the one below, which indicates the number of base changes between each pair:

	H	C	G	O
H	-	-	-	-
C	1	-	-	-
G	3	2	-	-
O	7	6	4	-
B	12	11	9	10

Following the instructions given in the text, develop the relationships in the following manner:

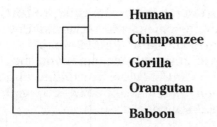

- **Human**
- **Chimpanzee**
- **Gorilla**
- **Orangutan**
- **Baboon**

25. The classification of organisms into different species is based on evidence (morphological, genetic, ecological, etc.) that they are reproductively isolated. That is, there must be evidence that gene flow does not occur among the groups being called different species. Classifications above the species level (genus, family, etc.) are not based on such empirical data. Indeed, classification above the species level is somewhat arbitrary and based on traditions that extend far beyond DNA sequence information. In addition, recall that DNA sequence divergence is not always directly proportional to morphological, behavioral, or ecological divergence. While the genus classifications provided in this problem seem to be invalid, other factors, well beyond simple DNA sequence comparison, must be considered in classification practices. As more information is gained on the meaning of DNA sequence differences in comparison to morphological factors, many phylogenetic relationships will be reconsidered, and it is possible that adjustments will be needed in some classification schemes.

26. Many sections of DNA in a eukaryotic genome are not reflected in a protein product. Indeed, many sections of DNA are not transcribed and have no apparent physiological role, while other nontranscribed regions can have considerable physiological impact. Regions without physiological impact are more likely to tolerate nucleotide changes compared with those regions with a physiological impact. Introns, for example, show sequence variation, which is not reflected in a protein product, yet certain sequences in introns may have a regulatory role. Exons, on the other hand, code for products that are usually involved in production of a phenotype and, as such, are subject to selection.

27. (a) Since noncoding genomic regions are probably silent genetically, it is likely that they contribute little, if anything, to the phenotype. Selection acts on the phenotype; therefore, such noncoding regions are probably selectively neutral.

(b) These polymorphism data indicate that all the Lake Victoria area (lake and contributing rivers) cichlids are related by recent ancestry, whereas those from neighboring lakes are more distantly related. In addition, since Lake Victoria dried out about 14,000 years ago, it is likely that it was repopulated by a relatively small sample of cichlids.

28. A number of studies using SINES, repetitive DNA, and neutral polymorphisms (see Problem 27) indicate that most, if not all, cichlid species in Lake Victoria evolved from a single ancestral species. If that is the case, then this finding would represent the most rapid evolutionary radiation ever documented for vertebrates.

29. The pattern of genetic distances through time indicates that from the present to about 25,000 years ago, modern humans and Cro-Magnons show an approximately constant number of differences. Conversely, there is an abrupt increase in genetic distance seen in comparing modern humans and Cro-Magnons with Neanderthals. The results indicate a clear discontinuity between modern humans, Cro-Magnons, and Neanderthals with respect to genetic variation in the mitochondrial DNAs sampled. Assuming that the sampling and analytical techniques used to generate the data are valid, it appears that Neanderthals made little, if any, genetic contributions to the Cro-Magnon or modern European gene pool.

It could be argued that the absence of Neanderthal mtDNA lineages in living humans is a consequence of random drift or lineage extinction since the disappearance of Neanderthals. However, the examination of mtDNA in ancient Cro-Magnon mtDNA shows no evidence of a historical relationship and suggests that Neanderthals were not genetically related to the ancestors of modern humans.

30. In general, there are two methods for calibrating molecular data, amino acid and nucleotide substitutions, to absolute times of divergence. First, molecular data are compared with the existing fossil record. Second, major paleontological events such as the Bryophyta/Tracheophyta split during the Ordovician (443–490 Mya) or the Actinopterygii/Mammalia split during the Devonian (354–417 Mya) can provide some clues for calibration. Both methods are subject to error due to the uncertainty of the fossil record and the uncertainty of the times of major paleontological events. In addition, different mutation rates, generation times, and population structures occur among different taxa.

31. (a) In general, animals are less tolerant to changes in ploidy than plants. Exceptions are some fish and amphibian groups where polyploidization is well documented.

(b) When two genomes combine, significant anatomical and physiological changes are expected. On occasion, such changes can exploit niches previously unavailable to the parental populations.

(c) Just as the initial event of polyploidization generates morphological and physiological changes, so does gene loss following polyploidization. Each genetic adjustment provides genetic variation upon which selection is based and adaptation is enhanced.

(d) One would expect that the function of essential genes would be preserved during the loss process. In addition, genes that function in conjunction with other genes would probably be retained compared with those that function independently. Differential loss might be based on mere chance or on the presence of similar systems that buffer changes in product amounts. In some cases, reduction in gene number down to the diploid complement may have no significant impact on the phenotype and may occur rapidly, while others may be of evolutionary consequence and remain polyploid.

(e) 1. Diploid genomes combine:

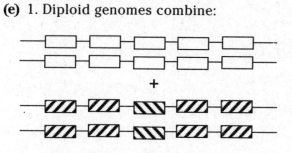

2. Allopolyploid formation

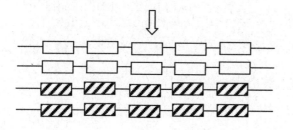

3. Selective gene loss (genetically diploid amalgam). Two models of loss are as follows.

Model 1.

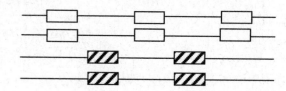

Model 2.

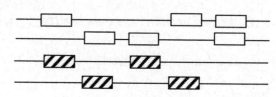

Chapter 29: Conservation Genetics

Concept Areas	Corresponding Problems
Population Dynamics	1, 3, 11, 16, 19
Genetic Assessment of Threatened Species	1, 12, 14, 15, 17, 18, 19, 23, 24, 26, 27
Management of Threatened Species	2, 5, 6, 7, 9, 10, 15, 20, 22, 23, 25, 28
Inbreeding and Drift in Small Populations	3, 4, 6, 8, 13, 21, 22, 25

Vocabulary: Organization and Listing of Terms and Concepts

Structures and Substances

Grey wolf (*Canis lupus*)

California condors

   Gymnogyps californianus

Antarctic fur seal (*Arctocephalus sp.*)

Cheetah (*Acinonyx jubatus*)

Red-cockaded woodpecker (*Picoides borealis*)

North American brown bear (*Ursus arctos*)

Polar bear (*Ursus maritimus*)

Fruit fly (*Drosophila melanogaster*)

Black-footed ferret (*Mustela nigripes*)

Native rock grape (*Vitis rupestris*)

IUCN Red List or Threatened Species

  FAO

Domesticated species

Allozyme

Short tandem repeats

Microsatellite

DNA profile

  nuclear

  mitochondrial

  chloroplast

Gene bank

Core collection

Metapopulation

Processes/Methods

Human population growth

Biodiversity

  human impact

Conservation genetics

Intraspecific diversity

  interpopulation

  intrapopulation

Interspecific diversity

Loss of genetic diversity

  reduced population size

  habitat loss

  population fragmentation

Detection of genetic diversity

Absolute population size (N)

  effective population size (N_e)

  $N_e = 4(N_m N_f)/(N_m + N_f)$

  $N_e = 1/(1/t)(1/N_1 + 1/N_2 + 1/N_3 \ldots)$

Population bottleneck

Founder effect

Genetic drift

Inbreeding

Concepts

Vulnerable and endangered species

Genetic diversity

Loss of genetic diversity

   population size

Population dynamics

   bottleneck

   founder effect

   genetic drift

   inbreeding

   gene flow

genetic erosion

Conservation strategies

Probability of fixation $p(A)$

Inbreeding coefficient

   $F = (2pq - H)/2pq$

   $H_t = (1 - 1/2N_e)^t H_o$

   inbreeding depression

Genetic load

   purging genetic load

Gene flow relates to migration

Genetic erosion (loss of diversity)

Ex situ and *in situ* conservation

   captive species

   gene banks

Population augmentation

   outbreeding depression

Solutions to Problems and Discussion Questions

1. (a) Apply the formula that computes the effective population size as the harmonic mean of the numbers in each generation:

$$N_e = 1/(1/t)(1/N_1 + 1/N_2 + 1/N_3 \ldots)$$

Substituting the values:

$$N_e = 1/(1/4)(1/47 + 1/17 + 1/20 + 1/35)$$

$$N_e = 25.21$$

(b) Apply the formula that computes the frequency of heterozygotes after *t* generations as a function of effective population size:

$$H_t = (1 - 1/2N_e)^t H_o$$

Substituting the values:

$$H_t = (1 - 1/2(25.21))^4(0.55)$$

$$H_t = 0.5073$$

(c) Apply the formula that relates the inbreeding coefficient to the frequency of heterozygotes in a population:

$$F = (2pq - H)/2pq$$

$$F = (0.55 - 0.5073)/0.55$$

$$F = 0.0776$$

2. The frequency of the lethal gene in the captive population ($q^2 = 5/169$ and $q = 0.172$) is approximately double that in the gene pool as a whole ($q = 0.09$). Applying the formula

$$q_n = q_o/(1 + nq_o)$$

one can estimate that it would take ten generations to reduce the lethal gene's frequency to 0.063 in the captive population with no intervention (random mating assumed). Since condors produce very few eggs per year, a more proactive approach seems justified.

First, if detailed records are kept of the breeding partners of the captive birds, then knowledge of heterozygotes should be available. Breeding programs could be established to restrict matings between those carrying the lethal gene. Such "kinship management" is often used in captive populations. If kinship records are not available, it is often possible to establish kinship using genetic markers such as DNA microsatellite polymorphisms. Using such markers, one can often identify mating partners and link them to their offspring.

By coupling knowledge of mating partners with the likelihood of producing a lethal genetic combination, selective matings can often be used to minimize the influence of a deleterious gene. In addition, such markers can be used to establish matings that optimize genetic mixing, thus reducing inbreeding depression.

3. Notice (in the text) that the probability of fixation through drift is the same as a gene's initial frequency. In this problem, the probability of *A* being fixed (and therefore *a* being lost) is 0.75. The probability of *B* being fixed (and *b* being lost) is 0.8, and the probability of *C* being fixed (and *c* being lost) is 0.95. Therefore, the probability that all the recessive alleles will be lost through genetic drift is

$$0.75 \times 0.80 \times 0.95 = 0.57$$

4. Both genetic drift and inbreeding tend to drive populations toward homozygosity. Genetic drift is more common when the effective breeding size of the population is low. When this condition prevails, inbreeding is also much more likely. They are different in that inbreeding can occur when certain population structures or behaviors favor matings between relatives, regardless of the effective size of the population. Inbreeding tends to increase the frequency of both homozygous classes at the expense of the heterozygotes. Genetic drift can lead to fixation of one allele or the other, thus producing a single homozygous class.

5. There are a number of dangers inherent in the management of such a small herd of endangered rhinos. Because of the small breeding pool, inbreeding depression is likely to lead to less fit individuals over time. To combat this problem, genetic markers (such as microsatellites) can be used to assess the general degree of relatedness and heterozygosity of each of the 16 rhinos. From such information, appropriate matings can be facilitated and would reduce inbreeding depression. However, additional efforts may be needed in this extreme case. It is possible to develop exchange programs whereby animals from other herds provide semen (either naturally or artificially), thereby reducing inbreeding. This practice can be successful if females are receptive and if no deleterious genes are brought into the population (outbreeding depression).

Population augmentation, where individuals are transplanted into a declining population, can be used to increase numbers and genetic diversity. However, as stated earlier, outbreeding depression accompanies this practice. Sometimes drastic measures must be taken in extreme cases such as the black rhino. Dehorning is often practiced to remove the incentive for poaching and reduce lethal wounding due to fighting. This practice is only useful in areas void of dangerous predators.

6. Inbreeding depression, over time, reduces the level of heterozygosity, usually a selectively advantageous quality of a species. When homozygosity increases (through loss of heterozygosity), deleterious alleles are likely to become more of a load on a population. Outbreeding depression occurs when there is a reduction in fitness of progeny from genetically diverse individuals. It is usually attributed to offspring being less well-adapted to the local environmental conditions of the parents.

Even though forced outbreeding may be necessary to save a threatened species, where population numbers are low, it significantly and permanently changes the genetic makeup of the species.

7. Cloning of some highly threatened species may be the only way to save that species from extinction. However, the long-term disadvantages of cloning for this purpose are often considered self-defeating. With cloning, one "short-circuits" normal processes (meiosis, gametic union, etc.) necessary to maintain genetic variation. With a loss of genetic variation comes difficulties with adaptation as environments change. It may be possible to identify certain conditions in which cloning would be useful to "save" a species. However, interbreeding provides benefits that allow a species to evolve. In addition, as members of a species become more uniform (through cloning), they are more likely to suffer more severe and widespread responses to disease and environmental stress.

8. Often, molecular assays of overall heterozygosity can indicate the degree of inbreeding and/or genetic drift. As inbreeding (and genetic drift, for that matter) occurs, the degree of heterozygosity decreases. An allele whose frequency is dictated by inbreeding and/or genetic drift will not be uniquely influenced. That is, other alleles would be characterized by decreased heterozygosity as well. So, if the genome in general has a relatively high degree of heterozygosity, the gene is probably influenced by selection rather than by inbreeding and/or genetic drift.

9. *Ex situ* conservation involves the removal of an organism from an original habitat to an artificially maintained habitat. *In situ* conservation attempts to preserve a species in its original habitat. Each confronts problems in that while it may be possible to maintain an organism in an artificial habitat, it is no longer subject to the same selective pressures as experienced in the wild. Thus, the population will change. Attempts to maintain original habitats for *in situ* conservation are often met with failure as factors beyond a conservationist's control may dominate (air pollution, encroachment, and other aspects of habitat deterioration).

10. Generally, threatened species are captured and bred in an artificial environment until sufficient population numbers are achieved to ensure species survival. Next, genetic management strategies are applied to breed individuals in such a way as to increase genetic heterozygosity as much as possible. If plants are involved, seed banks are often used to maintain and facilitate long-term survival.

11. Genetic diversity generally increases the likelihood of long-term survival of a species by providing multiple opportunities for adaptation to environmental change. The ability of an organism to exploit varied environments and withstand environmental modification is directly related to genetic diversity.

12. Allozymes are variants of a given allele often detected by electrophoresis. Such variation may or may not impact the fitness of an individual. The greater the allozyme variation is, the more genetically heterogeneous the individual. It is generally agreed that such genetic diversity is essential for long-term survival. All other factors being equal, allozyme variation is more likely to reflect physiological variation than RFLP variation because RFLP regions are not necessarily found in protein-coding regions of the genome. RFLP allows one to detect very small amounts of genetic diversity in a population and is unlikely to encounter an organism that is not in some way variable in terms of RFLPs with respect to other organisms (within and among species).

13. Apply the formula:

$$N_e = 4(N_m N_f)/N_m + N_f = 6.9$$

14. (a) The probability of being a heterozygote is $2pq = 2(0.99)(0.01) = 0.0198$. Multiplying this value by 20 gives the probability of being heterozygous:

$$0.0198 \times 20 = 0.396$$

(b) To determine N_e use the expression:

$$N_e/N = 0.42$$
$$N_e = 0.42 \times 50 = 21$$
$$H_t = (1 - 1/2N_e)^t H_o$$
$$= (1 - 1/42)^5 \times 0.0198$$
$$= 0.01755$$
$$H_t/H_o = 0.01755/0.0198 = 0.886$$

Therefore, there is a loss of approximately 11.4 percent heterozygosity after five generations.

15. The maximum genetic diversity of the population will be enhanced by using the largest possible number in the founding population and minimizing the number of generations in captivity. By keeping complete pedigree records, one can increase genetic variation by reducing inbreeding and exchanging breeding individuals among captive populations.

16. Data from *Antechinus* provide insight as to the significance of genetic diversity to the survival of a species. Because such mechanisms (i.e., sperm mixing) are in place, there must be considerable evolutionary rewards. In this case, maintaining diversity must offset the cost (if any) of evolving such a mechanism.

17. (a) Maintenance of heterozygosity in a population is dependent on a number of factors, including degree of inbreeding, population size, and mutational input through migration and/or mutation. If a population is small and isolated, inbreeding and genetic drift are likely consequences. Both decrease heterozygosity. Coupled with lessened connections with neighboring populations, reduced heterozygosity is expected.

(b) Urbanization usually leads to fragmentation of natural populations as highways, strip malls, and housing developments disrupt the natural habitat and, as a consequence, the movements of organisms. Even though two populations may be relatively close to each other geographically, they may be genetically distant because of restricted movement. Restricted movement between and among such populations will foster genetic diversity.

(c) In general, restrictions to movements must be greatly reduced or eliminated. Safe corridors for passage over or under highways and through populated areas must be developed. Unless population augmentation is to be employed, native populations must be able to maintain sufficient genetic diversity through interbreeding in order to survive.

18. (a) Since prairie dogs are the main food source for black-footed ferrets, a reduction in prairie dogs would likely stress black-footed ferrets. Unless alternate food sources are available and utilized by the ferrets, their numbers would decline.

(b) The fact that a population survives a population bottleneck does not mean that the population is in a healthy state. Usually, bottlenecks reduce genetic variability upon which survival and adaptation depend. A second bottleneck, while perhaps not having immediate ramifications, would likely have a negative impact on the long-term survival of the species. One would expect additional reductions in genetic diversity.

(c) Because extinction of an organism is irreversible, one might consider the fate of the ferret as the highest priority. If the prairie dog population is reduced very slowly, the ferret population may succeed in finding alternative food sources, but this is doubtful. Since the ferret population is the most fragile of the three (ferret, prairie dog, cattle) and represents one of America's most endangered mammals, this case will

test the strength of laws designed to protect such species. In some situations, compromise to the point of mutual agreement is not possible.

19. (a) Genetic diversity in a species can be determined in a number of ways that include both obvious visual and more cryptic molecular markers. Allozyme assessments and DNA fingerprinting using short tandem repeats or microsatellites provide indices of genetic diversity.

(b) Numerous examples from a variety of observations and experiments indicate that as genetic diversity decreases, chances of a population's long-term survival also decrease. Natural examples include the peppered moth (*Biston betularia*), lions, seals, and woodpeckers. Laboratory studies using *Drosophila melanogaster* indicate that a loss of genetic diversity reduces the ability of a population to adapt to changing environments. Such a loss of adaptability diminishes the chances of long-term survival.

(c) A variety of methods are often used to increase population numbers. These include preservation of habitat, *in situ* and *ex situ* conservation, and population augmentation. Each situation is unique and dependent on a number of factors, including available resources, economic impact, and degree of population stress. In many cases, there is no single approach, and multiple avenues are employed. In general, habitat erosion is a major cause of population collapse and therefore represents the most logical and immediate avenue of rehabilitation.

(d) In addition to attempts to maintain the genetic health of species by the conservation methods mentioned in (c), often as a last resort, gene banks are established to preserve reproductive components such as sperm, ova, and embryos.

20. First, it will be necessary to determine whether the native habitat in the Asian steppes of the 1920s is suitable to any introduction. If the original range is supportive of reintroduction, care must be taken to introduce horses with maximum genetic diversity possible. To do so, you might monitor AFLP (amplified fragment length polymorphisms) patterns or other indicators of genetic diversity. Since the founder breeding group included a domestic mare, it may be desirable to select those for reintroduction that are least like the domestic mare genetically. It might be desirable to release reasonably sized breeding groups in separate locations within the range to enhance eventual genetic diversity.

21. DNA profiles indicate the degree of heterogeneity in DNA sequences and, therefore, the degree of genetic variation. While noncoding DNA sequences represent the bulk of sequence diversity, such information can be helpful in determining gene flow, ancestry, and overall inter- and intrapopulation diversity. Since diversity per se appears to be essential for long-term species survival in natural environments, one would expect the assessment of diversity by any tool to be a useful predictor.

22. From a physiological standpoint, cryogenic preservation in liquid nitrogen can allow 100 years or more of seed storage for some species. However, such elaborate storage can only be offered to a small fraction of the world's seeds. Thus, seeds of most species undergo storage loss, which decreases genetic diversity. Seeds of tropical plants are somewhat intolerant to cold storage and must be regenerated frequently, a practice that is prone to a loss of genetic diversity arising from genetic drift. Only a finite number of seeds can be used in each regeneration procedure, and the restriction of sample size (often fewer than 100 plants) reduces genetic diversity. To somewhat counteract this problem, plants are grown under optimum conditions to reduce selection. Another problem with

preserved seeds is the accumulation of deleterious mutations as a result of both seed storage and regeneration. Some studies indicate increased frequencies of chromosomal and mtDNA lesions, chlorophyll deficiency mutations, and decreased DNA polymerase activity associated with long-term seed storage.

23. A census of population size and range would be needed to establish levels of habitat exploitation and probable number of effective breeding pairs. From this information, an estimation of long-term habitat support can be provided, along with the probability of genetic drift eroding genetic variability. Effective breeder estimates will also provide a method for estimating inbreeding depression. It would be helpful to conduct surveys on a season-to-season and year-to-year basis to decrease the possibility of sampling in an atypical season or year. It would be important to determine the age and stage-specific structure of the endangered population. Few young or juveniles might indicate that reproductive capacities are in decline. It would be important to determine the general biodiversity and carrying capacity of the habitat as well as the genetic diversity of the species in question. Nuclear, mitochondrial, and chloroplast DNA profiles can be used to assess intrapopulation and interpopulation variation, as well as aid in determining migration and breeding patterns.

24. The longest bottleneck-to-present interval occurred with cheetahs, and one would expect cheetahs to show the highest degree of microsatellite polymorphism. The shortest bottleneck-to-present interval occurred with the Gir Forest lions, so it would be expected to have the least polymorphism. Data from Driscoll et al. (2002 *Genome Research* 12:414–423) include the following estimates of microsatellite polymorphism in the three feline groups mentioned above: cheetahs (84.1 percent), pumas (42.9 percent), and Gir Forest lions (19.3 percent).

25. The following graph would incorporate the expected relationship between bottlenecks and microsatellite variation.

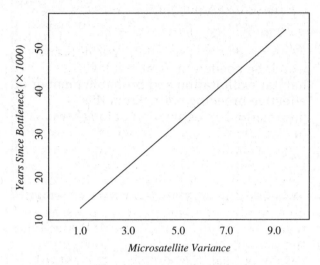

26. (a) The species with the greatest genetic variability, as estimated by these markers, is the domesticated cat. Domesticated cats share an immense and variable gene pool. Their staggering numbers and outbreeding behaviors allow them to maintain a high degree of genetic variability.

(b) The lion has the least genetic variability.

(c) Since allozymes code for proteins and proteins often provide a significant function in an organism, selection is stronger and mutations are less tolerated. Selection would be expected to be harsher on DNA segments that are related to function. In addition, by their very nature, microsatellites and minisatellites are more mutable.

27. Since there is less genetic variation in lions (according to these data), they are likely the species that underwent the population crisis mentioned above. That "bottleneck" apparently reduced allelic variation considerably.

28. While flagship species (often large mammals) may make it possible to gather considerable public support and funding, they may reduce support for species that may have a greater impact on a community of species. Primary producers (plants) are a necessary component of a diverse and supportive habitat. If one focuses on a flagship species within an area, it is possible that other areas will suffer more dramatically because foundational species are lost. Using umbrella species to protect a large geographic area in hopes of protecting other species in that area is a reasonable approach. However, the size of an area is not necessarily a primary factor in determining species success. Diversity and productivity of a habitat are major contributors to species success. Since land is at a premium, it may be wiser in the long run to select umbrella species in diverse and productive habitats rather than on the basis of land size. By selecting sets of species that show considerable biodiversity, one increases the likelihood of protecting a sufficiently rich habitat to support many species. Such habitats are often of considerable economic value, thereby making their availability limited.

Sample Test Questions

(detailed explanations of answers follow in next section)

How to use this section

The purpose of these *Sample Test Questions* is to present a slightly different style of question. Set aside several hours of study time, perhaps a week before each examination. Select two questions from each chapter covered on your upcoming test. Attempt to work selected questions, five or so per hour, under test conditions. **Write down your answers**; then, *after* you have finished the entire "test," check your answers.

If you are having difficulty, then you are weak in the concept areas listed for each question. If you have made mistakes, take comfort: there are many places to make mistakes on these problems. Some of the students who made the same mistakes are now practicing geneticists!

For the questions below from Chapter 1, there are few major concepts. This chapter serves as an introduction and gives you a general overview of the content of the text and its significance. Test questions are primarily oriented toward reading retention and study effort.

Ch. 1 Ques.1 What is meant by the phrase "the Chromosome Theory of Inheritance"?

Ch. 1 Ques.2 Name the individual who, working with the garden pea in the mid-1850s, demonstrated quantitative patterns of heredity and developed a theory involving the behavior of hereditary factors.

Ch. 1 Ques.3 What does the term *genetics* mean?

Ch. 1 Ques.4 Name the substance that serves as the hereditary material in eukaryotes and prokaryotes. Is your answer the same for viruses?

Ch. 1 Ques.5 When examining chromosomes from a single nucleus of an individual cell, it is often possible to match up chromosomes on the basis of overall size, centromere position, and sometimes other physical characteristics. Chromosomes that can be matched up or paired are called_____.

Ch. 1 Ques.6 What is the difference between deoxyribonucleic acid and ribonucleic acid?

Ch. 1 Ques.7 List three components of the genetic material, DNA.

Concepts: chromosome mechanics (mitosis, meiosis), symbolism, DNA content (cell cycles)

Ch. 2, 3 Ques.8 The mosquito, *Culex pipiens*, has a diploid chromosome number of six. Assume that one chromosome pair is metacentric and the other two pairs are acrocentric.

(a) Draw chromosomal configurations that one would expect to see at the following stages: primary oocyte (metaphase I) and secondary spermatocyte.

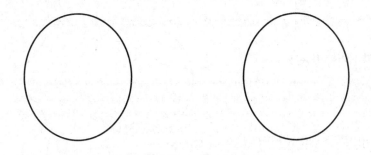

(b) Assuming that a G1 nucleus in *Culex* contains about 20 picograms (pg) of DNA, how much DNA would you expect in the following nuclei: primary spermatocyte, first polar body, secondary oocyte, and ootid in G1 phase.

(c) Assume that a female mosquito is heterozygous for the recessive gene *wavy bristles* (symbolized as *wb*) and this gene locus is on an acrocentric chromosome. Draw an expected mitotic metaphase with the appropriate genetic labeling pattern.

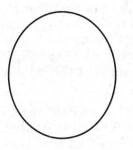

Concepts: chromosome mechanics (mitosis, meiosis), symbolism, DNA content (cell cycles)

Chs. 2, 3 Ques.9 In humans, chromosome #1 is large and metacentric, the X chromosome is medium in size and submetacentric (submedian), and the Y chromosome is small and acrocentric. Assume that you were microscopically examining human chromosomes at the stages given in the following graphic.

(a) Illustrate (draw) the above-mentioned (#1, X, and/or Y) chromosomes and/or pairs at the stages given (several different configurations may be applicable in some cases):

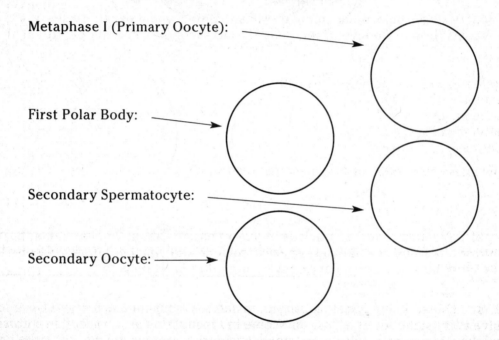

Metaphase I (Primary Oocyte):

First Polar Body:

Secondary Spermatocyte:

Secondary Oocyte:

(b) The Rh blood group locus is on Chromosome #1. Individuals are *DD* or *Dd* if Rh⁺ and *dd* if Rh⁻. The locus for glucose-6-phosphate-dehydrogenase deficiency (*G6PD*) is on the X chromosome. There are two alternatives at this locus, + and −. For each of the above cells, place genes (using the symbolism given) on chromosomes if the female is heterozygous at both the *Rh* and *G6PD* loci. Do the same for the secondary spermatocyte (above) assuming that the male is Rh⁻ and + for the *G6PD* locus.

(c) Assume that the average DNA content per G1 nucleus in humans is 6.5 picograms. For the nuclei (including the entire chromosome complement for each nucleus) presented, give the expected DNA content:

Metaphase I (Primary Oocyte): _____   Secondary Spermatocyte: _____

First Polar Body: _____   Secondary Oocyte: _____

Sample Test Questions

> **Concepts: chromosome morphology (telocentric, etc.), anaphase configurations, chromosome mechanics, meiosis, mitosis, DNA content in cell cycles**

Ch. 2 Ques.10 Assume that you are examining a cell under a microscope and you observe the following as the total chromosomal constituents of a nucleus. You know that $2n = 2$ in this organism, that all chromosomes are telocentric, and that each G1 cell nucleus contains 8 picograms of DNA.

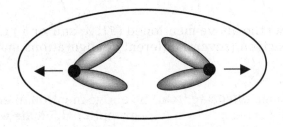

(a) Circle the correct stage for this cell:
   anaphase of mitosis
   anaphase of meiosis I
   anaphase of meiosis II
   telophase of mitosis

(b) How many picograms of chromosomal DNA would you expect in the cell shown above?

> **Concepts: chromosome mechanics (meiosis), symbolism, meiotic nondisjunction, sex-linkage**

Chs. 2, 3, 4 Ques.11 The genes for *singed bristles (sn)* and *miniature wings (m)* are recessive and located on the X chromosome in *Drosophila melanogaster.* In a cross between a singed-bristled, miniature-winged female and a wild-type male, all of the male offspring were singed-miniature.

   (a) Draw meiotic metaphase I chromosomal configurations that represent the X and/or Y chromosomes of the parental (singed-miniature female and wild-type male) flies. Place gene symbols (*sn, m*) and their wild-type alleles (sn^+, m^+) on appropriate chromosomes.

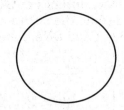

(b) Draw a mitotic metaphase chromosomal configuration that represents the X and/or Y chromosomes of the F_1 male. Place gene symbols (*sn, m*) on the appropriate chromosomes.

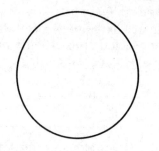

(c) Most of the female offspring from the above-mentioned cross were phenotypically wild type; however, one exceptional female was recovered that had singed bristles and miniature wings. Given that meiotic nondisjunction accounted for this exceptional female, would you expect it to have occurred in the parental male or parental female?

(d) Draw a meiotic, labeled (with gene symbols) circumstance and division product(s) that could account for the exceptional female described in part (c). (Confine your drawing to X chromosomes only.)

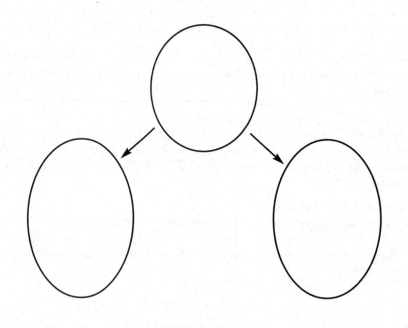

Sample Test Questions

Ch. 2 Ques.12 The red fox (*Vulpes vulpes*) has 17 pairs of somewhat long chromosomes. The Arctic fox (*Alopex lagopus*) has 26 pairs of somewhat shorter chromosomes.

(a) If a female red fox is crossed with a male Arctic fox, what will be the chromosome number in the somatic tissues of the hybrid?

(b) Assume that a somatic G1 nucleus of the Arctic fox contains 12 picograms of DNA, while a somatic G1 nucleus of the red fox contains 8 picograms of DNA. How much nuclear DNA could you expect in a G2 somatic nucleus of the hybrid?

Chs. 3, 4, 7 Ques.13 Red-green color blindness is inherited in humans as an X-linked, recessive gene. Using the symbols below, draw a pedigree that is consistent with the following statements:

A phenotypically normal woman is married to a phenotypically normal man. The woman's parents are phenotypically normal, but her maternal grandfather is color-blind. The woman's paternal grandparents, as well as her maternal grandmother, are phenotypically normal.

male = □
female = ○
Rg = normal color sight
rg = color-blind

What is the probability that the first son born to the woman will be phenotypically normal (not color-blind)?

Concepts: sex-linked inheritance (X-linked), chromosome mechanics, meiosis, conventional symbolism

Chs. 3, 4, 7 Ques.14 In a *Drosophila* experiment, a cross is made between a homozygous wild-type female and a tan-bodied (mutant) male. All the resulting F_1 flies were phenotypically wild type. Adult flies of the F_2 generation (from a mating of the F_1's) had the following characteristics:

Sex	Phenotype	Number
Male	wild	346
Male	tan	329
Female	wild	702

(a) Using conventional symbolism, illustrate the genotype, *on an appropriate chromosomal configuration*, of a secondary oocyte nucleus of one of the F_1 females. Be certain to distinguish the X chromosomes from the autosomes. Note: *Drosophila melanogaster* has a diploid chromosome number of eight.

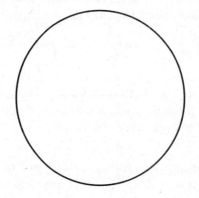

(b) Using the same conventional symbolism, give the genotype, *on an appropriate chromosomal configuration*, of a primary spermatocyte of the tan-bodied F_2 males.

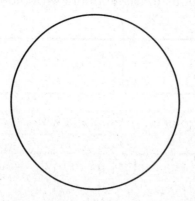

Sample Test Questions

> **Concepts: Mendelian genetics, monohybrid cross, dominance/recessiveness, 3:1 and 1:1 ratios**

Ch. 3 Ques.15 *Gray* seed color in peas is dominant to *white*. Assume that Mendel conducted a series of experiments where plants were crossed and offspring were classified according to the following table. What are the most probable genotypes of each parent?

Parents			Progeny	
			gray	white
(a) gray	×	white	81	79
(b) gray	×	gray	120	42
(c) white	×	white	0	50
(d) gray	×	white	74	0

(a) gray _____ × white _____
(b) gray _____ × gray _____
(c) white _____ × white _____
(d) gray _____ × white _____

> **Concepts: sex-linkage (X-linked), autosomal inheritance, dihybrid situation, incomplete dominance, complete dominance**

Chs. 3, 4, 7 Ques.16 Hemophilia (type A) is recessive and X-linked in humans, whereas the ABO blood group locus is autosomal. Assume that the following matings were examined for the transmission of these genes. Give the expected phenotypes and numbers assuming 800 offspring are produced.

Group A: Females heterozygous for hemophilia with blood type AB mated to normal males with blood group O.

Group B: Females heterozygous for hemophilia with blood type AB mated to males with hemophilia and blood group AB.

311

Sample Test Questions

> **Concepts: Mendelian patterns, 1:1:1:1 ratio, null hypothesis, expected values, χ^2 analysis, interpretation of χ^2**

Ch. 3 Ques.17 For the cross *PpRr* × *pprr* where complete dominance and independent assortment hold, assume that you received the following results and that you wished to determine whether they differ significantly (in a statistical sense) from expectation.

PR phenotypes = 40
Pr phenotypes = 10
pR phenotypes = 20
pr phenotypes = 30

(a) State the null hypothesis associated with this test of significance.

(b) How many degrees of freedom would be associated with this test of significance?

(c) Assuming that a Chi-square value of 20.00 is arrived at in this test of significance, do you accept or reject the null hypothesis?

Degrees of Freedom	p = 0.05
1	3.84
2	5.99
3	7.82
4	9.49
5	11.07

> **Concepts: sex-linked inheritance (X-linked), gynandromorph production, sex determination in *Drosophila*, insect development mitosis, nondisjunction**

Chs. 2, 7 Ques.18 Explain the processes—genotypic, chromosomal, and developmental— that would lead to a bilateral gynandromorph in *Drosophila melanogaster* in which the male half of the fly has white eyes and singed bristles, while the female half is phenotypically wild type.

Concepts: interaction of gene products, relationship between genotype and phenotype, multi-factor inheritance

Chs. 2, 3, 25 Ques.19 Describe and exemplify similarities and differences between *discontinuous* and *continuous* traits at the *molecular* and *transmission* levels.

Concepts: crossing over mechanisms, meiosis, gene mapping, chromosome mechanics

Chs. 2, 5 Ques.20 Assume that there are 18 map units between two loci in the mouse and that you are able to microscopically observe meiotic chromosomes in this organism. If you examined 150 primary oocytes, in how many would you expect to see a chiasma between the two loci mentioned above?

Concepts: linkage and crossing over, computation of map units, complete linkage, independent assortment, lack of crossing over in males

Ch. 5 Ques.21 Following are four dihybrid crosses between various strains of *Drosophila*. To the right of each are map distances known to exist between the genes involved. For each cross, give the phenotypes of the offspring and the percentages expected for each.

	Matings	
Female	*Male*	*Map distance*
(a) *AB/ab*	*ab/ab*	20
(b) *Pq/pQ*	*pq/pq*	50
(c) *DB/db*	*db/db*	0
(d) *ab/ab*	*AB/ab*	20

(a) *AB/ab* × *ab/ab* _____

(b) *Pq/pQ* × *pq/pq* _____

(c) *DB/db* × *db/db* _____

(d) *ab/ab* × *AB/ab* _____

Sample Test Questions

Ch. 6 Ques.22 Following are phrases that refer to various forms of recombination in bacteria. For each, clearly state whether you **agree** or **disagree**. If you disagree, briefly explain your reason(s).

(a) Transduction is the process in which exogenous DNA is drawn into bacteria as a single-stranded structure, then integrated into the bacterial chromosome. [   ]

(b) Temperate phages are capable of entering a lysogenic cycle such that their genomes are incorporated into the bacterial chromosome. [   ]

(c) During the lysogenic cycle, phages are capable of producing bacteria when exposed to U.V. light. [   ]

Ch. 9 Ques.23 Direction of shell coiling in the land snail, *Limnaea peregra*, is determined by alleles at a single locus: *dextral* (right) = *DD or Dd; sinistral* (left) = *dd*. However, a maternal effect is present such that the genotype of the mother determines the direction of coiling (phenotype) of the immediate offspring. Given the following crosses, write the genotypes and phenotypes in the spaces provided. Be certain to indicate which genotypes go with which phenotypes.

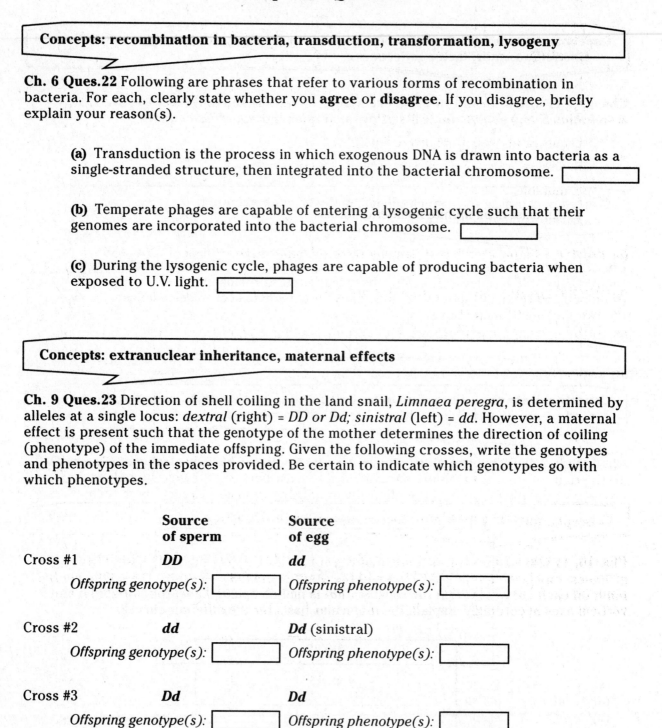

	Source of sperm	Source of egg
Cross #1	*DD*	*dd*

Offspring genotype(s): [   ]   *Offspring phenotype(s):* [   ]

Cross #2	*dd*	*Dd* (sinistral)

Offspring genotype(s): [   ]   *Offspring phenotype(s):* [   ]

Cross #3	*Dd*	*Dd*

Offspring genotype(s): [   ]   *Offspring phenotype(s):* [   ]

Sample Test Questions

Concepts: understanding of gene function, understanding DNA structure, function, mutation, variation

Chs. 10, 11, 12, 16 Ques.24 The foundations of molecular genetics rest upon the assumption that a genetic material exists with the following properties:

    a. autocatalytic (can replicate itself)

    b. heterocatalytic (can direct form and function)

    c. mutable

    d. can exist in an infinite number of forms

(a) Provide a simple sketch that demonstrates the replication scheme of DNA.

(b) Briefly describe how DNA provides form and function.

(c) At the level of nucleotides, what characterizes mutant DNA?

(d) Why may we say that DNA can exist in an infinite number of forms?

Concepts: nucleic acid hybridization, hybridization kinetics, C_0t curves

Chs. 10, 11 Ques.25 On the accompanying graph, draw C_0t curves for DNA from two genomes, one lacking repetitive DNA and the other containing repetitive DNA. Indicate the point on each curve at which the renaturation is half-complete. Label the horizontal and vertical axes accordingly. Explain the molecular basis for the different curves.

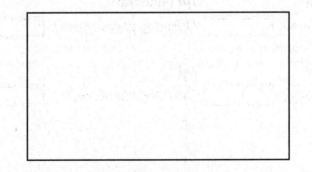

315

Concepts: DNA and RNA structure, complementarity 5′, 3′ orientations,
    degradation products

Chs. 10, 11 Ques.26 Given here is a single-stranded nucleotide sequence. Answer the questions that refer to this sequence.

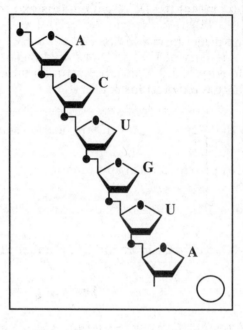

(a) In the circle at the bottom of this sequence, place a 5′ or 3′, whichever corresponds.

(b) Is the above structure an RNA or a DNA? State which_____.

(c) Assume that a complementary strand is produced in which all the innermost phosphates of the adenine triphosphonucleoside precursors are labeled with ^{32}P. What bases would be labeled if the complementary strand were completely degraded with spleen diesterase (cleaves between the phosphate and the 5′ carbon)?_____.

(d) What bases would be labeled if the complementary strand were completely degraded with snake venom diesterase (cleaves between the phosphate and the 3′ carbon)?_____.

Sample Test Questions

Concepts: semiconservative replication, labeling, centrifugation, denaturation

Ch. 11 Ques.27 Assume that you were able to culture a strain of *E. coli* in medium containing either "normal" nitrogen or a heavy isotope of nitrogen (^{15}N). You grow the bacteria for a time in ^{15}N-containing medium, which permits one complete replication of the bacterial chromosome. You extract the DNA, calling this extraction A. You continue to grow the bacterial culture in the ^{15}N DNA for a time, which permits one more complete round of chromosome replication. You again extract the DNA, calling this extraction B. Assuming that nonlabeled DNA has a density of 1.6 and that fully labeled DNA (that is with *all* the ^{14}N replaced with ^{15}N) has a density of 1.9, construct sedimentation profiles that reflect the expected densities of DNA from extractions A and B.

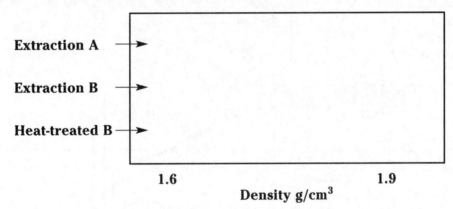

Knowing that heating DNA to 100° C causes separation of complementary strands, use a broken line (- - -) to indicate the sedimentation profile of heat denaturation of extraction B DNA.

Concepts: semiconservative replication, chromosome morphology, DNA structure, labeling, enzymatic digestion, 5′, 3′ orientations

Chs. 11 Ques.28 Assume that you are microscopically examining mitotic metaphase cells of an organism with a 2*n* chromosome number of two (both telocentric). Assume also that the cell passed through one S phase labeling (innermost phosphate of dCTP radioactive) just prior to the period of observation.

(a) Draw this cell's chromosomes and the autoradiographic pattern you would expect to see.

(b) Assuming that the A + T/G + C ratio of the DNA in this cell is 1.67 and that this DNA is digested with snake venom diesterase (cleaves at the 3′ position), what percentages of the total radioactivity would the following products have?

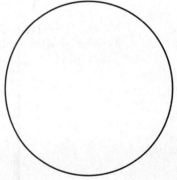

Adenine _____   Guanine _____
Thymine _____   Cytosine _____

317

Sample Test Questions

Concepts: overall DNA replication, 5′, 3′ polarity restrictions, enzymology, priming

Ch. 11 Ques.29 Drawn here is a diagram (not to scale) of DNA in the process of replication. Numbered arrows point to specific structures that you are to identify in the corresponding spaces.

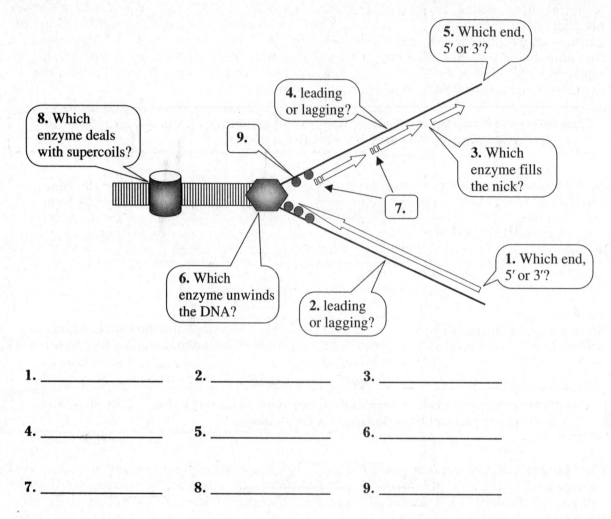

1. _____   2. _____   3. _____

4. _____   5. _____   6. _____

7. _____   8. _____   9. _____

Concepts: experimental strategies, action of nucleases, DNase, restriction endonucleases

Ch. 13 Ques.30 DNase is often used to map the locations where DNA-binding proteins (histones, RNA polymerases, transcription factors, etc.) interact with DNA. Restriction endonucleases are used to cut DNA for identification and cloning. Why are these two different enzyme classes used in these different ways?

Concepts: experimental strategies, cDNA probes, Southern blots, electrophoresis, restriction endonuclease analysis, hybridization

Ch. 13 Ques.31 Assume that you have a radioactively labeled cDNA probe for the gene causing retinoblastoma and that you prepare Southern blots probing DNA in cells from normal individuals and from a child with retinoblastoma. Genomic DNA is prepared using the restriction endonuclease *Hind*III (the *Rb* gene contains four *Hind*III fragments as indicated in the following graphic), and the following hybridization appears:

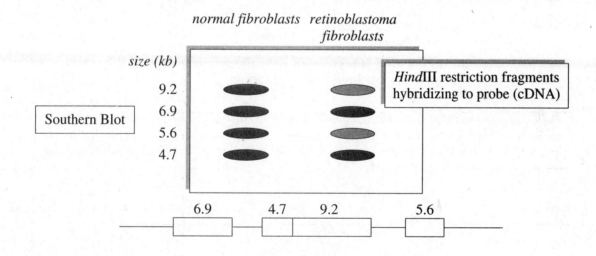

What does each band represent?

What conclusions can be drawn from these data?

Concepts: experimental strategies, electrophoresis, restriction digestion,
   fragment analysis

Ch. 13 Ques.32 The *thioredoxin* gene in bacteria aids in the necessary reduction of proteins. It encodes a protein of 108 amino acids and is contained in a 0.9 kb (*Pst*I/*Bam*HI) fragment. The gene for kanamycin resistance is contained in a 1.4 kb (*Bam*HI/*Pst*I) fragment. The restriction map (one orientation) of these two genes (flanked by *Bam*HI sites) in a plasmid vector is as follows.

(A)

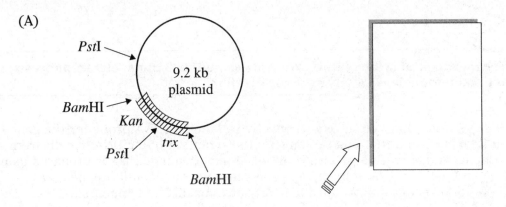

(a) Assume that the plasmid is restricted with the enzyme *Bam*HI. What would be the electrophoretic pattern of the cleaved fragments?

(b) Assume that the orientation given above is only a guess and that the *Bam*HI fragment containing the *trx* and *Kan* genes could possibly exist in the opposite orientation (B). What experiment would you perform to determine whether the orientation is as in (A) or (B)?

(B)

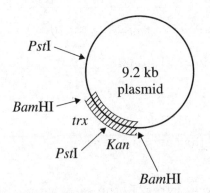

Chs. 14, 15 Ques.33 Following is a schematic of transcription and translation occurring simultaneously as described by Miller et al. (1970) in *E. coli*.

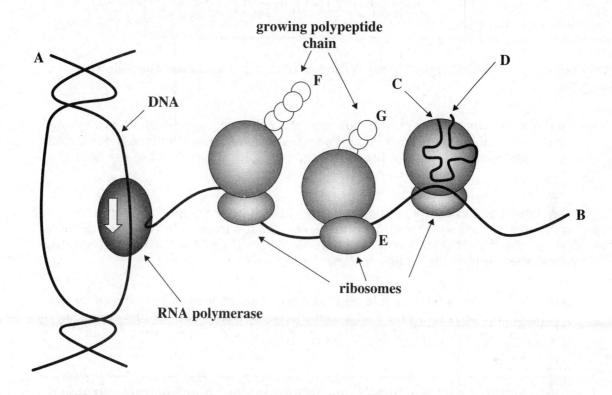

1. Is "A" at the 5′ or 3′ end (*state which*) of the DNA strand?_____

2. Is "B" at the 5′ or 3′ end (*state which*) of the RNA strand?_____

3. Is "C" at the 5′ or 3′ end (*state which*) of the RNA strand?_____

4. To what type of RNA does "D" point?_____

5. Would base sequences near letters "C" or "D" (*state which*) be expected to hold the amino acid?_____

6. What is the S value of the rRNA in the small subunit of the ribosome closest to letter "E"?_____

7. Is the amino acid nearest letter "F" the same type as the one nearest letter "G" (*yes or no*)?_____

Sample Test Questions

> **Concepts: translation, coding, mutation**

Chs. 14, 15, 16 Ques.34 Assume that the following sequence of amino acids occurs in a protein starting from the "N" terminus (with asp) of a large polypeptide chain:

> asp-glu-ile-leu-ser-thr-met-arg-tyr-try-phe-gly

Assume that gene *X* is responsible for synthesis of this gene. Answer the following questions.

(a) Which amino acid(s) would you expect to change if gene *X* is altered by the mutagen, 2-amino purine, such that a transition mutation occurred that caused a change in the ninth base of the mRNA (counting from the 5' end of the coding region)?

(b) Which amino acid(s) would you expect to change if gene *X* is altered by mutagen, for example, acridine orange, such that a frameshift mutation occurred that caused an insertion of a base between bases 3 and 4 of the mRNA (counting from the 5' end of the coding region)?

(c) Which amino acid(s) would you expect to change if gene *X* is altered by the mutagen, nitrous acid, such that a mutation occurred that caused a change in the eleventh base of the mRNA (counting from the 5' end of the coding region)?

> **Concepts: pathway analysis, Beadle and Tatum "set-up," biochemical (nutritional) phenotype**

Chs. 14, 15 Ques.35 Following is a set of experimental results relating the growth (+) of *Neurospora* on several media. Based on the information provided, present the biochemical pathway and the locations of the metabolic blocks.

Strain	Medium		
	MM	MM+A	MM+B
t4	−	+	+
t41	+	+	+
t3	−	−	+

Concepts: importance of primary structure, varieties of bonds, "higher level" folding, structure/function relationships

Ch. 15 Ques.36 Drawn here is a hypothetical protein that contains areas where various types of bonds might be expected to occur. For each area, a box is drawn, and in that box is a number. In the corresponding spaces, state which bond type (or interaction) is most likely illustrated **and** state how that particular type of bond (or interaction) is formed. *You may use a given bond type only once.*

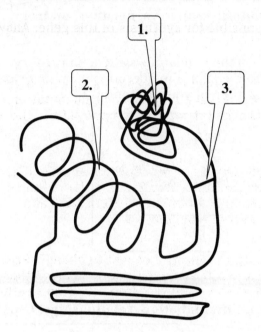

1.

2.

3.

4. What type of amino acids tend to be located on the outside (water side) of the molecule?

Sample Test Questions

> **Concepts: overlapping genes, differential hnRNA splicing**

Ch. 14 Ques.37 Some viruses, as well as eukaryotes, have evolved different mechanisms for obtaining more than one kind of protein from a single transcription unit (a transcription unit simply being a stretch of DNA that is transcribed into a single primary RNA transcript). Describe two different mechanisms.

> **Concepts: genetic regulation, positive vs. negative control**

Ch. 17 Ques.38 Depending on the regulatory system, in prokaryotes when the regulatory protein **is** or **is not** bound to the DNA, the operon may be **on** or **off**. Fill in the following chart and give a brief explanation of your reasoning.

Relationship of Regulator Protein to DNA	Operator	
	Positive control	*Negative control*
is bound		
is not bound		

> **Concepts: determination, differentiation, relationships, *Drosophila* development**

Ch. 19 Ques.39 Two terms, *determination* and *differentiation*, are consistently used in discussions of development.

   (a) Provide a brief definition of each term.

   (b) Which, determination or differentiation, comes first during development of *Drosophila*, for example?

> **Concepts: variable gene activity hypothesis, genomic equivalence, evidence for differential transcription**

Ch. 19 Ques.40 Development may be defined as the attainment of a differentiated state. Given that all cells of a eukaryote probably contain the same complete set of genes, how do we currently explain development in terms of gene activity? What evidence supports your explanation?

Sample Test Questions

Concepts: Hardy-Weinberg applications to X-linked gene, maintenance of gene frequencies over time

Ch. 27 Ques.41 Assume that in a particular population, approximately 8 percent of the males show red-green color blindness. Knowing that this form of color blindness is X-linked, what percentage of the females would be expected to be color-blind?

What would be the expected frequency of heterozygous females?

Assuming that the Hardy-Weinberg equilibrium assumptions pertain, what percentage of men will be color-blind in the next generation?

Concepts: factors which change gene frequencies, influence of inbreeding on gene frequencies

Chs. 27, 28 Ques.42 List and briefly describe factors that change gene frequencies in populations. Is inbreeding a factor in changing gene frequencies? Explain.

Concept: relationship between speciation and Hardy-Weinberg assumptions

Ch. 28 Ques.43 A *species* is often defined as a population of interbreeding, or potentially interbreeding, organisms reproductively isolated from other such populations. Given such an isolated population, will speciation (formation of a new species) occur if the Hardy-Weinberg assumptions are met?

Concepts: natural selection, speciation

Ch. 28 Ques.44 Assume there exists a group of organisms that is temporally or spatially isolated from other such groups. This group has evolved genetic differences from neighboring groups. Describe the process of speciation in terms of this genetically distinct group of organisms.

> *The following answers should be examined AFTER you have attempted to completely resolve (on paper) the problem on your own. You will learn more by struggling with a solution over a period of time than by immediately searching out the correct solution in the answer book.*

Ch. 1 Answer 1 Inherited traits, controlled by genes, are located on the chromosomes of an individual.

Ch. 2 Answer 2 Gregor Mendel

Ch. 1 Answer 3 Genetics is a subdiscipline of biology concerned with the study of heredity and variation at the molecular, cellular, developmental, organismal, and populational levels.

Ch. 1 Answer 4 DNA, or deoxyribonucleic acid, is the hereditary material in eukaryotes and prokaryotes. Either DNA or RNA (ribonucleic acid) serves in viruses.

Ch. 1 Answer 5 homologous

Ch. 1 Answer 6 In mitosis, chromosome number remains constant, while in meiosis, chromosome number is reduced by half in the final products. In meiosis, there is pairing of homologous chromosomes.

Ch. 1 Answer 7 nitrogenous bases, phosphate, deoxyribose sugar

Chs. 2, 3 Answer 8 This question is intended to determine your understanding of mitosis, chromosome morphology, symbolism, the positioning of genes on chromosomes, and the changes in DNA content through the cell cycles. **(a)** Since the diploid chromosome number is six, there will be three bivalents, one involving metacentrics, and two involving acrocentrics in a primary oocyte. We can draw the chromosomes of the primary oocyte as follows:

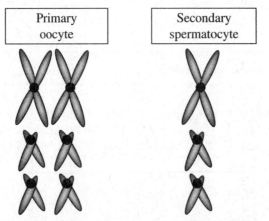

| Primary oocyte | Secondary spermatocyte |

Since secondary spermatocytes arise after meiosis I, there should be only dyads, one metacentric and two acrocentric, and they should be aligned end-to-end as indicated in the above drawing.

(b) Given that there are about 20 picograms of DNA in a G1 nucleus, we would expect there to be 40 pg in a G2 nucleus (after S phase) and 40 pg to the point where homologous chromosomes separate in meiosis I. Secondary spermatocytes and secondary oocytes (as well as first polar bodies) should therefore each have 20 pg of DNA. After meiosis II, the resulting nuclei should have 10 pg each. If you understand events at interphase and in meiosis, this question is easy to answer. Carefully examine the figure below to understand events during interphase, as far as DNA content is concerned. Then examine the figures in Chapter 2 in this book to see how chromosomes behave in meiosis. From this information you should see the answers as follows:

Primary spermatocyte	= 40 pg
First polar body	= 20 pg
Secondary oocyte	= 20 pg
Ootid (in G1)	= 10 pg

It might be helpful to view changes in DNA content in graphic form:

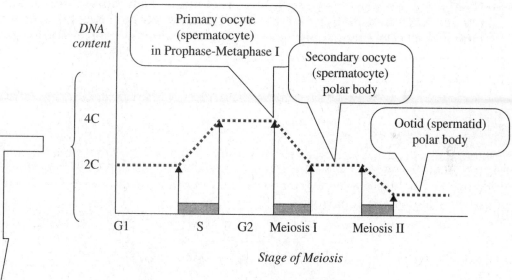

The "C" stands for "complements" of DNA.

Sketch chromosomes in the various stages listed above:

(c) If the mosquito is heterozygous for the recessive gene *wavy bristles* (*wb*), then it would have the genotype *Wb/wb*. Because there are four letters here representing the two genes, the slash between the symbols helps us to understand that only two genes are being discussed.

We are asked to draw an acrocentric, mitotic metaphase chromosome complement in this heterozygous insect. We are expected to place the gene symbols on the chromosomes. Recall that there is no synapsis of homologous chromosomes in mitotic cells; therefore, the homologous chromosomes should not be placed side-by-side. Since sister chromatids are *identical* and homologous chromosomes are *similar*, we should draw the figure as follows:

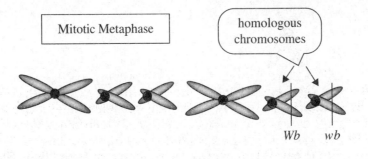

Common errors for Question 8: incorrect number of chromosomes, incorrect chromosome morphology, metacentric, acrocentric, poor relationship of DNA content to cells, inappropriate symbols, inappropriate placement of genes

Chs. 2, 3 Answer 9 (a, b) Recall that a metacentric chromosome has "arms" of approximately equal length, while submetacentric and acrocentric chromosomes have arms of unequal length.

Metaphase I (primary oocyte): Homologous chromosomes are replicated and synapsed. Two X chromosomes will be present because oocytes occur in females. On the metacentric chromosomes (#1), place the *Dd*, such that sister chromatids are identical. Place the + − alternatives on the X chromosomes.

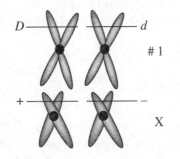

First polar body: The first polar body is a product of meiosis I, after homologous chromosomes have migrated to opposite poles. At this stage, dyads are present. Because females produce polar bodies, an X chromosome should be present. Because the female is

heterozygous, there are several possible answers. Note that there is only one representative of each allele for each gene pair.

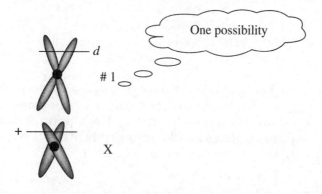

Secondary spermatocyte: A secondary spermatocyte will have the same chromosome configuration as a first polar body. Both are products of meiosis I, and dyads should be present. Because spermatocytes occur in males, either an X chromosome or a Y chromosome will be present. There are, therefore, two possible answers. Regarding the genetic constitution of these cells, as stated in the problem, we are to assume that the male is Rh⁻ and + for the *G6PD* locus. Since this locus is on the X chromosome, only one genotype (regarding the X chromosome) can be presented.

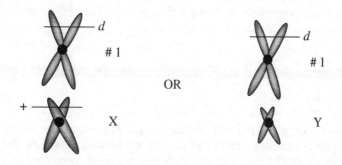

Secondary oocyte: Being a product of meiosis I, dyads will be present. Because oocytes occur in females, an X (not a Y) chromosome should be present. The genetic labeling pattern for the secondary oocyte will be the same as that for the first polar body.

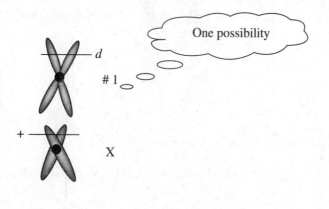

(c) If a G1 nucleus contains 6.5 pg DNA, then the following DNA contents are expected:

Metaphase I (primary oocyte):   13 pg
First polar body: 6.5 pg
Secondary spermatocyte: 6.5 pg
Secondary oocyte: 6.5 pg

Common errors for Question 9: **incorrect number of chromosomes, incorrect chromosome morphology, metacentric, acrocentric, poor relationship of DNA content to cells, inappropriate symbols, inappropriate placement of genes**

Ch. 2 Answer 10(a) Since the cell contains only two chromosomes (2n = 2) and two chromosomes are pictured, it cannot represent a cell in the second phase (II) of meiosis. The chromosomes are telocentric, which means that the centromere is at the end of the chromosome. When pulled at anaphase, two sideways "Vs" or "< >" would be expected and the cell would be at the anaphase stage of meiosis I. The only other possibility to produce the "< >" figure would be a metaphase chromosome at anaphase of mitosis or anaphase II of meiosis. However, these possibilities are negated because the chromosomes are stated as being telocentric.

(b) In order to get the correct answer for the second part, one must consider that, because of the S phase, at anaphase I the DNA complement is twice that of a G1 cell. Therefore, the correct answer is 16 pg DNA.

Common errors for Question 10: **confusion on: significance of *telocentric*, significance of chromosome number, many students consider the chromosomes to be metacentric**

Chs. 2, 3, 4 Answer 11 (a) The female parent would have the following labeled chromosomal symbolism (Remember that at meiotic metaphase I, chromosomes are doubled, condensed, and synapsed.):

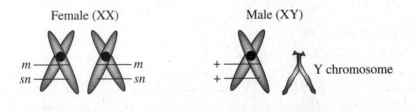

Female (XX)   Male (XY)

(b) In general, mitotic metaphase chromosomes are not synapsed, although in *Drosophila* mitotic chromosomes do pair. To avoid confusion and to be consistent with what is expected in other organisms, the mitotic chromosomes will not be drawn in the paired state.

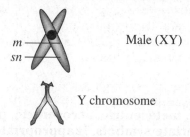

Male (XY)

Y chromosome

(c) All of the female offspring from the preceding cross should be heterozygous and phenotypically wild type. The one exceptional female could have resulted from maternal nondisjunction at meiosis I or II, thus producing an egg cell with two X chromosomes, each containing the *sn* and *m* genes. When fertilized by a sperm cell carrying the Y chromosome (along with the normal haploid set of autosomes), an $X^{sn\ m}X^{sn\ m}Y$ female is produced.

(d)

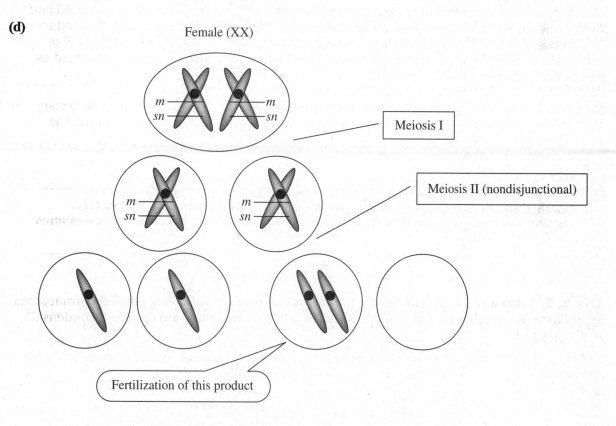

Female (XX)

Meiosis I

Meiosis II (nondisjunctional)

Fertilization of this product

Common errors for Question 11: incorrect chromosome morphology, X and Y chromosomes, inappropriate symbols, inappropriate placement of genes, problems with meiotic nondisjunction

Ch. 2 Answer 12 (a) Since the chromosome numbers are given in *pairs*, recall that during meiosis each gamete contains one chromosome of each pair. If the red fox has 17 pairs of chromosomes, then each gamete will contain 17 chromosomes. For the Arctic fox, each gamete should contain 26 chromosomes. A zygote is produced from the union of the parental gametes; therefore, it should contain 43 chromosomes (17 + 26). It turns out that some such hybrids are viable, but are usually sterile because of developmental and chromosomal alignment and segregational problems at meiosis.

(b) If G1 nuclei contain 12 pg and 8 pg DNA, then the gametes produced from these organisms will contain 6 and 4 pg DNA, respectively. Combining these gametes gives 10 pg for a G1 cell. For a G2 cell there should be 20 pg DNA.

> **Common errors for Question 12: confusion with pairs of chromosomes, gametic chromosome number, confusion with uneven number of chromosomes, confusion with *somatic* cells**

Chs. 3, 4, 7 Answer 13 Because the maternal grandfather was color-blind, the woman's mother is a carrier for this X-linked gene ($X^{Rg}X^{rg}$). The woman therefore has a 1/2 chance of inheriting the X^{rg} chromosome from her mother and a 1/2 chance of passing this X^{rg} chromosome to her son. The chance that the son will receive the X^{rg} chromosome is therefore 1/4 (1/2 × 1/2). However, the question asks for the probability that the son will be normal.

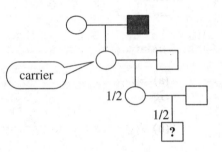

The answer is, therefore, 1 minus 1/4, which equals 3/4.

> **Common errors for Question 13: difficulty in setting up pedigree, inability to see independent probabilities, multiplication of independent probabilities, seeing that the *normal* is requested**

Chs. 3, 4, 7 Answer 14 (a) First, one must determine whether the gene for *tan body* is X-linked or autosomal (not on the sex chromosome). Because half of the F_2 males are mutant and half are wild type, and all the females are wild, the gene for *tan body* is behaving as X-linked. The F_1 female is heterozygous; therefore, she should have either of the alleles (t, t^+) on the one X chromosome (a secondary oocyte has one representative of each chromosomal pair) in the following arrangement. Because *Drosophila* has eight chromosomes, each secondary oocyte should have four chromosomes (including the X chromosome).

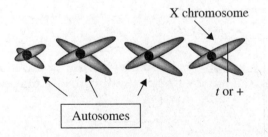

332

(b) A primary spermatocyte has the chromosomes in a doubled, condensed, and synapsed state. A tan-bodied male should have an X (containing a *t* gene) and a Y chromosome, as well as a diploid complement of autosomes.

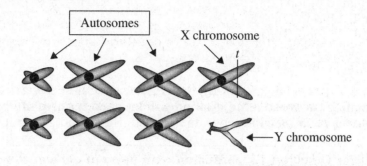

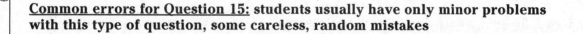

> **Common errors for Question 14:** difficulty in recognizing X-linked inheritance, problems with placing genes on chromosomes, problems with visualizing genome

Ch. 3 Answer 15 First, assign gene symbols: *G* = gray, *gg* = white.

(a) Since there is an approximate 1:1 ratio in the progeny, the parental genotypes are *Gg* × *gg*.

(b) A 3:1 ratio is apparent; therefore, the parental genotypes are *Gg* × *Gg*.

(c) Because there are no gray phenotypes and *gray* is the dominant allele, the parental genotypes must be *gg* × *gg*.

(d) Since there are no white types and the sample is sufficiently large, it is very likely that the parental genotypes are *GG* × *gg*.

> **Common errors for Question 15:** students usually have only minor problems with this type of question, some careless, random mistakes

Chs 3, 4, 7 Answer 16 Set up the crosses with an appropriate symbol set such as the following:

h = hemophilia H = normal allele $I^A I^B$ = AB blood group $I^o I^o$ = O blood group.

Group A

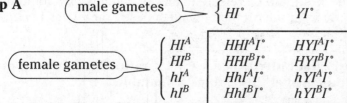

Collecting phenotypes gives:

1/4 female, normal, A blood (200)
1/4 female, normal, B blood (200)
1/8 male, normal, A blood (100)
1/8 male, normal, B blood (100)
1/8 male, hemophilia, A blood (100)
1/8 male, hemophilia, B blood (100)

Group B. In this example the forked-line method will be used. Consider what will be happening for the *hemophilia* locus independently from the blood group locus.

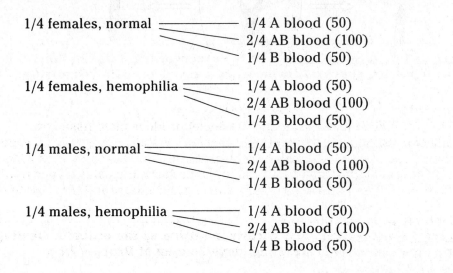

1/4 females, normal —— 1/4 A blood (50)
2/4 AB blood (100)
1/4 B blood (50)

1/4 females, hemophilia —— 1/4 A blood (50)
2/4 AB blood (100)
1/4 B blood (50)

1/4 males, normal —— 1/4 A blood (50)
2/4 AB blood (100)
1/4 B blood (50)

1/4 males, hemophilia —— 1/4 A blood (50)
2/4 AB blood (100)
1/4 B blood (50)

> **Common errors for Question 16: difficulty with any dihybrid situation, X-linked with autosomal inheritance, incomplete dominance, calculating frequencies, observed numbers**

Ch. 3 Answer 17 (a) An appropriate null hypothesis for this example would be that the observed (measured) values do not differ significantly from the predicted ratio of 1:1:1:1. One might also say that any deviation between the observed and predicted values is due to chance and chance alone.

(b) Because four classes are being compared, there will be three degrees of freedom.

(c) Given that the Chi-square value of 20.00 is considerably greater than 7.82 (for three degrees of freedom), the null hypothesis should be rejected and the conclusion should be that the observed values differ significantly from the predicted values based on a 1:1:1:1 ratio.

> **Common errors for Question 17: inability to see a 1:1:1:1 ratio, development of the expected ratios, interpreting probability values from table**

Chs. 2, 7 Answer 18 In order for this type of fly to occur, the zygote must start out as a heterozygote in which both mutant genes are on one homolog and wild-type alleles are on the other. In addition, one of the wild-type chromosomes must get "lost" at the first mitotic division, thus making the female half $X^{+\ +}X^{w\ sn}$ and the other half $X^{w\ sn}$ O. The following diagram explains this situation.

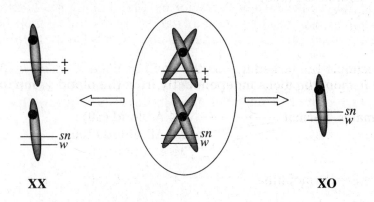

XX		XO

Because XX nuclei produce female tissue and XO nuclei produce male tissue, the phenotypes of the two sides are thus described. Developmentally, once the cleavage nuclei reach the peripheral areas of the egg to form a blastoderm, they become committed to their adult fate. Because there is little "wandering" of nuclei either during their migration to the egg periphery or after they reach the periphery, the male/female boundary is quite clean.

<u>**Common errors for Question 18:**</u> **difficulty in setting up the problem, dealing with mitotic nondisjunction, embryonic development of *Drosophila***

Chs. 2, 3, 25 Answer 19 At the *molecular level,* one would consider that in discontinuous inheritance the gene products are acting fairly independently of each other, thereby providing a 9:3:3:1 ratio in a dihybrid cross, for example. Genotypic classes

$$A\_B\_,\ A\_bb,\ aaB\_,\ and\ aabb$$

can be clearly distinguished from each other because the gene products from the *A* locus produce distinct influences on the phenotypes as compared with those gene products from the *B* locus. Exceptions exist where epistasis and other forms of gene interaction occur. In discontinuous inheritance, one would consider each locus as providing a *qualitatively* different impact on the phenotype. For instance, even though the *brown* and *scarlet* loci interact in the production of eye pigments in *Drosophila*, each locus is providing qualitatively different input.

In continuous inheritance, we would consider each involved locus as having a quantitative input on the production of a single characteristic of the phenotype. In addition, although it may not always be the case, we would consider each gene product as being qualitatively similar. Under this model, the *quantity* of a particular set of gene products, influenced by a number of gene loci, determines the phenotypic characteristic.

At the *transmission level* one sees "step-wise" distributions in discontinuous inheritance, but "smoother" or more bell-shaped distributions in continuous inheritance. For instance, in a dihybrid situation (*AaBb* × *AaBb*) where independent assortment holds, one would obtain a 9:3:3:1 ratio (assuming no epistasis, etc.) under a discontinuous mode, but a 1:4:6:4:1 ratio where genes (or gene products) are acting additively (continuous inheritance). Both patterns are formed from normal Mendelian principles of segregation, independent assortment, and random union of gametes. It is the manner in which the genes (or gene products) interact that distinguishes discontinuous from continuous inheritance.

> **Common errors for Question 19: difficulty with "molecular level" of the question, confusion over differences and similarities relating discontinuous and continuous patterns**

Chs. 2, 5 Answer 20 The basis of the solution is to recall that crossing over occurs at the "four-strand stage" (after the S phase) and each chiasma involves only two of the four chromatids present in each tetrad. Therefore, for each chiasma only two of the four, or 1/2, of the chromatids are crossover chromatids.

Gene mapping basically is the process of dividing the number of crossover chromatids by the total number of chromatids. Since each chiasma involves only two of the four chromatids, the map distance must be half of the chiasma frequency. If there are 18 map units between two genes, then the chiasma frequency would be 36 percent. If one examined 150 primary oocytes, one would therefore expect to see 0.36 × 150, or 54, cells with a chiasma between the two loci.

> **Common errors for Question 20: problem seeing relationships of chiasma and map units, problems "seeing" meiosis, visualization of crossing over**

Ch. 5 Answer 21 The key to solving these types of "reverse mapping" problems is to keep in mind that a map unit is computed by the equation [# crossover types/total number (×100)] and that if the map distance is given, it is easy to determine the percentages of parental and crossover offspring. Remember that there are two classes of crossovers and two classes of parentals from each cross.

(a) *AB/ab* = 40%, *ab/ab* = 40% (parentals)
Ab/ab = 10%, *aB/ab* = 10% (crossovers)

(b) *Pq/pq* = 25%, *pQ/pq* = 25% (parentals)
PQ/pq = 25%, *pq/pq* = 25% (crossovers)

Notice that this is independent assortment.

(c) *DB/db* = 50%, *db/db* = 50% (all parentals)

(d) *AB/ab* = 50%, *ab/ab* = 50% (all parentals)

The reason that there are all parentals and no crossovers in this cross is that there is no crossing over in male *Drosophila*. With no crossing over, the *AB/ab* chromosomes in the male are passed to gametes without crossovers.

> **Common errors for Question 21:** difficulty going from map units to offspring frequencies, failure to see that there are two parental and two crossover classes, careless mistakes

Ch. 6 Answer 22 (a) Disagree: The process being described refers to *transformation,* not transduction. Transduction is *phage-mediated* recombination, whereas in transformation exogenous DNA is taken up as indicated in the statement.

(b) Agree: Viruses that can enter either the lytic or lysogenic cycle are called *temperate* viruses. During the process of lysogeny, the viral chromosome is integrated into the bacterial chromosome as stated.

(c) Disagree: This statement is fairly silly in that it asserts that phages are capable of producing bacteria. Regardless of the exposure to UV light, phages cannot produce bacteria. Ultraviolet light can cause induction of the lytic cycle, therefore phages, when lysogenic bacteria are exposed.

> **Common errors for Question 22:** carelessness in reading statements, confusion as to what terms mean: transduction, transformation, conjugation, lysogeny, temperate viruses

Ch. 9 Answer 23 The definition provided initially in the problem can be applied directly to the solution of this problem. The *genotype* of the mother determines the direction of coiling (phenotype) of the immediate offspring. In this case, one merely assigns first the genotypes on the basis of normal Mendelian principles and then the phenotypes based on the genotype of the mother.

Notice that in Cross 2, the *Dd* has a sinistral phenotype. While this may confuse some students, remember that the phenotype is determined by the *maternal* genotype. When early developmental events are involved, often the maternal genotype will have a significant influence over those events because the mother makes the egg.

	Offspring genotype(s):	*Offspring phenotype(s):*
Cross #1:	*Dd*	all sinistral
Cross #2:	*Dd*	all dextral
	dd	
Cross #3:	*DD*	all dextral
	Dd	
	dd	

Chs. 10, 11, 12, 16 Answer 24 (a) DNA replicates in a semiconservative manner such that each daughter strand is "half-new" and "half-old" in a particular pattern.

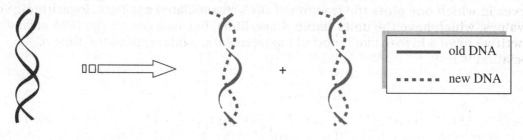

(b) The *Central Dogma of Biology* is based on the production (through transcription) of an RNA messenger from a DNA template and the subsequent "decoding" of that messenger by the process of translation.

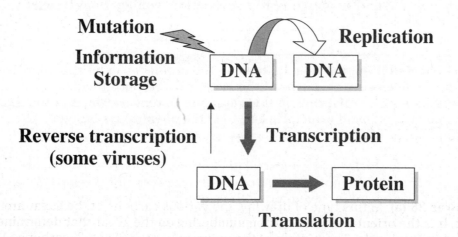

(c) The DNA template contains a sequence of nitrogenous bases that specifies a code from which amino acids are ordered in proteins. Through tautomeric shifts and a number of other natural factors (radiation, chemicals), changes can occur in that sequence of bases. Indeed, the mechanisms by which genes replicate themselves generate errors and leave us with the conclusion that DNA is an inherently unstable molecule.

(d) Given the variety of organisms and the variation within organisms, there must be numerous, hundreds of millions, elementary factors that are inherited. DNA can provide for this variety by differences in the length and sequence of bases for each inherited functional unit. Given that there are four different types of bases, a sequence having merely 10 bases would be capable of 4^{10} (over 1 million) different sequences.

Common errors for Question 24: There are usually very few problems with this type of question, except that students often have difficulty clearly explaining that which they know in model form. Written descriptions tend to be more lists of examples rather than explanations of structures and/or processes.

Chs. 10, 11 Answer 25 As discussed in the text, the rate of reassociation of melted DNA increases as the proportion of repetitive DNA increases. Such relationships are reflected in C_ot curves in which one plots the fraction of DNA reassociated against a logarithmic scale of C_ot values, which have the units (mole × sec/liter). Because denatured DNA strands that are repetitive have a higher likelihood of complementary interaction, the time of reassociation is less.

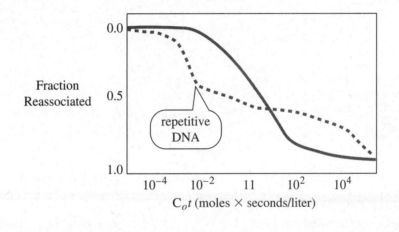

Common errors for Question 25: orientation (coordinates) of graph, significance of curve components, repetitive DNA fraction, unique fraction

Chs. 10, 11 Answer 26 (a) In this type of drawing, the various carbons of the sugar are readily apparent. It is the orientation and carbon numbering on the sugar that determines the 5′-3′ orientation of the molecule. The bottom of the polymer has the 2′ and 3′ carbons projecting, while the top has the 5′ carbon projecting. Therefore, the bottom, near the circle is the 3′ end of the molecule.

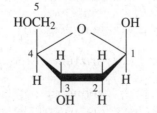

(b) Notice that there is no vertical line protruding from the 2′ carbon position in the drawing and that uracil (U) is present. The molecule must therefore be an RNA.

(c) It is best to start this portion of the problem by roughly drawing the complementary strand, remembering that it will be antiparallel.

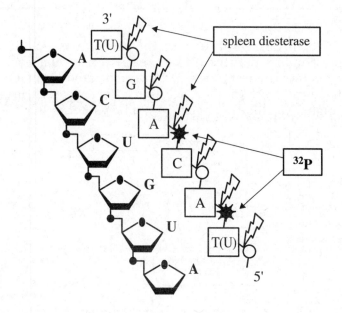

If it is a DNA complement, it will have thymine in place of uracil. There is no indication as to the complementary strand being RNA or DNA. Since all ATPs (or dATPs) have at their innermost phosphate a ^{32}P, make certain that they are properly labeled. Since spleen diesterase cleaves between the phosphate and the 5′ carbon, the 5′ neighbors (C, T or U) will be labeled with the ^{32}P.

(d) Since snake venom diesterase cleaves at the 3′ position (between the phosphate and the 3′ carbon), the originally labeled ATP (or dATP) will retain the label.

Common errors for Question 26: 5′ to 3′ orientations, labeling of complementary strand, understanding enzyme cleavages

Ch. 11 Answer 27 Even though circular, in the context of this question, DNA from *E. coli* can be viewed in the following manner. Replication will occur semiconservatively and give the following sedimentation profile.

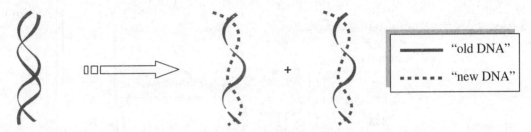

The heat treatment will cause the double-stranded structures to separate, giving the following strands and the profile as shown above.

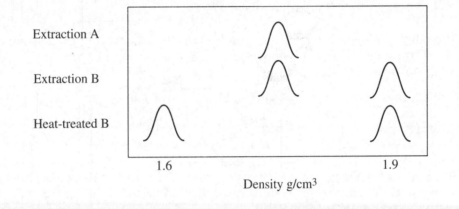

Common errors for Question 27: confusion with the labeling experiment, difficulty in seeing sedimentation profiles, application of semiconservative replication

Ch. 11 Answer 28 (a) There will be two telocentric metaphase chromosomes in the drawing, and each chromatid will be labeled.

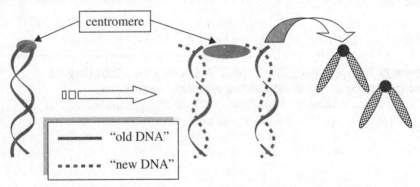

This autoradiographic pattern results because of semiconservative replication. Any cell that contains labeled chromosomes will have had its chromosomes pass through an S phase in the presence of a label.

(b) Consider that the DNA was labeled with a dCTP having the innermost phosphate labeled. As this triphosphonucleoside is incorporated into the DNA, it will have the following relationship to its neighbors. *Snake venom diesterase* cleaves DNA at the 3′ position, meaning that it breaks the bond between the phosphate and the 3′ carbon.

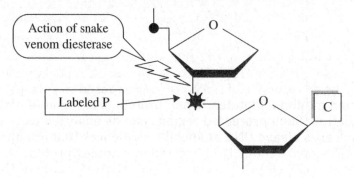

Therefore, the labeled phosphate remains attached to the 5′ carbon of the cytosine nucleotide. The A + T/G + C ratio of 1.67 is of no consequence in answering this problem because all of the label remains attached to the cytosine.

    Adenine_____   Guanine_____

    Thymine_____   Cytosine <u>100%</u>

> **Common errors for Question 28:** inappropriate labeling pattern, inability to draw telocentric chromosomes, understanding cleavage at 3′ position, eliminating extraneous information

Ch. 11 Answer 29

1. This must be the *5′ end* of the polymer because all synthesis of polymers is 5′ to 3′ and the head of the arrow is at the other end of the polymer.
2. The *leading strand* is that strand which is synthesized continuously.
3. A *DNA ligase* will join the nicks.
4. The *lagging strand* is the discontinuous strand.
5. The free end that is complementary to the 5′ end at arrow #1 must be the 3′ end. That being so, the complement to that 3′ end would be 5′. Therefore, the *5′ end* is at arrow #5.
6. A *helicase* is involved in unwinding the DNA helix.
7. An *RNA primer* is synthesized to initiate DNA synthesis.
8. *DNA gyrase* functions to remove supercoils generated by unwinding the DNA helix.
9. *Single-stranded binding proteins* stabilize the template that is to be replicated.

Common errors for Question 29: determination of 5′- 3′ polarity, naming of enzymes involved

Ch. 13 Answer 30 DNase is a general term that includes a variety of exo- and endonucleases that cleave DNA from the ends or internally, respectively. Such cleavage is often irrespective of base sequence. If naked DNA is exposed to DNases, it is rapidly degraded to oligo- and mononucleotides. When protein is associated with DNA, it protects regions from degradation. Such protected regions can be analyzed as to base content. Restriction endonucleases cleave DNA at specific sequences that are often hundreds or thousands of base pairs apart. If one is interested in mapping protein-binding sites, one will want to use an enzyme (a DNase) with frequent, yet relatively random, cleavage characteristics, not restriction endonucleases.

Common errors for Question 30: understanding overall strategy, differences between DNases restriction endonucleases

Ch. 13 Answer 31 Notice that the fragment sizes (in kb) on the left side of the figure match the *Hind*III restriction fragments that are hybridizing to the radioactive probe. Each band, therefore, represents a region where the radioactive probe sticks by complementary base pairing to single-stranded DNA fragments, which are bound to the filter of a typical Southern blot. The smaller fragments migrate faster in the gel and are in the bottom portion. See that the intensity of the bands from the normal individual is somewhat uniform, indicating that all the restriction fragments are found in equal amounts. However, the intensity of two of the bands from the patient with retinoblastoma is about half as in the normal. Two bands (6.9 and 4.7 kb) apparently have the same intensity as in the normal. Because humans are diploid organisms, with normally two copies of each gene, these data support the hypothesis that the individual with retinoblastoma has a heterozygous deletion of a portion of the retinoblastoma gene. The deletion includes *Hind*III fragments (9.2 and 5.6 kb). It is likely that such a deletion is setting up a situation whereby mutation of the normal allele in a single cell of the eye may cause retinoblastoma.

Common errors for Question 31: understanding of experimental design, cDNA probes, Southern blots, electrophoresis, restriction endonuclease analysis, hybridization, recognition of deletion

Ch. 13 Answer 32 Following is a drawing of the expected product if either of the above plasmids (A) or (B) is restricted to completion with *Bam*HI. There should be a 2.3 kb fragment (1.4 + 0.9 kb) and the remainder (9.2 − 2.3 = 6.9). Notice that the 6.9 kb fragment migrates more slowly (higher in the gel) than the 2.3 kb fragment. Also notice that the intensity of the stain is less in the smaller band because there is less DNA to bind the stain.

(a)

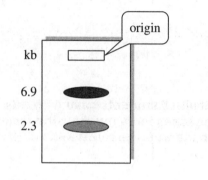

(b) To distinguish between the (A) and (B) orientations, one could make use of the change in position of the *Pst*I restriction site in the two orientations. First, estimate the number of kb in the two fragments resulting from *Pst*I restriction of orientation (A). Notice that in orientation (A) the *Pst*I fragments are approximately 2.4 (1.4 for the *Kan* gene + about 1.0) kb and 6.8 kb. In orientation (B) the sizes would be approximately 1.9 (0.9 for the *trx* gene + about 1.0) and 7.3 kb. With appropriate standards, these size differences could be distinguished on agarose gels.

Common errors for Question 32: electrophoretic analysis, restriction enzyme analysis, experimental design

Chs. 14, 15 Answer 33 Overall, this is a drawing of simultaneous transcription and translation in which the RNA polymerase is moving from top to bottom, making an mRNA that is complementary to one of the two strands of DNA. Ribosomes have added to the nascent (newly forming) mRNA, and what appear to be polypeptide chains are protruding from the ribosomes.

(1, 2) In answering this question, remember that all synthesis of nucleic acids starts at the 5′ end and finishes at the 3′ end. Therefore, immediately label the end near point "B" with a 5′. The projecting strand is the nascent mRNA. Recall that all orientation of complementary strands is antiparallel and since the RNA polymerase is going from top-to-bottom (according to the arrow) the end of the DNA strand from which the mRNA is copied is the 3′ end. Now, since the 3′ end of the DNA template strand is identified, its DNA complementary end (at point "A") must be the 5′ end.

(3) The codon-anticodon relationship is also antiparallel (based on hydrogen bonding), and since the 5′ end of the mRNA is identified, letter "C" must be at the 5′ end.

(4) While the diagram is *not to scale*, given the folded structure of the molecule and its position in the ribosome, consider the RNA nearest to letter "D" as tRNA.

(5) Remember that the 3′ end of the tRNA holds the amino acid; therefore, letter "D" is where the amino acid would be attached.

(6) The tRNA binds mainly to the large subunit of the ribosome, while the mRNA binds mainly to the small subunit of the ribosome. The question asks for the S value of the rRNA in that small subunit. Simultaneous transcription and translation occurs in prokaryotes only (not eukaryotes). The S value for the small subunit of a prokaryotic ribosome is 30S, but that value includes both rRNA and protein. The rRNA molecule, however, has an S value of 16, which is the correct answer.

(7) Since all of the ribosomes are moving along the same mRNA, the amino acid sequences are the same. Therefore, the amino acids nearest the letters "F" and "G" are the same.

> **Common errors for Question 33:** polarity of DNA and RNA strands, structure of ribosomes, overall understanding of translation

Chs. 14, 15, 16 Answer 34 One of the most frequent difficulties students have with this problem is remembering that the code is triplet and three bases in the mRNA code for each amino acid in a protein. The 5′ end of the mRNA corresponds with the N-terminus of the amino acid chain.

(a) Transition mutations will cause amino acid substitutions. Counting over by "threes" from the N-terminus, the amino acid ile should be altered.

(b) Inserting a base between positions 3 and 4 will change the second amino acid; however, recall that acridine orange is a frameshift mutagen and insertion of a base will alter the reading frames for all "downstream" amino acids. Therefore, all amino acids in positions two (glu) through twelve will be influenced (excluding degeneracy).

(c) Nitrous acid causes base substitutions; therefore, a mutation in the eleventh base would influence the amino acid leu.

> **Common errors for Question 34:** counting amino acids as bases, not understanding what base changes do to amino acid sequences

Ch. 14 Answer 35 Notice that there are two mutant strains (cannot grow on minimal medium) and one wild-type strain (*t41*). The best way to approach these types of problems, especially when the data are organized in the form given, is to realize that the substance (supplement) that "repairs" a strain, as indicated by a (+), is after the metabolic block for that strain. In addition, and most importantly, the substance that "repairs" the highest number of strains either is the end product or is closest to the end product. Looking at the table, notice that supplement B "repairs" both of the mutant strains. Therefore, it must be at the end of the pathway or at least after all the metabolic blocks (defined by each mutation). Supplement A "repairs" the next highest number of mutant strains (1); therefore, it must be second from the end. The pathway therefore would be as follows:

Precursor →║→ A →║→ B (with *t4* and *t3* over the blocks)

To determine the locations at which the strains block the pathway through mutation, apply a similar logic. A block that is "repaired" by all the supplements must be early in the pathway. A block that is "repaired" by only one supplement must be late in the pathway. A supplement that does not "repair" a strain is before that strain's metabolic block. Be certain not to introduce any "blocks" for the wild-type strain.

Common errors for Question 35: inability to construct a pathway, failure to see how additives "repair" mutant phenotypes, difficulty in assigning metabolic blocks in pathways

Ch. 15 Answer 36

1. hydrophobic cluster formed by interaction of hydrophobic amino acids

2. α helix formed from hydrogen bonds between components of the peptide linkage

3. covalent, disulfide bonds formed between cysteine residues

4. The polar amino acids will tend to orient to the outside of the protein where the charged R groups will interact with water.

Common errors for Question 36: nature of hydrophobic clustering, understanding of α and β structures, polar side chains, and hydrophilic interactions

Chs. 14, 15 Answer 37 In some viruses, overlapping genes present a mechanism for providing two and sometimes more protein products from a single stretch of DNA. In eukaryotes, different sets of introns may be removed, thus providing for a variety of protein products from a single section of DNA. This process is often called *differential* or *alternative splicing.*

Common errors for Question 37: Students often have difficulty in orienting *specific information* they have learned to a general question. If asked about overlapping genes, or differential hnRNA splicing, they would be able to develop an answer. Students sometimes confuse overlapping genes with the nonoverlapping code.

Ch. 17 Answer 38 Any time a regulatory protein interacts with DNA and transcription is stimulated, it is called *positive* control. Any time a regulatory protein interacts with DNA and represses transcription, it is called *negative* control. In completing the chart, apply these simple rules.

Relationship of Regulator Protein to DNA	*Operator*	
	Positive control	*Negative control*
is bound	**on**	**off**
is not bound	**off**	**on**

Common errors for Question 38: confusion with positive and negative control, confusion with repressible and inducible systems

Ch. 19 Answer 39 *Determination* is a significant, complex, yet poorly understood process whereby the specific pattern of genetic activity is initially established in a cell. This pattern will direct the developmental fate (differentiation) of that cell.

(a) *Differentiation* is the process of cellular expression of the determined state. It is the complex series of genetic, morphological, and physiological changes that characterize the variety of adult cells.

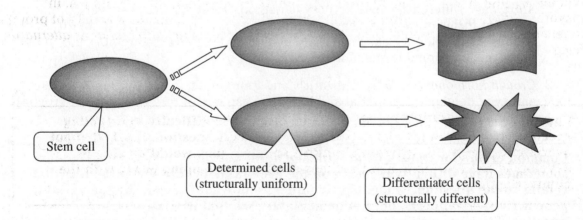

Stem cell

Determined cells
(structurally uniform)

Differentiated cells
(structurally different)

(b) *Determination* occurs before *differentiation*. In *Drosophila*, determinative events are thought to occur about the time of blastoderm formation, when nuclei encounter the peripheral regions of the egg. *Differentiation* of most of the adult cells occurs during metamorphosis, some five to six days after embryogenesis (determination).

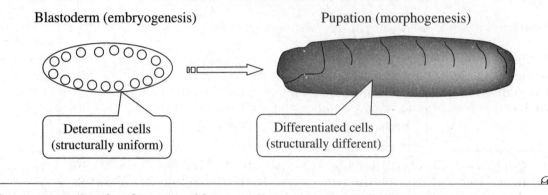

Blastoderm (embryogenesis)

Pupation (morphogenesis)

Determined cells
(structurally uniform)

Differentiated cells
(structurally different)

Common errors for Question 39: providing accurate definitions, failure to relate determination and differentiation to each other temporally

Ch. 19 Answer 40 The *variable gene activity hypothesis* of differentiation acknowledges the genomic equivalence of cells within an organism and assumes that of all the genes in a given cell type, only certain ones produce products, while the others are shut down and are not transcribed. Certain genes will be active in all cells, those *housekeeping* genes coding for vital cellular functions, while others will be differentially regulated in various cell types. Differential gene transcription occurs in both spatial (different cells of an organism) and temporal (different times during development) dimensions.

Support for this model is provided by several observations and experiments.

1. *Chromosome puffs*: Specific puff patterns, representing differential gene activity, are observed in dipteran polytene chromosomes at different times during development.

2. *Allozymes*: Differential gene activity is demonstrated by the observation that different forms of the same enzyme (allozymes) are present in cells of different tissues. This evidence assumes that such allozyme patterns are not caused by post-transcriptional forms of genetic regulation.

3. *Growth hormone*: *In situ* hybridization and immunochemical studies in mouse embryos demonstrate spatial and temporal aspects of the regulation of growth hormone transcripts in the anterior pituitary gland.

Common errors for Question 40: With a general question such as this, students sometimes have difficulty focusing on the area in their notes or in the text that relates to the question. Students may understand what is meant by the variable gene activity hypothesis, but not immediately see that it relates to the question. Students also have difficulty in relating a variety of experimental findings to a general theme.

Ch. 27 Answer 41 Since 8 percent of the males express the trait and males have only one X chromosome, the frequency (q) of the recessive gene would be .08 and p would be .92. Since females have two X chromosomes, the expected frequency of females that are homozygous for the color blindness gene would be q^2 or .0064 (.64%).

The frequency of females that are heterozygous would be $2pq$ or 2(.08)(.92) = .1472 or 14.72%.

Because the population is in equilibrium, the frequency of men with color blindness will not change from generation to generation. Eight percent of the men will be color-blind in the next generation. Students should be aware of many deviations of these types of questions. The basic scheme is the Hardy-Weinberg equilibrium and the equations that apply.

Common errors for Question 41: application of the Hardy-Weinberg equations to an X-linked gene, failure to apply the Hardy-Weinberg equations in determining the frequency of heterozygous females; students often make the question harder than it is by forgetting that under equilibrium conditions, gene frequencies do not change

Chs. 27, 28 Answer 42 *Mutation*, while being an original source of genetic variability, is not usually considered to be a significant factor in changing gene frequencies.

Migration occurs when individuals move from one population to another. The influence of migration on changing gene frequencies is proportional to the differences in gene frequency between the donor and recipient populations. Organisms often migrate as a result of some stress. Those organisms suffering from the most stress are often those that leave. Therefore, they do not represent a random sample of the individuals in that home range.

Selection can be a significant force in changing gene frequencies. It results when some genotypic classes are less likely to produce offspring than others. Selection may be directional, stabilizing, or disruptive.

Genetic drift can be a significant force in changing gene frequencies in populations that are numerically small or have a small number of effective breeders. In such populations, random and relatively large fluctuations in gene frequency occur by "sampling error."

Inbreeding is not a significant factor in changing gene frequencies in populations; however, it will change zygotic or genotypic frequencies. The number of homozygotes will increase at the expense of the heterozygotes.

Common errors for Question 42: failure to provide a complete list, failure to briefly and adequately describe each term, failure to see that inbreeding does not, in itself, change gene frequencies

Ch. 28 Answer 43 Reproductive isolation can occur because of the introduction of geographic barriers or other dramatic changes in the environment that subdivide a population. Such factors facilitate speciation because gene flow is eliminated or at least restricted. With gene flow restricted, isolated populations can experience changes in gene frequencies when the Hardy-Weinberg assumptions are not met. Under Hardy-Weinberg equilibrium conditions where there is *random mating, no genetic drift, no selection, no mutation*, and *no migration*, gene frequencies will remain the same and speciation will not occur.

Common errors for Question 43: confusion as to what the question is asking, difficulty in relating information from one chapter to information contained in a different chapter

Ch. 28 Answer 44 Any circumstance or process that favors changes in gene frequencies has the potential of generating a new species.

Factors such as selection, migration, genetic drift, or even mutation may be important in species formation. One would certainly include geographic and/or temporal isolation as major barriers to gene flow and, thus, an important process in such formation.

Natural selection occurs when there is nonrandom elimination of individuals from a population. Since such selection is a strong force in changing gene frequencies, it should also be considered as a significant factor in species formation.

Common errors for Question 44: explanations of terms, general relationships among diverse phenomena